sensory experience

sensory experience

SECOND EDITION

Raymond J. Christman

Utica College

Harper & Row, Publishers

New York, Hagerstown, Philadelphia, San Francisco, London

Sponsoring Editor: George A. Middendorf
Project Editor: Renée E. Beach
Designer: Robert Sugar
Senior Production Manager: Kewal K. Sharma
Compositor: American Book–Stratford Press, Inc.
Printer and Binder: Halliday Lithograph Corporation

SENSORY EXPERIENCE, Second Edition

Library of Congress Cataloging in Publication Data

Christman, Raymond John, 1919–
   Sensory experience.

   Bibliography: p.
   Includes indexes.
   1. Senses and sensation.   I. Title.
BF233.C48   1979   612'.8   78–15276
ISBN 0–06–04128–4

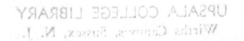

contents

preface

Sensory Experience was written in response to a need for a textbook that would meet several overlapping requirements. Indeed, the very idea for the first edition arose out of the author's experience in teaching an undergraduate class for which no single available text was adequate. In essence, this book was meant to be an undergraduate level text, providing the student with a broad, general introduction to the entire area of human sensory phenomena, without the necessity of turning to a multitude of original reports and highly technical writings aimed primarily at the professional in the field. Material of a highly perceptual nature was intentionally avoided. There is enough material available on purely sensory phenomena to keep the average student busy and interested. Perception can be better presented in a separate course or, if desired, with supplemental readings.

I have tried to make the book readable and interesting, avoiding wherever possible highly technical references and reports of original research. I have also attempted to include everyday examples and to present complex sensory phenomena in a manner understandable to the student with a limited mathematical and biological background. I hoped the book would be relevant to the needs of the average student. For the student or instructor who wishes to delve into a topic at greater depth, references and additional bibliographic listings are provided; many highly technical references are to be found in the bibliography. In addition, each chapter has a short list of suggested readings, many from easy-to-read secondary sources. Most of these are from books of readings, other textbooks, semiprofessional journals, and easily obtained reference books. A conscious effort was made to include, where possible, only readily available sources for the suggested readings.

I had also hoped that, through the use of this book, at least some students of general and experimental psychology might become interested in specific areas of sensory-perceptual psychology that might lead ultimately to successful careers in the discipline.

My experience has shown that a course based on this book can also be of considerable value for a broad spectrum of nonpsychology students, as well as psychology undergraduates. Students in premedicine, occupational therapy, physical therapy, and other biologically oriented sciences often remain quite naive about and sometimes oblivious to the importance of sense organ functioning unless they take individual, advanced courses in several separate disciplines. This book is aimed at providing such a broad, general introduction to the sense organs and thereby helping to fill this gap.

Graduate students have a strong inclination to concentrate their efforts in one narrow area; indeed, since this is often a necessity, I hope that the material presented here is of value to students concentrating solely on visual research, and who might otherwise have little opportunity to gain even a passing familiarity with such sensory areas as audition or the chemical senses. For such students, concentrating in one narrow discipline, the book should provide at least the language of the related disciplines. This thought was foremost in its preparation—to provide the student with the "language" of sensory psychology, its terms and constructs, and some of its methodology. The student doing doctoral research in vision will probably find little of value in the chapters on vision; they are not aimed at his level. But the non-vision chapters may be of great value to such a student.

Most graduate students must take examinations in several areas as a requirement for advanced degrees. For such nonexperimental, nonsensation-perception students as those in clinical or social psychology, examinations in such areas present a formidable barrier. With its emphasis on the "language" of sensory experience, the text should provide at least some of the background information required by such students.

With a similar purpose and format, this revised edition does not differ extensively from the original edition. Errors in the first edition that were called to my attention have been corrected. Many users of the book offered valuable suggestions concerning the inclusion of some new material and the revision and clarification of some of the original material. I have tried to follow their suggestions where this was possible. One noticeable result of this is the extensive revision of the material on the chemical senses, which involved adding one more chapter.

I have also included more recent bibliographic material. To be sure, such well-established principles as Rico's and Piper's laws cannot be radically updated in a text of this nature. But I did try to increase coverage of such topics as Stevens's power function, the McCullough phenomenon, and the ubiquitous subject of chemical pheromones, so basic to an understanding of the development of the human chemical senses. The suggested readings have also been revised and updated.

I should like to extend my appreciation to the administrative staff of Utica College of Syracuse University, who, by providing time and facilities, made the completion of this book possible. I would also like to thank the numerous professional colleagues who were so generous in providing access to copyrighted material, original photographs, and other vital materials. Finally, I should like to extend my deepest gratitude to my wife, Dorothy, who cared for me at such a sacrifice to herself during my recent serious illness. To her I dedicate this edition.

R. J. Christman

1 / introduction

The study of the human senses, the determination of their essential character, their capabilities and limitations, represents the oldest area of interest in modern psychology. Long before interest arose in the application of psychology to such practical problems as learning and the measurement of intelligence, the study of the sense organs* had reached an extreme pinnacle of academic popularity and methodological sophistication. Why should this have been true?

Although philosophical approaches to the mind-matter problem had existed at least since the time of the ancient Greeks, the establishment of a distinct psychological discipline, with its own unique methods and interests, had to await the development of related areas whose methods, technology, and apparatus could be adapted to fit the new science. The general scientific awakening commonly associated with the seventeenth and eighteenth centuries provided this opportunity. Heralded by developments in classical physics, chemistry, and the newly discovered "electricity," and spurred on by the uprising of an insatiable curiosity, it was natural that those interested in the human organism should turn to the sense organs as a most obvious and easily accessible contact with the physical world. After all, weren't the eyes the "windows of the soul"?

The psychology of sensory-perceptual phenomena was not originated by psychologists. Indeed the very label *psychologist* was not given to students of the sense organs until many years after the interest in the subject was

---

* Although the terms *sense organ* and *receptor* may be used somewhat interchangeably throughout the book, there is an accepted distinction between them. Sense organ refers to the overall physical entity, such as the eye, ear, or semicircular canals; a receptor is some *part* of the sense organ that transduces the external energy. A receptor, for example, changes mechanical energy such as sound waves into neural energy—or in the case of taste, chemical energy into neural energy.

1

spawned. Rather, physiologists and medical doctors, on the one hand, and physicists, on the other, developed the new discipline. Men like Frances Glisson, who in 1677 contributed the concept of irritability as an attribute of animate tissue, and Giovanni Borelli, who in 1680 suggested that something is transmitted through the spongy ducts (nerve fibers) to "inflate" the muscles, were necessary before others could work out the intricate details of neurosensory functioning (Boring, 1942).

The invention of the Leyden jar in 1745, Benjamin Franklin's experiments in electricity published in 1774, and Galvani's experiments in stimulating a frog's leg and later constructing a battery of the muscle all were important contributions to the rapprochement of the physiological and physical disciplines necessary for the development of a science of sensory phenomena (Boring, 1942). By the beginning of the nineteenth century the ground work was well laid for the concerted attack on the mind-body problem—or as it was popularly known, *psychophysics*.

Related Disciplines

Although the genesis of sensory-perceptual knowledge can be traced to the alignment of the broad physical and physiological disciplines, other and more narrowly defined areas of study suggest themselves as vehicles for obtaining an understanding of the relation between "what goes on out there" and "what goes on in here." Most of the data used to describe the relation between the outside world and the world of experience can be categorized within one or more of these areas. Some knowledge of all these areas is necessary for a proper grasp of the place of the sense organs in the behavior of man. Let us look at a few of these specialized approaches, bearing in mind that they are neither highly definitive nor mutually exclusive. They are merely examples of interrelated disciplines that play a part in the understanding of sensory-perceptual experience.

PHYSICS OF THE EXTERNAL WORLD

The word *psychophysics*, which will be encountered often in this book, is indicative of the importance of physics as an associative discipline. It is probably a truism that one cannot hope to understand the relation between experience and the outside world unless one first *understands* the outside world.* Although this statement may at first appear to be too obvious for comment, it does describe a situation not always met and not always completely possible in the light of our limited knowledge of things physical. In the case of one of our sensory experiences, the olfactory sense, or sense of smell, the actual physical stimulus for the experience is not known with absolute certainty. It is generally but not universally agreed that small particles of the odorant material must make physical contact with the epithelial lining of the nasal passages for a chemical reaction to take place, but

* "Understanding the outside world" is a relative expression, and one can only hope to approach such an Olympian ideal.

the specific nature of the sensory excitatory action is not known. Indeed, it is thought by some persons that there may be some sort of radiation involved, as well as a primary chemical reaction. Neither the chemists with their involved formulas nor the physicists with their knowledge of radiation can provide us with definitive answers.

If you glanced through this book before starting to read (a wise procedure before reading any book), you may have noticed that before any detailed examination of the various sense modalities is made, a fairly extensive section is devoted to the nature of the physical stimulus for each.

In vision, for example, it is important to know of the "wave theory" of light, as contrasted with the "corpuscular theory." One should be aware of the nature of intensity, the location of visible light in the broad electromagnetic spectrum, and various other properties such as refractivity and speed of transmission. Simple physical optics involving spherical, cylindrical, and prismatic refraction are encountered in any but the most superficial treatment of vision. Such things need not be understood at the level of sophistication required of the physicist, or the professional optometrist or ophthalmologist, but at least a working knowledge of the gross properties of visible radiation is important.

Similarly, understanding of the auditory sense cannot be achieved without a working knowledge of the physics of sound. Loudness, pitch, and timbre all have their physical counterparts, and a knowledge of one without the other is incompatible with a firm grasp of sensory-perceptual relations. A complete understanding of any experience—warmth, cold, equilibrium, and so on—cannot be obtained without some detailed insight into the physical world that elicits it. We *must* understand the external world if the inner world of experience is to make any sense to us.

A primary requisite of any discipline is to develop its own methodology and techniques. The psychology of sensory-perceptual processes has borrowed heavily from physics in the development of its "tools of the trade." Unlike the psychology of testing, which had to begin from scratch, the study of sensory processes was helped by the availability of equipment and research methodology. Many psychologists today are experts in the use of complex equipments that to the uninitiated might appear the exclusive interest of the physicist. An experimental psychologist working in sensory-perceptual research would be hard pressed to get along without a knowledge of such equipment as photometers, spectroscopes, audio oscillators, and cathode-ray oscilloscopes. Furthermore, no person today can entirely escape the influence of our computerized society, and an experimental psychologist with no knowledge of computer technology is almost as hard to find as a hospital intern without a stethoscope.

CHEMISTRY

Man has long recognized that he is made up of a lot of chemicals, combined in ways that defy the imagination. The full impact of knowledge concerning the influence of chemical reactions on sensory behavior has, however, been somewhat more recent. One landmark occurred in 1876 when Franz Boll of the University of Rome isolated a brilliant red pigment from the eye of the frog. This substance, which Boll called *visual red* (now known as visual purple or rhodopsin), has since been the focus of an almost unbelievable amount of attention. In addition to this light-sensitive substance, other pigments with selective color sensitivities have been isolated and studied. Much of what we now know about color vision can be attributed to the work of men who must list their occupations as "chemist."

It would appear that all the senses, with the possible exception of those that clearly respond to mechanical changes in the environment, are highly dependent on chemical reactions for their existence. Even experiences like hearing and touch most certainly require chemical mediation at the junctures between individual nerve fibers.

No one can doubt the significance of chemical mediation in taste and probably smell. And at higher neural levels the importance of such substances as RNA and DNA is gaining widespread recognition. Certainly chemistry pervades the entire field of sensory-perceptual experience.

ANATOMY OF THE SENSE ORGANS

Although it is indeed true, as Lorenz has pointed out (1974), that an erroneous approach to analogy of structure among different species may lead us down the primrose path, there is much we can learn from the anatomy of the sense organs. The gross anatomy of the sense organs is in many cases a valid indicator of how they function. When people abandoned the idea that the eye works by squirting out "corpuscles" and decided that it was really a sensing device, utilizing external energy in its modus operandi, they were taking advantage of their knowledge of its gross structure (Wald, 1950). The similarity between the camera obscura and the mammalian eye must have been impelling to some early investigators. It must have been apparent that the eye had the parts necessary to gather light and focus an image on its rear surface. Although it may have been unclear just how this was done, the fact that it *was* done must have been almost indisputable. Today many aspects of visual functioning can be inferred on the basis of gross anatomical observation. The function of such structures as the lens, the cornea, and the iris can be assigned rather confidently from their gross structure.

In like manner the design of the external ear and the bones of the middle ear clearly reveal their function. The external ear must serve as a sound-collecting device, and the articulation of the ossicles points to the actual conduction of vibratory or sound motions.

Microanatomical approaches have made it possible to examine individual neural elements, individual cells, and the structural relations between them. Without such techniques the vast knowledge of the retina would be largely lacking. Neural structures in the central nervous system, the skin, and the inner ear are particularly amenable to study by microscopic techniques.

Unfortunately, attributing a function to an organ on the basis of its gross anatomy or microanatomy alone can be extremely hazardous. Additional information of a functional nature is necessary. As an example, textbooks for many years described the nature of the end organs in the skin, their distribution, and their presumed purpose. To the chagrin of the early microanatomists, modern experimental techniques have not been able to verify the functions assigned to many of these so-called sensory nerve endings. Even today, with the vast amount of microanatomical study that has been directed at the skin, our knowledge of just how such experiences as warmth, cold, tickle, and pain are mediated is woefully inadequate.

Another example might be mentioned of anatomical description leading us down the wrong path. The changing of pupil size as a result of activity of the iris is a familiar experience. A logical explanation of this effect might result in the conclusion that the purpose of the pupil constriction is to limit the amount of light entering the eye and thereby protect the sensitive surface inside. This is about what the author learned in high school many years ago. Actually this is not the situation at all. The maximum range of pupillary area is only about 20 to 1, but light intensity varies in a ratio of millions. The constriction serves quite another purpose: to permit, under conditions of adequate illumination, utilization of the central path of the optical system, thereby minimizing various optical aberrations and providing maximum acuity and resolution.

Although some knowledge of structure is essential to an understanding of function, it is clear that structure by itself is not enough. The other disciplines we have discussed must play their roles.

PHYSIOLOGY OF THE SENSE ORGANS

Physiological information is the basis of our entire discipline. Most of the early investigators in the field were physiologists, and the distinction today between a physiologist and a physiological psychologist may often be difficult to make.

With respect to the major contributions of physiology, I suspect the key word may well be electricity. Physiologists have provided us with an immense collection of data describing the electrical activity of the neural elements, actvity at the juncture of two neurones, and activity within a mass of cell bodies, such as in the various ganglia and in the largest ganglion of all, the brain. In addition, electrical activity at the receptors has been studied and we now have a knowledge of how sensory cells are activated which was not possible before the widespread application of electric and electronic equipment and methods.

A great deal of what we know about the role of the brain in sensory-perceptual processing can be attributed to developments in physiological instrumentation and physiology in general. As suggested earlier, instrumentation and techniques developed by physiologists have contributed immensely to the advancement in sensory-perceptual psychology.

The relatively modern development of the high-speed computer has, by so-called modeling, suggested how complex neural-sensory systems *might* work. Although many persons, this author among them, deplore the simplistic analogy of the brain as a high-speed digital computer, investigative approaches involving just such hypotheses may prove to be valuable in our ultimately learning just how the nervous system does function. However, making the assumption that the brain works like a computer may be dangerous. We might unwittingly fall into the trap: "After all, God is just as smart as man, isn't He? And since man can make a device that 'thinks,' wouldn't God have used a similar technique in designing the brain?" God also made creatures that fly, but when man devised flying machines he had to abandon the flapping wings in favor of propellers and jets. We cannot logically conclude that birds fly by means of propellers and jets just because man-made "birds" have them. However, if we are careful to avoid such logical inconsistencies, the apparent analogies between brain functioning and high-speed computer operations may indeed help us gain a better insight into sensory-perceptual processes.

COMPARATIVE AND MAMMALIAN EMBRYOLOGY

The serious student of sensory-perceptual psychology would do well to spend a little time studying the organism from a developmental point of view. Probably no occurrence in the author's past so impressed him with its relevance to sensory psychology as a course he once took in comparative embryology. Tracing the development of the sense organs ontogenetically from the gamete to the adult, and phylogenetically from the amoeba to *Homo sapiens* can be an extremely interesting and rewarding experience. Much of our understanding of the sense organs is based on such analyses. Did you know, for example, that the previously mentioned bones of the middle ear are derived from the gill arches of the primitive shark? That an evolutionary process of many eons has resulted in the migration of these structures from the gill area to their present location in the middle ear? Are you aware that the human eye, or at least that part known as the retina, is actually, in the true sense of the word, an extension of the brain? That in ontogenetic development a bulge in the embryological "brain" results in a bulb on the end of a stalk, the former turning inside-out to form the inside rear surface of the eye, the latter forming the optic nerve?

Such facts as these are of more than passing interest. They are fascinating, true. But more than that, they reveal to us how the structures in question probably work. When we know that the retina is actually an extension of the brain we are not at all surprised to discover what a large amount of information processing goes on there.

DIRECT ANALYSIS OF CONSCIOUSNESS

An approach not often encountered today, but popular during the latter part of the nineteenth century, involved the direct observation of one's "sensations." Because it did make major contributions and does have some applicability today, it should be mentioned.

Introspective analysis of one's innermost psychological behavior was a favorite tool of such workers as O. Külpe, Wilhelm Wundt (who founded the first psychological laboratory in Leipzig), and E. B. Titchener, who brought the new discipline to this country via Cornell (Boring, 1942). They believed that the proper way to study sensory processes was to study sensations. Such a statement should not, on the surface, evoke much criticism, but the manner in which they proceeded to study them *did* leave much to be desired. They felt that sensations were merely one of the components, or elements, of consciousness, the other two being simple images (like memory pictures), and feeling or affective tone. All consciousness, then, was made up of sensations from the sense organs, images from the memory, and affective tone or feeling (the latter generally being assumed to be either pleasant or unpleasant, or some such dichotomy). In the language of Wundt, sensations were the basic elements of consciousness; perception was the combination of sensation and affection.

Research consisted primarily in studying the content of one's consciousness, and in a more analytical manner, the nature of one's sensations. By the time of Titchener, all sensations were allegedly describable in terms of four characteristics, called *attributes*. These essential attributes were *quality* (for example, hue or pitch), *quantity* (brightness or loudness), *temporal* (duration), and *spatial*—or as it was sometimes called, *extensity*. An additional attribute of *clarity* was added later.

The idea that one can learn all about the sensory processes by simply "introspecting" and examining one's innermost thoughts has not been considered seriously for many years. One can't understand the basis for afterimages by simply spending many hours looking at them and trying to figure out their genesis. In like manner, the breaking down of theoretical constructs such as *consciousness* into hard-and-fast "structures" is repugnant to our modern approach to science. However, in spite of their defects, these approaches were not as sterile as a modern scientist might have been led to predict. The *attributes* of sensation are still to be found in every book on sensation and perception. Only now we call them by a different name, such as *characteristics* or *modes of discrimination*. Although the structuralist theory of these early pioneers has died with them, they did leave a legacy of knowledge and methodology that is still of great importance.

RELATION OF OUTSIDE WORLD, SENSATIONS, AND EXPERIENCE

One of the most fruitful approaches, and that of this book, is the examination of the relationship between what our sense organs do and what we think happened to make them do what they did. In simple language, we "see" a light; what did our eyes *do* as a result of some outside event (presumably electromagnetic radiation) that we interpret as "light"? And, of course, what sorts of outside events will produce the effect in the sense organ that we have come to call "light"? We have all experienced so-called illusions, in which the event we think we experience does not occur at all.

Some misinterpretations occur because of errors in the transition from the outside world to the world of the sensory organs; others must occur in the transition from sensory organ activity to conscious awareness. While your friend is romping in the "warm" water, you are gingerly testing the "cold" water with your toe. How is it possible that the same water feels warm to the person entirely immersed and cold to an individual not yet wet? Such adaptation phenomena are discussed in later chapters of this book. There is also an instance of so-called inadequate stimuli. If you bump the back of your head, you may "see stars" even though the eyes are in no way directly involved.

Psychophysics, in its broadest sense, attempts to disclose the relations between the physical world and the world of experience. It is such a fundamental part of sensory-perceptual experience that we are going to devote two entire chapters to its methods.

Table 1–1 presents in summary form the three aspects of sensory experience for a few of the better-understood sensory modalities, both for broad stimuli ranges (e.g., the first entry) and for more specific energies

TABLE 1–1
Relation of Outside World, Sensory Function, and Experience

Outside World	Sensory Functon	Experience
Electromagnetic radiation from about 400 to 750 mμ	Chemical-electrical response of rods and cones in retina	Light
Electromagnetic radiation of 700 mμ	Chemical-electrical response of *some* cones in retina	Red light
Acoustic vibration from 20 to 15,000 Hz (cycles/sec)	Mechanical-electrical response in cochlea	Sound
Acoustic vibration at 10,000 Hz	Mechanical-electrical response of one part of cochlea	High-pitched sound
Presence of certain dissociated ions in solution	Chemical-electrical response of receptor cells on tongue	Taste of salt
Tilting of the body	Mechanical-electrical response of cells in semicircular canals	Position of head
Flexing of the arm	Mechanical-electrical response of sensory cells in the joint	Bent elbow
Moderate temperature rise	Thermal(?)*-electrical response of cells in the skin	Feeling of warmth
Lack of water in the body	Mechanical(?)†-electrical response of cells lining the mouth	Thirst

* A so-called vascular theory suggests that warmth may be mediated by pressure-sensitive nerve endings in the walls of the small blood vessels.

† This is only one basis of thirst. Receptors in the brain are stimulated by lowered water content in the body fluids and this probably serves as the primary indicator of water need.

(such as the second entry). Note that in all cases, although the sense organ input may be in the form of mechanical, chemical, or thermal energy, the output is always in the form of "electricity." As we shall see later, this electrical output of the receptor is not an electrical current as we know it; rather it is a train of more or less coded impulses, apparently produced by chemical means.

Classifying the Senses

How many senses are there? Your answer is as good as mine, because it really depends on how you classify and name them. What about the classical five senses: vision, audition, touch, olfaction, and taste? Aren't all the senses included under these five categories? Hardly. These are merely convenient categories based on gross observation. Equilibrium and position of the head as sensed by the organs of the inner ear appear to be unique senses. The skin is sensitive to warmth, cold, pain, and touch. Are these not separate senses? And what about color perception? Inasmuch as there are probably separate receptor cells (cones) in the retina for each primary color, are these not separate senses? Experience and gross observation are not satisfactory bases for classifying the senses.

The structuralists referred to earlier discovered that sensations are indeed quite personal, and what one person might call red, another would see as yellow, or perhaps simply as a shade of gray. If we cannot classify our sensory experiences in terms of their inner nature, is there not some other, more acceptable way of distinguishing them?

One answer lies in the nature of the outside stimuli that produce them. Thanks to the efforts of physicists, chemists, and other natural scientists, a large body of knowledge bearing on the nature of natural phenomena is available. We simply refer to a sense modality in terms of the stimulus that produces the experience, and everyone knows what we are talking about. We do not have the problem of the gross nature of the morphological entities nor the sensory interpretation problems of the structuralists.

Let us look at some of the different forms of energy which are capable of producing effects in the organism which might be referred to as sensations.

CHEMICAL ENERGY

A generalized chemically induced response in irritable tissue is probably the oldest and most primitive forerunner of our now complex sensory functioning. In lower animals at the level of the amoeba, for instance, it is possible that the only environmental change which has the potential for stimulating the animal is chemical in nature. You may find many lower organisms which do not respond to sound or electromagnetic energy, but I know of no organisms entirely insensitive to chemical changes.

Higher animals' dependence upon chemical energy is likewise well known. Both the sense of smell and the sense of taste* are clearly mediated by chemical energy; smell by stimulation of nerve endings in the epithelial lining of the nasal passages and taste by the chemical nature of particles which evoke responses in the sensory cells of the taste buds. As we will see in Chapters 17, 18, and 19 we do not understand these functions adequately, but it is a safe bet to attribute their responses to a chemical reaction of some sort.

While energy other than chemical may produce activity in the sense organs, it does appear to be a fact that for every response to the environment by an organism, a chemical reaction takes place somewhere. Living organisms are chemical machines. Electromagnetic energy may stimulate the elements of the retina to action, but the intermediary condition which produces the neural response is chemical in nature. Even when neural energy is released by direct mechanical energy, such as sound waves or tactual vibration, the neural impulse itself, is, basically, a chemical reaction.

Adaptation is an important aspect of the chemical senses, and appears to be a factor in all of them. Most chemical reactions are reversible, but a finite amount of time is required to produce the reverse reaction. In the meantime, the depletion of one or more of the contributors to the reaction results in a general slowdown of the reaction, and hence, an apparent adaptation. Sensory adaptation may be more than this, but at a superficial level, a slowing-down of the reaction due to the depletion of that constituent of the reaction supplied by the organism appears to be a satisfactory if not completely adequate explanation.

In addition to the senses of taste and smell, numerous other "senses" are of a chemical nature. Quotation marks are used for the word *senses* here because these receptors may not result in sensations in the popular sense. We have receptors lying deep in the brain which detect conditions in the blood stream that warrant attention. The recognition of water need, oxygen shortage, or blood temperature must be classed as a form of sensory activity. These sensory functions frequently do not reach a level of conscious awareness, and we do not ordinarily think of them in terms of sensations or perceptions. When things are going along correctly, we are not even aware of the existence of most of these functions. Yet hunger, thirst, and body temperature changes are conditions meriting attention at a level of insistence equal to or greater than those arising wholly from the outside environment. Although we can be certain that these internal sensory organs work in many cases as chemical receptors, their nature is still somewhat of a mystery—a mystery, incidentally, that is being attacked with considerable vigor by our friends in physiology.

In summary, chemical reactions are the basis of most receptor activity,

---

* As indicated earlier, the "sense of taste" is undoubtedly several senses if we are to be precise in our language. However, for the purpose of simplicity, the word "sense" may at times be used with its popular, loosely defined meaning: sense of smell, sense of taste, sense of vision, etc.

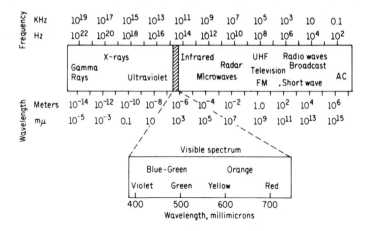

Figure 1-1
The electromagnetic spectrum. Note the overall width of the total spectrum, more than
twenty log units. Note, too, the relatively narrow portion that is visible to the human
eye. (Adapted from the IES Lighting Handbook by permission of the Illuminating
Engineering Society.)

and even in the case of those receptors that clearly respond to nonchemical
events, some chemical mediation must play a role somewhere, certainly in
the neuron itself if not before.

ELECTROMAGNETIC ENERGY

Most living organisms also appear to be sensitive, in one way or another,
to one or more forms of electromagnetic energy. In general, the portion of
the spectrum to which most animals are sensitive respresents only an infinitesimal part of the whole. As shown in Figure 1–1, the visible spectrum
for man ranges from approximately 400 to 750 nanometers (nm), also
called millimicrons (mμ), but the total known spectrum has a range of some
24 log units, that is, a range of 1,000,000,000,000,000,000,000,000 to 1. In
comparable units the total known spectrum contains waves with wavelengths from 10^{-7} to 10^{16} mμ or nm. Expressing it in another way, if the
total spectrum were divided into octaves, that is "doublings" of frequency
or wavelength, nearly 80 octaves would be required to encompass it. In
contrast, the visible portion of the spectrum would be included in less than
one of these octaves.

Figure 1–1 also shows the position of various other functions in the electromagnetic spectrum. In addition to showing wavelengths in meters, this
figure also includes corresponding frequencies in cycles per second, now
referred to as hertz (Hz).The position of diverse forms of radiation such as
X rays, ultraviolet, infrared, and radio, radar, and TV waves are also indicated. The schematic expansion of the visible portion of the spectrum is

considered in much more detail in the chapters devoted to vision and the discrimination of hue or color.

The visual sense, especially in higher-order animals, has achieved a remarkable level of development. The sensitive elements of the human eye have reached such a peak of perfection that they can respond, it is said, to one quantum of radiant energy—the absolute minimum that can be shown to exist (Wald, 1950). The visual sense of lower animals is no less impressive. A broad variety of receptor types and configurations adapt the various species to their environments, in many cases often exceeding the capabilities of *Homo sapiens*.

In general, most animals with sensitivity to electromagnetic energy confine their sensitivities to the restricted portion of the spectrum that produces the sensation "light." There is variability among species, and of course some animals may be sensitive to portions of the spectrum well outside the limits of the normally visible portion. We do not know with certainty just what portions of the spectrum may affect some living organisms.

At one extreme, however, marked sensitivity to radiant heat, or infrared radiation, appears to be a capability of some forms of animal life. Numerous cold-blooded animals that feed on small warm-blooded creatures can presumably detect their prey by means of specialized infrared detectors. Several types of snakes have receptors for radiant energy which are of sufficient sensitivity to enable them to capture their prey with a minimum of assistance from the other senses. (Harris, 1971 and Hartline et al., 1978)

Although it is still within the normally visible spectrum, polarized light can be discriminated by some insects. Honeybees, for example, owe much of their navigational ability to a differential sensitivity to the direction of light polarization. (See, for example, Wellington, 1974, and Wehner, 1976, as well as an interchange of letters between Wehner and Jaffe in the November issue of *Scientific American*.) For centuries superstitious people have attributed supernatural powers to the moon, specifically to moonlight. The word *lunacy* came from the old idea that people behave differently under the light of the moon, or as a function of the phase of the moon. Inasmuch as moonlight tends to be polarized differently from sunlight, perhaps the old superstition is not quite as fantastic as one might think. Perhaps moonlight does affect some animals differently from daylight. Certainly, within his state of awareness, however, discrimination of direction of light polarization is a capability denied man; he must equip himself with special polarizing filters even to determine the direction of the polarization.

Some animals can sense ultraviolet—that is, wavelengths lying further along the short-wavelength end of the spectrum. The capability of insects to utilize light in the ultraviolet region has been well documented (Mazokhin-Porshuyakov, 1969). We even have a good idea of how the visual stimulus might appear to the creature (Eisner et al., 1969). Various flowers that to the human eye appear identical may perhaps be discriminable to the eye of the honeybee, which can allegedly distinguish the ultraviolet content of the electromagnetic radiation.

There are also slight differences within the human species. Some people can also see colors well out on either the violet or red ends of the normally visible spectrum. The retina of the eye itself is sensitive to wavelengths in the near ultraviolet that cannot be detected by the eye as a whole. This is due to the yellow coloring in the crystalline lens, which, by absorption, prevents some of the shorter wavelengths from reaching the retina. (Insects presumably do not have this filtering capability.) Persons who have had their lenses removed in the course of cataract operations can often see colors in the violet or near ultraviolet that are invisible to the normal eye. Many former patients of cataract operations wear tinted lenses in their spectacles to replace the ultraviolet absorption function.

As was true for the chemical senses, adaptation plays an important role in the electromagnetic-sensitive senses, at least in those having a chemical reaction as an intermediate stage. Adaptation in color vision has long been recognized, is familiar to everyone, and is usually explained as the result of the chemical breakdown of the color-sensitive pigments in the cones. Negative afterimages, on the other hand, are generally attributed to the reverse anabolic process in the receptor, although the possibility of some central nervous system contribution cannot be denied.

THERMAL ENERGY

Most organisms, certainly all those relatively high on the phylogenetic scale, react to thermal energy or temperature. As indicated in the previous section, some of this sensitivity is probably due to an extension of the electromagnetic sensitivity into the infrared end of the spectrum. Most sensitivity to electromagnetic energy involves the chemical change of some pigment, not entirely unlike the events occurring in a sensitive photographic emulsion. Indeed, at least one investigator has succeeded in taking the pigments from an animal's eye, crushing them into an emulsion, and making a "photographic plate" that actually works (Wald, 1950). I suspect that the sensitivity of some reptiles to heat from an anticipated dinner may involve a breakdown of pigment in their skin or tongue receptors produced by the heat from the body of the warm blooded victim.

On the other hand, there appears to be some sensitivity to temperature change, both increasing and decreasing temperature, mediated by other, perhaps more direct, means. The skin is sensitive to both warmth and cold, and that these sensations are mediated in the same manner as vision, or the snake's infrared sensitivity, appears highly unlikely. Early investigators suggested that there were indeed separate end organs for the receiving of warmth and cold (heat has usually been attributed to a combination of warmth and pain) and they proceeded to "map" them on the skin with an abandon later to be regretted. Now we are not so sure. *Some* end organs do appear to mediate one or the other sensation, but the microanatomical description of the temperature sensitivity of the skin is far from complete.

The temperature of the blood, as another example, is regulated largely as a feedback mechanism from sensors located within the blood vessels. Just how this is accomplished we do not know. Perhaps it is simply a sensitivity to expansion and constriction; but then what about changes in blood pressure? How can the sense organs "know" which it is? It would appear that there must be some direct mediation, but its nature escapes us.

One particular problem is the amount of accommodation or adaptation in the temperature senses. If you immerse your hand in ice-cold water and then place it in water of a neutral temperature, it may feel quite warm, perhaps even hot. Conversely, adapting to warm water will result in subsequent cool water feeling quite cold. The lukewarm water following a hot shower often feels just like ice water.

It would appear too that the temperature sense is not really a temperature sense at all. It is in fact a *change-in-temperature* sense. As implied in the previous paragraph, prolonged subjection to any temperature extreme (within rather obvious limits) results in adaptation, such that the original sensation of warmth or cold gradually diminishes and a more nearly neutral feeling takes its place. It has been said that if a live frog is placed in a pan of cold water and the pan placed on a stove, the temperature can be slowly raised to the boiling point, cooking the frog without his ever being disturbed. Certainly you can recall instances where you adapted to bath water, gradually getting it hotter and hotter until you emerged from the tub looking like a boiled lobster. And the last sunburn you got—you probably were not even aware you were being burned.

Much is yet to be learned about the temperature sense (or senses?); it is one of the most fascinating and challenging areas in sensory-perceptual psychology.

MECHANICAL ENERGY

Most organisms respond to jabs, jolts, and almost any type of physical contact. The skin rather obviously is a favorite location for these receptors, whatever they might be. Although considerable attention has been paid to the sense of touch by classical psychophysicists, their interest was primarily in the nature of the sensation, especially such aspects as accuracy of localization and the determination of minimal distances between two points on the skin that could be just barely discerned as being two points, rather than one. The identification of the physiological event that indicates to the organism, "I have been touched," has proved to be quite elusive. Free nerve endings and various encapsulated end organs have at various times been credited with mediating tactual sensitivity. Nerve endings in the hair follicles are probably activated whenever a hair is disturbed. Much remains to be learned about cutaneous tactual sensitivity.

Mechanical energy is important in other than the skin senses. The position of our limbs is known to us, at least partially, through the stimulation of proprioceptors in the joints and movement sensors within the muscles. The proprioceptive and kinesthetic senses tell us when we have moved a limb, and in general just where it is at a given point in time and space. In locomotor ataxia, a disorder commonly the result of an untreated syphilitic infection, the ascending (leg-to-brain) paths of the sensory nerves have been destroyed. The patient walks as if he had some serious impairment to his motor function, hence the name. Actually the problem is not motor, but is due to the lack of feedback from the lower limbs. The patient appears to have difficulty in walking because he has to use other cues, such as vision, to indicate where his feet are.

As was true for the temperature senses, there are undoubtedly many internal functions mediated by mechanical receptors at a level below conscious awareness. It is likely that the automatic control of pressure functions such as blood pressure, and air pressure within the lungs, are at least partially regulated by stretch receptors in the walls of the involved organs. We alluded in the last section to the possibility that some temperature sensitivity might very well be a sensitivity to mechanical stimulation. Small blood vessels could constrict or dilate as a function of the temperature, and this change could be sensed by means of free nerve endings associated with the vessel walls.

Adaptation also plays a role of great importance in the tactual senses. A tight collar, or clothing that at first appears uncomfortable, can often be adapted to so that its presence is not only ignored but even completely forgotten. As was true for thermal receptors, "change" appears to be the key word for the mechanical receptors.

ACOUSTIC ENERGY

In essence, acoustic energy is simply mechanical energy of a high frequency. Although even at its highest frequencies it might still be considered as mechanical energy, there is such an amazing degree of specialization and evolutionary development in acoustic sensitivity that it clearly merits inclusion as a specialized sense. There is little evidence that unicellular animals show any appreciable sensitivity to acoustic energy, but almost all organisms higher in the phylogenetic scale have some sensitivity to acoustic or vibratory stimulation within broadly specified limits. (Did you ever wonder how earthworms can "hear" you coming if you walk too hard?)

Phylogenetic evidence tends to indicate, as might be expected, that the acoustic senses have developed primarily from the primtive mechanical energy sensors. The lateral line organs of the shark, for example, are basically cutaneous endings that have acquired a sensitivity to vibratory frequencies impinging on the fish's outer surface. Many arthropods have acoustic sensors in their body and leg regions that are only slightly different from conventional mechanical receptors. Brownell (1977), for example, studied the ability of desert scorpions to utilize compressional and surface waves in sand in locating their prey. By sensing slight movements in the sand they were able to locate and capture small insects at distances as great as 2 in.

Higher organisms have achieved a level of sophistication in the development of their acoustic sensitivity that is nothing less than miraculous. The sensitivity of the human ear is so great that, were it increased by an infinitesimal amount, the results would be disastrous. Brownian movement of the air molecules would be heard as a constant "whishing" sound. Just this sort of thing does arise occasionally in some auditory disorders, and the effects on the afflicted person are indeed serious.

Both the range of acoustic sensitivity and the uses to which it is put vary from species to species. Although the frequency range of auditory sensitivity for humans is generally found within the extreme limits of 20 to 20,000 Hz, there is a marked variability between individuals. Very few persons reach the upper limit of 20,000 Hz, and once beyond the middle teens, a person's sensitivity to the higher frequencies decreases rapidly. The range of sensitivity for an adult is probably closer to 40 to 12,000 Hz, or even lower at the upper end of the frequency spectrum. Increasing age results in continued lowering of the upper frequency limit.

Many infrahuman animals demonstrate a capability of hearing frequencies much higher than those sensed by man. The familiar Galton whistle, used to call dogs, produces a frequency too high to be heard by humans but is well within the sensitivity range of the dog. Bats not only are sensitive to frequencies in the ultrasonic (above normal human limits) range but are also able to produce "sounds" at these frequencies. (They are sounds to bats but silence to man.) Their remarkable hearing ability enables them to utilize the returning echoes much like a primitive form of radar, providing information about obstacles in their path. Anticollision radar has only recently been developed for airplanes and boats; bats had it millennia ago.

The auditory sense is extremely complex. In contrast to the other senses (except for vision), the amount of information that can be obtained and processed by the auditory sense is almost limitless. Lower animals may simply respond in a general way to acoustic energy or sound. An earthworm, for example, may pull itself back into its hole as a result of a vibration or an intense sound. Man and the higher animals, however, have reached such a state of development, with such a sophisticated analyzing capability, that an almost infinite amount of information can be accepted and processed.

GRAVITY

Probably there is no such thing as a "sense of gravity." However, whether it is mediated by a mechanical sense or whatever, the force of gravity does influence behavior. Because of gravity, fluid and small granules (*otoliths*) in the vestibular apparatus of the inner ear tend to assume a normal resting position when the organism is stationary. As the head moves, centrifugal forces move the fluid and granules about in their cavities, stimulating hair cells; this eventuates in neural signals indicating movement, and ultimately, the position of the head. To be sure, because this experience is similar to the use of accelerometers in aerial navigation, only *changes* in position are indicated, and other sensory experiences are needed to verify position at any given time.

Fortunately, there are other ways in which gravity tells us "which end is up." Our bodies and our internal organs have considerable mass, and pressure on various internal sensors in the customary direction (downward) probably indicates to us that we are right side up. Blood is influenced by gravity, and everyone is aware of the experience of blood leaving the feet and flowing to the head when one is upside down for any length of time. Actually, of course, the blood does not entirely leave the feet and flow to the head, but there are changes in relative pressure that can be sensed, probably by some of the same pressure-sensitive receptors we referred to before.

As is true for many other "internal" senses, response to gravity more often than not occurs below the level of conscious experience. Reflexive behavior is basic to much of our equilibratory sense and automatic adjustments are made without our being aware of them. Persons who have lost the use of their semicircular canals do not have this efficient, automatic feedback system. They must rely more on the proprioceptive pressure senses and the sense of vision to maintain their balance.

Astronauts, of course, survive with no ill effects in an environment completely lacking in gravity. They can determine their body position only through their internal proprioceptive and kinesthetic sense, and, of course, vision. Yet they are able to perform physical and mental feats that might tax the capabilities of many of us earthbound folk.

ELECTRICAL AND MAGNETIC ENERGY

In light of our present-day knowledge it is probably safe to say that man has no capability of sensing external electrical or magnetic energy directly. (An electric shock is most likely the result of stimulating receptors such as those for touch, pain, etc., and not the setting off of any special receptors "tuned" for electricity.) Some people believe that ESP (extrasensory perception) is made possible by the reception of some sort of magnetic or electromagnetic energy produced by the sender's brain. Until the existence of ESP can be demonstrated, claims for such sensory processes can scarcely be taken seriously.

Sensitivity to electrical and magnetic energy does, however, appear to be a basic characteristic of some forms of life, and perhaps a fundamental feature of undifferentiated protoplasm. Responses to magnetic or electric currents, often called *tropisms*, are displayed by many lower animals. If parameciums are placed in a watch glass with positive and negative electrodes placed a short distance apart, the little creatures can be seen to move, almost as one, toward the negative electrode. Or if an earthworm is placed on a sheet of paper within an electromagnetic field (plane electrodes above and below it), reversing the polarity of the field will cause the earthworm to roll over. It makes a startling experiment to alternate the fields rapidly and see the worm roll right off his paper platform. Neither of these examples can be likened to what happens when a permanent magnet attracts iron filings, because the movement of the animals seems to result from their own propulsive behavior.

Although such responses may be called tropisms (which of course doesn't explain anything), and not true sensory experience, they are evidence that the animal does have some sort of a sense that can discriminate between the positive and negative extremes of a magnetic or electromagnetic field.

It has been suggested that some birds utilize the influence of the earth's magnetic poles as navigational aids. Although man must carry compasses and delicate sensing instruments to even be aware that such phenomena exist, some forms of life may rely on their ability to sense variations in electrical potentials and magnetic fields to insure their existence. As a simple example, it has been demonstrated that low-frequency electrical fields produce changes in the shape and motility of amoebas (Friend and Finch, 1975). Furthermore, orientation to DC magnetic fields of low strength has been demonstrated for honeybees and birds. Larkin and Sutherland (1977) showed recently that migrating birds changed their altitudes as a result of flying over a large AC (72 to 80 Hz) antenna system.

A more sophisticated form of electrical field sensitivity, also at a higher phylogenetic level, has been reported. In addition to killing or stunning its prey, the discharge of the electric eel apparently serves as a form of "radar." Other fish seem to have a similar capability, although in a more modest way (Wooldridge, 1963). Receptors in the skin of the fish are sensitive to the patterns of the electric field, resulting from the emitted pulses interacting with surrounding objects. It is said that field changes as small as one-millionth of a volt can be detected!

The ancient art of astrology is based on the belief that the sun and the planets influence our behavior in a relatively direct and predictable manner. Although no serious scientist regards astrology as more than entertaining nonsense, there are those who do believe that electromagnetic fields can influence earthly creatures and that these fields may be produced by the sun and by the earth and other planets. Frank A. Brown of Northwestern University has conducted experiments indicating that living organisms may be sensitive to exceedingly weak variation of such phenomena. However, until more is known concerning the nature of their influence we need not pay any concerted attention to them.

What about the gravitational pull of the moon and major planets? Is it reasonable to believe that a force capable of piling ocean water 30 ft high along some coastal areas should have no effect on insignificant living creatures? I know of no animals which can sense the pull of the moon, but that is not to say that some do not exist. We may indeed find that some forms of migratory behavior, for example, are dependent on the moon and its attractive force.

Deviating somewhat from our original classification of forces, is it possible that some organism can detect other natural phenomena, such as meteorological changes, long before they are detected by humans? The fall in barometric pressure before serious storms may very well be detected by some animals, thereby enabling them to seek shelter before the full fury of the storm strikes.

Summary

In the first chapter we tried to become familiar with that broad area of sensory-perceptual psychology. We attempted to do this in two ways: First we tried to gain insight into the relationship among the various disciplines that contribute to an understanding of sensory-perceptual psychology. As an admittedly incomplete list, we considered physics, chemistry, anatomy, physiology, embryology, direct analysis of consciousness, and the relation of the outside world to experience. This latter, we learned, is "psychophysics." Second, we examined a method for classifying the sense organs, based on the nature of the stimuli that produce the experiences. Although we must admit that the list is somewhat arbitrary, we recognized chemical, electromagnetic, thermal, mechanical, acoustic, electrical and mechanical energies, and gravity as possible physical sources of sensory experience.

Suggested Readings

1. From J. J. Gibson. *The Senses Considered as Perceptual Systems.* Boston: Houghton Mifflin, 1966. Chapter I, "The Environment as a Source of Stimulation," chap. II, "The Obtaining of Stimulation," and chap. III, "The Perceptual Systems" are suggested as possible readings for the student with particular interest in these areas. These 59 pages suggest an approach more oriented toward an understanding of perceptual problems than toward an understanding of the physics and physiology of the senses. Although they are not especially difficult pages, the serious student will be rewarded by being introduced to an interesting approach to the classification of receptors and perceptual systems.
2. A. C. Crombie. "Early Concepts of the Senses and the Mind," *Scientific American,* May 1964. This article of about nine pages deals with a subject not covered in the text and is written in a manner that should prove to be of interest to the intermediate and advanced student. It is not a complete history of knowledge related to the senses and the mind; primarily it is an attempt to explain the nature of the development of scientific inquisitiveness of the seventeenth century with respect to mental functioning.
3. From E. G. Boring. *Sensation and Perception in the History of Experimental*

Psychology. New York: Appleton, 1942. This entire book is related to the material in this chapter. However, Boring's chap. 1, "Sensation and Perception," and chap. 2, "Physiology of Sensation," are of more specific interest. These 94 pages contain the most complete history of the development of sensory-perceptual psychology that I know of. The casual student will find this source somewhat detailed, but the serious, more advanced student can greatly gain in understanding of the field by reading these two chapters carefully. The importance of comprehensive and detailed background knowledge cannot be overemphasized.

4. John Thorson and Marguerite Biederman-Thorson. "Distributed Relaxation Processes in Sensory Adaptation," *Science* 183, (1974):161–172. This is not an easy article and is not recommended for the casual undergraduate. It does, however, contain a wealth of material on general adaptation phenomena and might be of value to the instructor who wishes to go somewhat more into depth.

5. N. R. F. Maier and T. C. Schneirla, *Principles of Animal Psychology.* New York: McGraw-Hill, 1935. As indicated by its title, this reference is directly applicable to only a small part of this book, but it does have such a wealth of information and at least a general applicability that I must recommend it for the interested student. Of equal importance, it is a very interesting and highly readable book.

6. M. Wilson, and the editors of *Life, Energy.* New York: Time, Inc., 1963. This is a fine book, written in an easy style, profusely illustrated and worthwhile reading for anyone, not just persons interested in sensory-perceptual psychology.

7. From William R. Uttal, *The Psychobiology of Sensory Coding.* New York: Harper & Row, 1973. Chapters 1 and 2 are particularly applicable to the material included in this chapter. Read chap. 2 for an interesting presentation of the physical stimuli involved in sensory activity.

8. From *Scientific American.* In addition to the Crombie article referred to above, there are a great number of articles in this colorful, well-written journal that are applicable to the material in this chapter. Many of these articles have been assembled in bound form under such titles as *Psychobiology, Physiological Psychology,* and *Perception,* and published by W. H. Freeman and Co., San Francisco.

9. Roger Eckert. "Bioelectric Control of Ciliary Activity," *Science,* 176 (1972): 473–481. This is an interesting, somewhat advanced article on the sensitivity-responsiveness of ciliated protozoa to electrochemical influences. It is recommended for the serious student or instructor who wishes to delve deeper into the subject. The nearly 60 references at the end of this article should be of considerable value.

10. Edward C. Carterette and Morton P. Friedman (eds.). *Handbook of Perception, vol. I, Historical and Philosophical Roots of Perception.* New York: Academic Press, 1973. This volume should be of great value to the serious student. It greatly extends the information presented in later chapters of this book, as well as this first chapter. This series of books is, in essence, the successor to Stevens' *Handbook of Experimental Psychology* and should be in every serious student's library.

2 / development of sensory organs

We will be better able to understand the complex functioning of our sensory organs if we examine them against a background of evolutionary as well as individual development. Were we to plunge into the mysteries of vision and audition, for example, without adequate background preparation we might find ourselves lost in a sea of apparently unrelated information, complex relations, and unresolved differences of opinion. To comprehend fully the functioning of our sensory organs we need information on both the development of the species and the development of the individual within the species. Indeed, a preliminary consideration of both phylogenetic and ontogenetic development appears essential to our understanding of the area.

Although the old saying "ontogeny recapitulates phylogeny" is valid only in a general way, an understanding of differences among species, both laterally (for similar levels of development) and longitudinally (for levels of increasing complexity of development), can be of extreme usefulness in gaining an understanding of how an organism is influenced by his external world. A subsequent comparison of individual development with phylogenetic development can be extremely rewarding. The remarkable similarity between the embryos of higher animals and the adult stages of many lower members of the animal kingdom appears more than coincidental and is certainly helpful in improving our understanding of both development of structure and function. It is fascinating that a man and a frog start life in an extremely similar manner. At a sufficiently early stage of development it is hard to distinguish which is which. Man, however, continues to develop long after the frog has realized its predestined potential and taken its place in the neighborhood swamp.

The sense organs develop in a manner reflecting the overall development cycle. The newborn infant can, like the adult frog, perceive movement. The ability to track a moving object skillfully and to perceive form is presumably a later development. But the frog? It never progresses much beyond the movement-perception stage. In the grand scheme of things this ability is adequate for catching a normal quota of insects, and the frog is indeed ideally suited for its lily-pond existence.

A major portion of this chapter will be devoted to species-related differences and evolutionary development. Ontogenetic development is considered to a greater extent in the chapters devoted to specific sensory-perceptual functioning.

The Place of Sensory Functioning in Life

As we learned in elementary biology, living matter differs from nonliving matter in several respects.

1. Assimilation. All living matter has the ability to take in and use other, often nonorganic material. A fundamental property of protoplasm, and hence all living organisms, is the capability to ingest food and perform some sort of chemical reaction on it such as digestion and respiration or photosynthesis, eventually resulting in the release of one or more forms of energy. Assimilation is probably the most fundamental distinction between animate and inanimate matter, the specific form of which serves as the primary distinction between the plant and animal kingdom.

2. Growth. Only living matter grows, in the true sense of the word. River deltas seem to "grow," but actually they merely accumulate more individual grains of sand, and no individual grains increase in bulk as is necessary to qualify as true growth. Living organisms change other, foreign material into protoplasm, and it is this phenomenon we refer to as growth, the creation of additional protoplasm. It may be as simple (on the surface, at least) as an amoeba getting larger or as complex as mitosis with the formation of new, presumably identical cells.

3. Reproduction. A third characteristic that distinguishes animate matter is reproduction—a form of growth, perhaps, but more than simple growth. In reproduction a new organism is formed, similar in many respects to the parent, but different in some slight detail, thus allowing for the progress of evolution and the continuous perpetuation, and at the same time, renewal of the species.

4. Irritability. Whether it is "as the sunflower turns on her god, when he sets, the same look which she turn'd when he rose" (Moore) or a youthful demonstrator tossing a brick through a window, protoplasm has the capability to react to changes in its surroundings. It is this capability we refer to as *irritability*. And it is the primitive irritability that has developed (through the fortunate genesis of the nervous system) into the magnificently varied capabilities of sensory processes and ultimately to the pin-

nacle of higher-level neural functioning that higher animals now enjoy. The subtitle of this chapter, of perhaps the entire book, might well have included the word *irritability*, for it is at the base of all sensory-perceptual functioning.

How did this simple function develop into the complex world of sensation-perception we now know?

The key word is *evolution*. Starting with a generalized "irritability" background, the process of evolution has produced such a variety of sensitivities and discriminabilities in the various species that a mere listing of conditions to which animals are responsive is probably impossible. Each species has developed a sensory capability ideally suited to its own pattern of behavior. (Perhaps the converse is more nearly true; that the animal developed a behavioral pattern consistent with its sensory capability.) Whichever we accept, the fact remains that the differences among species are tremendous, and the fact that so many different kinds of animals *have* survived really points to vast differences in sensory abilities. For example, some birds can locate and recognize small rodents on the ground at distances of hundreds of yards. The normal *Homo sapiens* cannot do this without the aid of powerful binoculars. But this keenness of vision represents the key to survival for the hawk; we do not need to see mice at a hundred yards in order to get our dinner and perpetuate our species. Our sensory capabilities *are* adequate for our needs, or *Homo sapiens* would not have outlasted so many of his contemporaries. Similarly, we do not need the dog's keenness of smell, nor the bat's auditory sensitivity to high-frequency squeaks.

Evolution has resulted in a considerable stratification of the various types of animals; some probably survived because of their visual capabilities, some because of their sensitivity to chemical stimuli, and some because of their auditory abilities. Man probably survived for an entirely different reason: the superb development of his central nervous system, especially that part known as the cerebral cortex. As we progress through this book we will learn of the pronounced limitations of man's sensitivity to changes in his external world and the manner in which his brain compensates for these limitations.

There is another aspect of man's sensory experiences that should be mentioned at this time. Probably because of his higher central nervous system development, man is much more selective than lower animals in his response to external stimuli. Lower animals are generally invariant (to some degree at least) in their responses to environmental changes. A frog will always flick out his tongue at a moving object in his field of vision if it approximates the size of a fly. My son once had a small manitor lizard with what appeared to be a dreadful temper. Whenever a mouse was placed in the cage with the lizard the behavior of the latter was entirely predictable. He would pounce on the poor mouse and dash it violently against the floor and sides of the cage until it was little more than a bloody pulp. If the lizard was hungry (as evidenced by not having eaten recently) it would proceed to eat the mouse; otherwise it would pay no more attention to the bloody remains. The lizard's reaction to the specific visual and perhaps olfactory stimulus was entirely predictable. Whether or not the mouse was then eaten apparently depended entirely on different sensory patterns: those from its organic "hunger" receptors.

In higher animals, and especially man, behavior as a result of external stimuli is much less predictable. We can "tune in" on desired external events, and we can often "tune out" those we wish to avoid. In the so-called cocktail party effect, we can pay attention to one conversation while excluding the effects of dozens of other conversations all around us. A mother who is "tuned in" to her infant's cries can be awakened by a slight whimper that doesn't disturb the normally sleeping father. Such a capability of selective *attention* greatly increases the flexibility and adaptibility of the sensory-perceptual world of the higher-order creatures. Although it is beyond the scope of this book, much progress is being made in acquiring an understanding of the neural mechanisms responsible for selective attention, inhibition, and even total repression of the sensory event.

Development of Sensory Structures

The sensory organs of man have come a long way from the extremely simple, general irritability of protoplasm. This evolution can, to a great extent, be traced from the simplest form of life in organized, logical steps.

PROTOZOA

The amoeba is probably the simplest form of life in which generalized irritability has begun to be specialized. It has no structures that can be properly classed as neural tissue, yet an amoeba is influenced diffentially by different forms of energy and different levels of stimulation to an extent that belies its low level on the phylogenetic scale. It reacts to chemical changes, temperature changes, and mechanical stimuli as well as to gravity and some forms of electromagnetic energy. Within wide limits, and subject sometimes to serious errors, it can withdraw from noxious stimuli and wrap its pseudopods around potential food. An amoeba also reacts differentially as a function of the magnitude (intensity) of a stimulus, showing temporal summation (several stimuli, none of which by itself would elicit a response, may when combined in time produce a response) and adaptation (when a stimulus capable of eliciting a response may over time be simply adapted to and lose its capacity for producing the response). The simple amoeba is not as simple in its behavior as its morphological structure might lead one to believe. The basic irritability of its protoplasm has developed into a capability for rather remarkable sensitivity and discrimination, and all this without anything that could be called neural tissue.

SIMPLE MULTICELLULAR ANIMALS

In the early multicellular animals a greater degree of coordinated behavior may be found, still without true nervous tissue. In the sponge each cell is an entity in itself, little more than a closely knit bundle of protozoa), but because of their physical juxtaposition, a response in one cell produces by physical contact a response in its immediate neighbor. Thus a very primitive form of "neural" transmission takes place without the need for the presence of true neural tissue.

When we reach the level of the hydras and jellyfish we find for the first time a differentiation in tissue to go along with the differentiation in behavior. Primitive receptor cells are found that are more sensitive to mechanical, thermal, and chemical changes than undifferentiated protoplasm. To go along with the animals' increased response capability (many of these animals have greatly enhanced mobility), fibrous extensions of the receptors may lead to primitive muscle cells. Such neurosensory cells actually combine the sensory and neural functions so clearly differentiated in higher animals. Some of the organisms in this group have their neurosensory cells arranged in a netlike configuration, thus appreciably increasing their potential for coordinated behavior.

Some highly specialized receptor organs can be found in animals at this level. For example, jellyfish are able to maintain their upright positions, in spite of considerable mobility, as a result of the presence of gravity-influenced granules resting on sensitive hair cells in sensory organs called *statocysts.*

BILATERAL ORGANISMS

The next stage in development is of extreme importance. As exemplified by the flatworms and the roundworms, for the first time a potential for maximum differentiation and flexibility in behavior is to be found. The replacement of radial symmetry with bilateral symmetry provides a framework for encephalization and concentraton of neural functioning at one "end" of the animal. It is difficult to imagine a highly developed organism with no head end. Only in television fantasies do we hear of the "blob" that captured New York.

The presence of a head end permits maximum orientation ability, optimal movement, and the potential for a concentration of specialized receptor organs where they would be most useful. As a result of this shift from radial to bilateral symmetry, worms were able to develop far more variability in their behavior and modes of adaptation than occurs in any lower forms of life. Indeed, some of the more courageous critters even left their protective liquid environment and crawled out onto dry land. Without the shift from radial to bilateral symmetry in such animals as the flatworms we might all be floating around today as jellyfish!

Of great importance to all of us is the fact that at this level the first evidence can be found of simple learning or conditioning based on modifications in a true nervous system. Perhaps modifiability is a characteristic of all protoplasm, but not until the development of a true nervous system do we find anything approaching learning as we understand it.

SENSORY ORGAN AND NEURAL DOMINANCE

As we move up the phylogenetic scale we cannot but be amazed at the variety and degree of sense organ development we encounter. The development of specialized vibration-sensitive hair cells, compound eyes, and remarkable chemical sensitivities are typical of these animals. Arthropods, such as insects, arachnids (spiders), crustaceans, and myriapods, are particularly impressive with their wide range of sensory organ specialization. In addition to a fantastic proliferation in kind and complexity of sensory organs, a remarkable increase in the amount and complexity of neural tissue is to be found. Animals at these levels for the first time exhibit a wide range of behavior, not nearly as stereotyped and invariant as the lower animals. We find a high level of development of motor behavior. Rapid movements and flying are characteristic of animals at this level. Finally, we find the first evidence of truly social behavior in many of the insects; in insect colonies the welfare of the group depends on the behavior of the individuals, and the welfare of the individual depends on the behavior of the group.

CENTRAL NERVOUS SYSTEM DOMINANCE

In some respects the chordata achieve the epitome of sensory development, but not without qualification. As indicated earlier, sensory organs for the lower animals have been developed for specific purposes, and they perform these purposes admirably—in many cases better than those of their higher-level relatives. Although many animals from fish through mammals do indeed exhibit remarkable upper limits in their sensory capabilities, we should recognize that much of this advantage must be attributed to central nervous system development rather than sense organ development. For the first time animals at this level reveal an extreme degree of encephalization and corticalization. Nearly all the neural capability is concentrated at one end of the animal, and the resultant brain with its higher-level cortex provides for an almost unlimited variability in sensory capacity and overt behavior.

As the same time, divergent developments among species have resulted in the remarkable sensory developments with which we are familiar: the olfactory sense of the dog, the vision of the hawk, and the high-frequency auditory sensitivity of the bat are only a few examples.

Simple Neural Action

Through the long process of evolution the simple neuron as an elementary building block for sensory-perceptual functioning has undergone tremen-

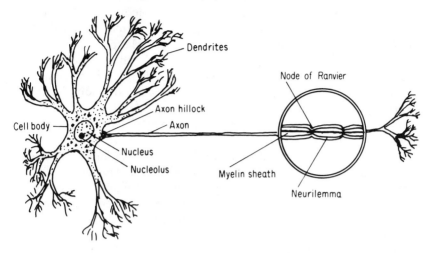

Figure 2-1
Idealized diagram of a neuron. The principal parts of a typical neuron are shown. The drawing is highly stylized and is more typical of a motor than of a sensory neuron.

dous change. Indeed, some specialized neurons such as those found in the retina bear almost no outward resemblance to the classical depictions. Nevertheless, although evolution has wrought great changes in the superficial appearance of many neurons their basic structure remains essentially unchanged.

DESCRIPTION OF THE NEURON

A neuron is a single cell, consisting of three basic parts: a sensitive end called a *dendrite*, a *cell body* or *perikaryon* containing the cell nucleus and other related structures, and an *axon*, which serves as the output portion of the cell. Figure 2–1 shows a stylized neuron with its axon, dendrite, and cell body as well as several other structures that may be of interest to us. These include a myelin sheath—a white, segmented, fatty covering found on many axons, and whose presence leads to the identification of the "white matter" of the brain. Other features of importance include the neurilemma, a thin membranous covering superficial to the myelin sheath, occurring even where no myelin is found; and numerous constrictions in the axon known as the nodes of Ranvier. Many neurons, particularly the motor, have branching termini at the ends of their axons, known as end brushes. These structures make neural contact with muscles, glands, or dendrites of other neurons. In the following pages we consider only those parts of the neuron that appear to be of importance for an understanding of sensory-perceptual phenomena. The interested reader is encouraged to dig deeper into the functioning of the neuron and the nervous system in general.

In size, the variability of neurons is tremendous. At one extreme, in the thin membrane of the retina a chain of several microscopic-sized neurons may be found lying end to end, over a distance no greater than the thickness of a sheet of tissue paper. Each neuron may be only a few microns (millionths of a meter) in length. At the other extreme some fibers of neurons may be several feet long, extending the length of the spinal cord, or from the digital extremities to ganglia (clusters of cell bodies) within the torso proper.

As a matter of fact, few neurons look like the stylized example of Figure 2–1, which is a *motor* neuron.

Figure 2–2 indicates better than words the extreme difference in external appearance of various neurons as indicated earlier. This figure illustrates diagramatically just a few of the many forms that fully developed neurons may take. Note the extreme diversity in their overall configurations. Even this figure is deceiving when we consider some of the more highly specialized receptor endings such as those found in the retina (rods and cones) and some of the encapsulated end organs found in the skin that are not included in the figure.

HOW THE NEURON FUNCTIONS

The neuron, like all protoplasm, exhibits irritability. Indeed this is almost its sole function, and evolutionary development has made it ideally suited for its sole raison d'être. Although we do not yet fully understand the functioning of the neuron, we have come a long way from the ancients who though of the neural fibers as tubules, carrying "humors" between the various parts of the body.

We now understand, in a gross way at least, the electrical activity of the neuron and its chemical basis. The neuron is *not* an electrical conductor like a wire, it does *not* conduct a current of electricity as we understand this useful phenomenon. Rather, it produces, by chemical means, an electrical charge, an increase in negative potential, which traverses the fiber in the form of a "spike" potential until it reaches the end of an axon. The relatively slow transmission speeds of from roughly 2 to 150 m per second are scarcely consistent with the normally encountered transmission speeds of conventional electric currents.

At the tip end of the axon, a chemical reaction takes place across a short distance (synapse) activating a dendritic structure in another neuron. Although it was once supposed that the neural impulse "leaped" across the gap from the tip of one axon to the dendrite of an adjacent cell, we now know better. In fact, a chemical reaction at the synapse, involving the release of *acetylcholine*, results in some manner in a depolarization of the postsynaptic neuron and a spontaneous firing of it. We shall come back to this action and its accompanying "generator" potential later in the chapter. In the case of motor neurons, activity may be evoked in muscle fibers or glands, rather than other neurons.

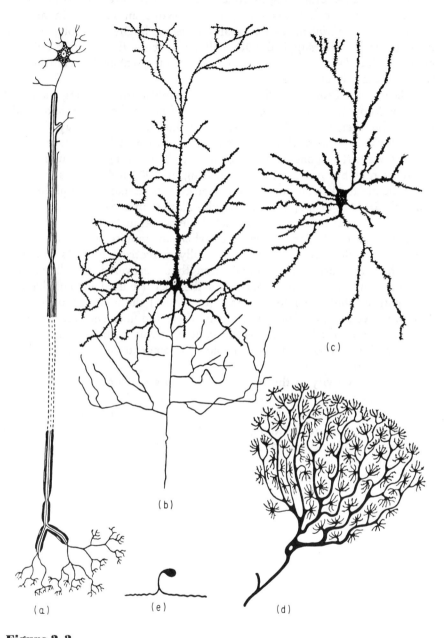

Figure 2-2
Some characteristic types of neurons. (a) Multipolar motor neuron of spinal cord. (b) Pyramidal cell of cerebral cortex. (c) Bipolar cell of spinal ganglion. (d) Purkinje cell of cerebellum. (e) Bipolar cell of spinal ganglion. (From C. L. Evans, *Principles of Human Physiology,* 14th ed. London: Churchill Livingstone, 1968.)

In some cases, branching or collateral axon structures are to be found. Frequently these collaterals serve, not to evoke an impulse in another neuron, but to *inhibit* the action of an adjacent cell. One level of the retina is particularly well supplied with collateral fibers that inhibit adjacent neurons, thus (as we shall see in a later chapter) enhancing contrast between adjacent visual areas.

All-or-None Principle. What sort of an impulse travels along the fiber? We now know it has a constant level, depending on the nature and condition of the fiber, rather than the stimulus that set it on its way. In 1871 Henry Pickering Bowditch discovered that a heart muscle fiber responds in just one way: It responds entirely or not at all. A strong stimulus may increase its rate, but not its strength of firing. In 1905 Keith Lucas extended the principle to skeletal muscle and later gave it its name, the *all-or-none principle*. In 1912 his pupil Edgar Douglas Adrian, in one of the most highly imaginative experiments ever conducted, demonstrated the same principle for neural fibers. Adrian showed that when an impulse passes through a portion of a fiber that has been partially narcotized and its apparent strength is decreased, the original strength is recovered in full when it passes beyond the narcotized portion of the fiber. He used a small chamber filled with alcohol vapor to eliminate (or reduce) the neural impulse midway in the course of a fiber. At a point where the fiber emerged from the alcohol chamber the impulse was the same as it was in the fiber before the chamber. Thus the all-or-none principle was demonstrated for neural fibers (Boring, 1942).

Electrical Activity in the Neuron. At the present time we have a good idea of what goes on in the neuron during transmission of an impulse. As early as 1890 the chemist Wilhelm Ostwald proposed a membrane theory for neural transmission. Although he did not actually use living tissue, his hypothesis, involving the transfer of ions through the semipermeable walls of the fiber membranes, was brilliant. Later work by A. Bernstein, who demonstrated temperature effects consistent with the behavior of permeable membranes, was followed by a series of supporting publications by R. S. Lillie early in the twentieth century. Largely through the work of Lillie the membrane theory of neural transmission is almost universally accepted today (Boring, 1942).

The membrane theory of neural conduction can be understood more easily from a study of Figure 2–3. Presumably, the resting neuron has a preponderance of sodium (Na^+) and chlorine (Cl^-) ions outside the membrane and a preponderance of positive potassium (K^+) ions inside. The result is a condition (resting potential) in which the interior of the neuron is some 70 millivolts (mV) negative with respect to the exterior surface. Under the proper conditions, the permeability of the membrane increases to such an extent that the outer sodium ions are permitted to flow inward, destroying the resting potential "balance." The immediate result is a decrease in the outside positive charge (or an increase in its negativity, as it is usually

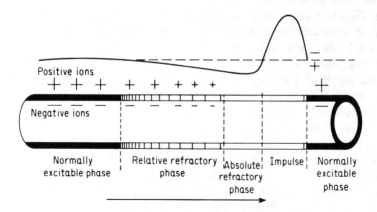

Positive ions
+ + +   + + + + +   +

Negative ions

| Normally excitable phase | Relative refractory phase | Absolute refractory phase | Impulse | Normally excitable phase |

Figure 2–3

Membrane theory of nerve conduction. Arrow indicates direction of neural impulse shown at top of drawing. (Adapted from E. Boring, *Sensation and Perception in the History of Experimental Psychology.* Appleton-Century-Crofts, 1942; based on an original drawing from Forbes, *A Handbook of General Experimental Psychology,* 1934.)

described). When a neuron "fires" in this manner the resting potential is replaced by a condition wherein the difference between the outer surface and the inside of the fiber can change about 90 mV—that is, to a point where the outside surface may be 20 mV negative with respect to the interior instead of the original 70 mV positive. This roughly 90-mV "spike" forms the nerve impulse as it moves along the axon.

On conclusion of the brief "spike" discharge, a second change in permeability permits positive ions to return from the inside of the fiber to the outer surface, thus restoring the resting potential. This reaction is somewhat slower than that referred to as the discharge or spike potential. The two permeability changes together, in rapid sequence, result in a moving "spike" of negativity that depolarizes the fiber as it moves along and restores the resting potential behind it.

Several characteristics in the behavior of individual neurons are understandable in light of the preceding physiological description. First, a single fiber cannot by any direct means indicate the magnitude of the stimulus that caused it to fire. It has only one level of output—determined by its size, chemical makeup, and perhaps the condition of the organism. It can however fire at different rates, and indeed this appears to be just what happens. Immediately after firing a neuron is in an *absolute refractory stage;* it cannot fire again, since there is no resting potential to be upset by an external stimulation. In a short time the reverse permeability condition allows for a return of the positive ions and the reestablishment of the normal resting potential. The neuron is now ready to fire again. In the meantime, before the normal resting potential has been reached, *some* partial return to normalcy has occurred and the neuron is said to be in a *relative refractory phase.* That is, a stronger-than-normal stimulus may result in a "spike" potential. It is simple to see then how strong stimuli might be discriminated from weak ones. The spike would be the same—complete neutralization of the resting potential, whether it has or has not reached its normal state. The ultimate result of a strong stimulus would be to produce more pulses in a given period of time. In fact, some neurons that can normally fire at a rate of 100 impulses per second may be made to fire at a rate of 1,000 per second with a sufficiently strong stimulus.

In anticipation of later discussions, it should be pointed out that much of our discrimination ability of intensity may also be due to the *number* of fibers being fired, as well as the rate of firing. A hard pinprick, for example, will set off more fibers than a gentle prick. An intense sound will activate more hair cells in the inner ear than a weak sound.

Generator Potential. In most laboratory experiments neurons are fired by direct electrical stimulation. But this is not what happens in the living organism. Where does the electricity from light on the retina come from? Or sound waves in the ear? Or impulses across synapses? It is clear that a receptor must in some way diminish the resting membrane potential of its associated neuron in order to induce it to fire.

The presence of local potentials in sense organs has been recognized for some time, leading Ragnar Granit of the Royal Caroline Institute in Stockholm to suggest, with remarkable foresight, that they be called generator potentials (Granit, 1935). Later, H. K. Hartline at the University of Pennsylvania found what appeared to be a generator potential from a single fiber of the *Limulus* (horseshoe crab) eye, and in 1950 Bernhard Katz of University College, London, demonstrated the presence of a generator potential in vertebrate muscle spindles. When the spindle was stretched a slight depolarization occurred that could be viewed on an oscilloscope. Superposed on the shifted local potential were the actual "spikes" or nerve impulses. The stronger the mechanical strain on the fibers, the greater the shift in the local potential and the greater the frequency of the spikes. It was also found that if a local anesthetic (remember Adrian and his alcohol chamber?) was applied to a fiber, thereby eliminating the spikes, the potential shift remained. Katz concluded that this potential shift was a generator potential, that it was an essential link between the stretching of the fibers and the evoking of the nerve impulse (Miller et al., 1961).

But how does the external stimulus produce a generator potential that can in turn evoke the firing of a neuron? For visual receptors some light can be shed on this difficult question. Based on the work of Hubbard and Wald at Harvard, and others, it seems apparent that the absorption of light in the eye results in a photochemical reaction that does indeed produce a change in the resting potential of the sensitive elements. When this generator potential achieves a sufficient level, the receptor elements fire (Miller et al., 1961). With similar logic, we may guess that the action of acetylcholine at the synapse, in some way alters the resting potential of the second-order neuron, thus causing it to discharge.

With respect to the nonvisual senses, we have less evidence concerning the manner in which the neuron is set into action. But all evidence does point to the necessity for some shift in the resting potential as induced by a generator potential. Perhaps some generation of a weak electrical current is produced by mechanical means as well as chemical, as appeared to be the case in Katz's muscle spindle preparations.

Utilization of Sensory Information

Sensory information can be used by the organism in a number of different ways and for somewhat different purposes. Let us examine some of these uses for data produced by the sensory organs, bearing in mind that the classification is highly arbitrary and perhaps artificial, being proposed primarily for purposes of convenience and pedagogy.

DEVELOPMENT

The importance of sensory stimulation for the physiological development of the sense organs has been recognized for some time (Riesen, 1947, 1961). What was once thought to be "learning to perceive" turned out, by and large, to be a requirement for stimulation of the sensory organs to ensure their proper development. The eyes, for example, do not develop properly unless stimulation with light occurs at an early stage in development. Curiously enough, the advantage of early sensory stimulation is not limited to the development of the corresponding receptors. Woolf and Bixby (1976), for example, have shown that auditory stimulation can accelerate the hatching of quail eggs. According to these authors, audible clicks, correlated with the embryo's respiratory cycle, provide the basis for interegg communication. Synthetic clicks provided by the experimenter can advance the hatching, and perhaps of equal importance, under some temporal conditions, delay hatching time. The authors offer evidence to substantiate the belief that these effects are indeed changes in the rate of embryonic development.

Actually, auditory stimulation is only one of several sensory stimuli that can influence prenatal development. Light, temperature, and vibration have also been shown to have the capability of accelerating development (Woolf and Bixby, 1976). The extent to which sensory stimulation may influence mammalian prenatal development is largely unknown, but it may be much more important than we suspect.

MAINTENANCE OF AROUSAL LEVEL

Considerable attention has been given recently to the need for stimuli impinging on the organism in order to maintain a currently ill-defined condition known as the "arousal level" (French, 1960). Experiments with human subjects in specially constructed chambers under conditions where they were isolated from all external stimulation have been revealing. To function properly, the human, at least, must be constantly bombarded with stimuli from the outside world. In an environment of total darkness, devoid of all sound stimulation and with essentially no tactual stimulation, the normal human is in sad shape. He becomes disoriented and restless and may even experience hallucinations and more serious symptoms of maladjustment.

We now have some fairly good ideas concerning the physiology involved in the arousal-level problem. A portion of the subcortical brain, known as the *reticular activating system* (RAS), as a result of varied stimulation from the sense organs, maintains a general level of functioning that keeps the organism in a waking state. Adequate functioning of the RAS is, indeed, necessary for a normal electroencephalographic pattern.

We have long known that external stimuli do not suddenly *start* activity in an inactive sense organ; rather, they tend to increase a process already in operation to a point where conscious awareness results. Without this ongoing background stimulation the organism is not ready to respond to changes in its environment. More recent work has demonstrated the possibility of manipulating the arousal level by carefully located electroshocks and/or surgery. A cat can be put to sleep in the presence of a mouse by adequately reducing the neural activity from its brain stem "arousal center." In the normal animal some minimal activity in the afferent (sensory) neural channel is necessary to maintain an adequate arousal level (French, 1960).

Although the arousal-level concept is of relatively recent interest to psychologists and is generally attributed to a fairly high-level neural structure, it is probably much more basic and widespread than is generally recognized. An all-pervasive arousal level is probably a condition for survival in all organisms possessing true neural tissue, even where a true brain or complex neural ganglion does not exist. In the lowest animals where no true nervous tissue can be found, there is still some sort of arousal level or condition of irritability, dependent on external stimulation.

DIRECT SURVIVAL

Many senses operate at a subconscious, reflexive-behavior level. Our internal senses are, by and large, of this nature. We may be aware of hunger, thirst, and internal pain, but the great bulk of our internal receptors, which aid in the regulation of blood pressure, body temperature, and water transfer, perform their functions quietly and efficiently, and without fanfare. Probably they reach a state of awareness only by indirect means; in some cases it is the adjustment to the imbalance that we perceive.

Much of sensory functioning in lower animals is of this unlearned, reflexive nature, involving in many cases structures analogous to our smooth muscles and associated autonomic nervous system. In addition to simple reflexes like the human knee jerk, which certainly reaches a conscious level, and the pupillary response, which does not evoke a conscious experience, countless other sensory phenomena with a direct survival value can be enumerated.

The simple tropisms of lower animals are an excellent example of such functioning. As we have noted earlier, if you place a number of paramecia in a watch glass and locate two oppositely charged electrodes near the edge of the glass, and across from each other, the little animals will swarm toward the negatively charged pole. This is not the same as a magnet attracting iron filings; the organisms appear to be traversing the distance under their own power. Why they go in this direction we do not know. What is even more strange, you will always find several of the little rascals going in the opposite direction! Theories of electrically differing potentials in growing protoplasm might account for the behavior of *most* of the paramecia, but not those contrary individuals. We have a lot to learn about "simple" behavior.

As another simple example, the unicellular Euglena responds to light and is also attracted to certain chemicals (Diehn, 1973). But animals at a phylogenetic level much higher than the single-celled paramecium or Euglena also exhibit tropistic behavior. Moths fly toward a light, salmon (when their reproductive cycle is at the appropriate stage) swim upstream, and some fishes navigate by means of magnetic fields. Newly hatched turtles of at least one species find their way to the ocean for the first time as a result of a positive phototropism. The sky over the water is brighter than that over the land, and the newly hatched reptiles are attracted by the light, thereby finding their way, for the first time, to the ocean.

Many animals, such as the earthworm, are negatively phototropic. Light, and especially moving shadows produced by the light, cause them to withdraw into their holes.

As an additional example of the unlearned, complex forms of behavior we call tropisms, or if complicated enough, instincts, we should consider the polarized light sensitivity of honeybees and the echolocation behavior of bats. For interesting reading on the echolocation capability of bats the curious should consider Simmons (1971, 1974).

All the preceding, and there are countless other examples, demonstrate ways in which nature has provided her creatures with simple yet highly specialized sensory capabilities to enable them to compete successfully with their environments and other, often equally highly specialized predators.

INDIRECT SURVIVAL

For want of a better term a number of other sensory uses have been lumped into the indirect survival category. Our senses enable us to avoid many potentially destructive difficulties. We can see (and hear) the approaching truck in time to step aside. We can spit out the foul-tasting substance that might be poisonous. The deer can smell the dog or wolf in time to take evasive action, and the dog can often locate his next meal by smelling the trail left by the fleeing rabbit.

At a much higher level of sophistication and development we can hear our neighbor when he tells us that our local emporium has a special today on Scotch. Without communication based on such sensory capabilities, we would have to drink water from the nearest rippling brook, like our sub-human animal friends or our primate ancestors.

When, by evolution, an organism has developed to the point where his tropistic behaviors are inadequate—that is, where much of his invariant behavior has been replaced by a capability for more highly varied behavior—the need for such sensory-perceptual flexibility is apparent. The dog must learn (or know by some means) that one animal (a rabbit) is a delicacy and another similar one (a skunk or a porcupine) is inedible and can be quite troublesome.

It should be obvious to the reader that sensory functions that serve such purposes will be of predominate or almost exclusive interest in this book.

CREATION OF PLEASURE

Some sensory stimulation appears to evoke a reaction we might, for want of a better term, call pleasure (Pfaffman, 1960). Music, rhythm, some odors and tastes, and in some cases gentle physical contact produce feelings of pleasure or joy. Although much human pleasure is undoubtedly the result of learning, there is recent evidence that the concept of "pleasure" goes much deeper (Cabanac, 1971).

It may be anthropomorphic to say that a lower animal experiences pleasure; certainly no animal has so reported. We can, however, define the word operationally: An animal is said to experience pleasure if he does nothing to terminate some activity or if he performs in such a way as to continue the activity. One of the oldest parts of the brain, the limbic system, has been found to be of importance in the experiencing of pleasure (MacLean, 1954). If a positive brain area (there are also negative areas) is stimulated electrically as a result of bar pressing, even a hungry rat will often continue pressing the bar that stimulates its limbic system in preference to another bar that would result in its obtaining food (Olds, 1966).

Certainly human infants seem to experience pleasure as a natural result of some forms of simple stimulation. Gentle rocking, stroking, and caressing, and soft, rhythmic sounds result in behavior on the part of the infant that gives every indication of being the result of pleasure. Babies may coo, gurgle, and at a later age smile in such a way that we are forced to say they are enjoying themselves. Some of this apparent pleasure *may* arise from simple conditioning, but some is surely of a more direct nature.

Summary

In this chapter we have considered a little more of the background leading to the study of the individual senses. We examined the role played by the sense organs and their general location in the grand scheme of things. We also examined, in some detail, the phylogenetic development of sense organs from amoeba to man, from single to multicellular organisms, and from radial to bilateral symmetry. We tried to learn, in a simplified form, the nature of the underlying neural activity and how it relates to sensory organ functioning. We considered how the nervous system is set into action by an external source of energy and considered the efficacy of a generator potential in setting off the neural impulse. Finally we examined the uses the organism may make of sensory-perceptual information in proper developing of the sense organs, maintaining an activity level, meeting the exigencies of life, and sometimes obtaining pleasure.

Suggested Readings

1. W. H. Miller, F. Ratliff, and H. K. Hartline, "How Cells Receive Stimuli," *Scientific American,* September 1961. This fine 12-page article traces the development of knowledge concerning the underlying behavior of sensory cells. It is excellent reading for those interested in the concept of the generator potential and how it has been studied. References to the work of Granit, Katz, Hartline, MacNichol and others give the article historical significance.

2. C. Bell. "Idea of a New Anatomy of the Brain," in W. Dennis, *Readings in the History of Psychology.* New York: Appleton, 1948. This article is recommended for its historical interest. Written in 1811 by one of the truly great anticipators of modern sensory physiology, this article summarizes much of what was known about the nervous system at that time that is of interest to our subject. The twelve pages are at times a little tedious in style, but for the reader interested in historical perspective they are certainly worth reading.

3. From E. G. Boring. *Sensation and Perception in the History of Experimental Psychology.* New York: Appleton, 1942. I suggested chaps. 1 and 2 of Boring's classic for the preceding chapter. Chapter 2 of this reference (pp. 52–90) is of particular interest now, and should be read by the serious student. After 37 years the presentation by Boring still has excellent historical perspective and is a must for the serious student. Topics of nerve conduction, sensory conduction, specific nerve energies, projection, and isomorphism are all of importance as a groundwork for later, more narrowly directed emphases.

4. J. Pfeiffer. *The Cell.* New York: Time, Inc., 1954. The 200 pages of this reference are well worth reading, although direct application to the subject matter of sensation and perception is not great. This book provides one of the finest, most painless approaches to an overall understanding of life and the living cell. It is profusely illustrated, written in a relatively simple style, and is above all interesting. It can be read profitably by anyone in the biological sciences.

5. From N. L. Munn. *Psychological Development.* Boston: Houghton Mifflin, 1938. This older book is worthwhile reading from cover to cover. However, chap. VI, "Development of Behavior from Conception to Birth," pp. 165–211, is particularly relevant to our consideration of embryological development. It elaborates on several of the topics discussed in this chapter in a highly interesting and readable manner.

6. S. S. Stevens (ed.). *Handbook of Experimental Psychology*. New York: Wiley, 1951. See chaps. 2 and 3, "Excitation and Conduction in the Neuron and Synaptic Mechanisms" by F. Brink, Jr. These 70 pages are probably the most technical of the references suggested to this point. They provide a wealth of information for the serious student and must be highly recommended. This entire volume should be familiar to the serious student who plans to emphasize sensation-perception in his professional future.

7. DeForest Mellon, Jr. *The Physiology of Sense Organs*. San Francisco: Freeman, 1968. This is the most technical and topical of the readings suggested for this section. With chapters such as "Principles of Stimulus Coding," the "Depolarizing Nature of the Trigger," and "Origins of the Receptor Potential," this book of 100 pages is especially intended for the serious student of the nature of the sensory event.

8. J. D. French. "The Reticular Formation," *Scientific American*, May 1957. This is a highly simplified, yet accurate presentation of a complex subject matter. It is written for the educated layman and is extremely interesting as well as informative. The reader should recognize, of course, that much more is known concerning the reticular formation than can be included in such a short article.

9. Michel Cabanac. "Physiological Role of Pleasure," *Science* 173 (1971):1103–1107. This reference may be considered to be somewhat diversionary, dealing with the inducement of pleasant or unpleasant feelings as a function of the individual's internal state. It is certainly a specialized topic but may be of more general interest than its title indicates.

10. Edward C. Carterette and Morton P. Friedman. *Handbook of Perception, vol. III, Biology of Perceptual Systems*. New York: Academic Press, 1973. Like the preceding volume recommended at the end of Chapter 1, this volume is a must for the serious student. It contains a wealth of information on energy and neural transducers, the property of neurons, primitive sense organs, evolution, and embryology of the nervous system. Like Volume I, this volume can be used throughout this book for additional, more specialized reference.

11. D. E. Koshland, Jr. "A Response Regulator Model in a Simple Sensory System," *Science* 196 (1977):1055–1063. This reading is recommended for the serious student who is interested in the early development of sensory experience. The author suggests that the behavior of bacteria can provide insight into aspects of more complex behavioral systems. The mechanisms of bacterial sensing are considered, bacterial memory (a comparison of past and present conditions), adaptation, and several higher neural processes such as "choice," "discrimination," and "judgment" are considered to be properties of the bacterium. A fascinating reading for the serious student.

3/methods for studying the senses–I

Background

The classical definition of *psychophysics*, "the science of the functional relations, or relations of dependency, between the body and the mind," stems from the great landmark of experimental psychology, G. T. Fechner's *Element der Psychophysik* (Boring, 1942). Published in 1860, this important book brought together, summarized, and elaborated on the new science of mind-body relations. Fechner did not invent psychophysics, but he did describe the existing methods, modify some, and mold the varying viewpoints of the times into a coherent discipline. For this reason Fechner is often referred to as the father of psychophysics.

Like most scientific progress, psychophysics developed as a child of the times, a product of a broader, general evolution in knowledge, as one aspect of the developing Gesellschaft. The early part of the nineteenth century saw a tremendous upswing in science. Astronomers were discovering sophisticated observation and mensuration techniques, physics was growing by leaps and bounds, and physiologists were starting to measure everything in sight. An attempt to quantify the heretofore philosophical discipline of psychology was inevitable.

The study of sensation as a separate discipline owed much of its early impetus to the Bell-Magendie law. Although it was not a completely new idea that sensations and responses should have separate neural bases, it remained for Charles Bell to show, in 1811, that sensory and motory nerves at the spinal cord are indeed separate. With Magendie's more convincing experiment in 1822, the groundwork for studying sensory processes was well laid. Johannes Mueller's expansion (1826) of the Bell-Magendie principle into the doctrine of specific energies of nerves was another important step leading to the development of a science of sensations, and its principal tool, psychophysics.

In 1834 E. H. Weber established what Fechner was later to call Weber's law: that two sensations are just noticeably different as long as the intensities of their stimuli bear a constant ratio to each other. Although we now know better, Weber believed that the same ratio between two stimuli would always result in a just noticeable difference. The skin, for example, according to Weber, could always appreciate the difference in two weights if said difference had a ratio of one-thirtieth, regardless of the absolute values of the weights. We normally encounter Weber's law written in the form $\Delta I/I = k$; where I is a stimulus value, ΔI is a barely noticeable increment of I, and k is a constant for a given observer and a specified condition.

Another milestone occurred when Fechner proceeded to modify and extend Weber's law into what has come to be known as Fechner's law. Fechner's law can be stated: $S = k \log I$, where S stands for a sensation, k is a constant, and I is a measure of stimulus intensity in threshold units. Like Weber's law, Fechner's law works to some extent, but it would be grossly gratuitous to say that Fechner succeeded in actually measuring a pure sensation as he originally believed.

In spite of the relative inadequacies of Weber's and Fechner's laws, and the criticism of those who objected to the measurement of the "incorporeal mind," the new science did grow rapidly (Boring, 1942).

Three basic psychophysical methods were described in great detail by Fechner in his now famous book. In addition to the original three, today there are numerous other measures that may be obtained by conventional and near-conventional psychophysical techniques, along with as many modifications as there are experimenters using them. Moreover, modern scaling techniques and the application of methodologies borrowed from mathematics and engineering have greatly enhanced the potential for sensory measurement. For a further description of additional, more recent approaches, the interested reader would do well to consult Carterette, vol. II (1974).

Applications

Before describing several psychophysical techniques and the measurements obtainable from them, we might reflect a bit on what may appear to the uninitiated to be merely a sterile carryover from the ninteenth-century mind-matter controversy. Psychophysical research is *not* a dead horse to be constantly beaten. In practice, every judgment you make, when you heft the package of hamburger and question the butcher's honesty, when you notice a traffic light some distance away, and even when you read this page, you are involving yourself in phychophysics. You are interpreting your experiences from your arm muscles as weight; you are seeing "color" when the only difference between the red and green traffic lights is one of wavelength; and you are utilizing the ability of your visual mechanism to discriminate among various forms on the printed page.

But for the scientist employing controlled research, more definitive, more precise experimental procedures are needed. To *determine* the acceptability of a new brand of breakfast cereal, to *determine* the ideal color for a new television picture tube, and to *determine* how large the characters must be on a traffic sign, something akin to psychophysics is needed. So, with the knowledge that psychophysics is still a viable, useful enterprise, let us gain historical perspective by examining some early methods.

Fechner's Methods

Let us take a brief look at Fechner's three methods. Later in this chapter we will describe them in more detail and include some additional approaches.

METHOD OF LIMITS

In the method of limits or *minimal change*, a stimulus is changed in successive, discrete steps until a point is reached where the subject changes his response. One can start with a stimulus that cannot be detected and, in discrete, usually equal steps, increase the intensity until the observer changes his response to "I see *it*," "I hear *it*," or what have you. Or the stimulus can be above *threshold* to start with and be decreased in successive steps until the observer indicates it can no longer be detected. Such a procedure results in an *absolute threshold*, usually abbreviated AL for *absolute limen*, or more traditionally, RL for *reiz limen*.

The method of limits can also be used to evaluate stimulus differences, as in Weber's procedure. In this case "differences" between two suprathreshold stimuli are manipulated in serial steps until the subject reports "same" or "different," depending, of course, on the direction of the change. Also called the method of just noticeable differences, this method results in a DL or difference limen.

METHOD OF RIGHT AND WRONG CASES

The method of right and wrong cases was the second method promulgated by Fechner. More commonly called the *constant* or *constant-stimuli method*, this technique involves the presentation of the stimuli in random or quasi-random order. The subject merely expresses his response in terms of "experience it' or "do not experience it," usually simplified to "yes" or "no." This method results in a psychometric function, a curve of percentage "yes" (or "no") plotted against stimulus magnitude. In a modification of the method, known as the *constant stimulus-difference method*, differences of varying size are presented in random or quasi-random fashion, the subject reporting on the existence or nonexistence of a difference. The stimuli for which differences are judged may be presented simultaneously, as for visual stimuli, or sequentially, as for auditory signals. This method is one of the most flexible and useful of all the psychophysical methods. It can be used for the obtaining of numerous additional measures as well as for absolute and difference thresholds. Because of its broad application it has been the subject of considerable controversy with respect to details of its use and interpretation of its results.

METHOD OF AVERAGE ERROR

In this method the subject is provided with a standard stimulus and some means of manipulating a comparison stimulus. It is also called the *production method,* and rather appropriately the *method of adjustment.* The subject himself, in adjusting the comparison stimulus, produces any error that may occur. Most of the psychophysical measurements obtainable by the previously described methods can be obtained by the method of average error. One advantage of the method is that reliance on verbal behavior, such as "yes," "no," "larger," "smaller," or "equal," is eliminated. On the other hand, sensory experiences are probably confounded with motor activities, and just what is being measured may be subject to some dispute.

Although these methods may result in measures with similar names, it should be emphasized that they are not completely interchangeable. A threshold determined by an adjustment method may not be the same as one derived from a constant method. Similarly, such indexes as *intervals of uncertainty* and *difference thresholds* are influenced by the method used to obtain them. The final determination of which method is to be used must depend on the nature of the situation and the use to which the results are to be put. To understand the various techniques fully as presented in detail in the following pages, this fact must be borne in mind.

Uses for Psychophysics

A great number of different measures can be obtained by conventional psychophysics, and more recently developed techniques have greatly expanded this potential. Let us examine briefly some of the measures psychophysical techniques make available to us.

ABSOLUTE THRESHOLD (AL)

This was one of the three measures of primary interest to Fechner and the other early workers in the field and can be obtained either directly or indirectly by most of the major psychophysical methods. The absolute threshold is that point where a stimulus reaches the level of consciousness as evidenced by positive response on the part of the subject. An example might be the minimum intensity of a spot of light (wavelength and spot size would have to be held constant) that can just be detected. A mariner searching for a very dim star is utilizing his absolute threshold for light intensity.

There are numerous ways in which the absolute threshold can be determined. It can be calculated mathematically, as in the constant methods (a level observed 50 percent of the time); directly, as in the method of limits; or manually, as in a production or adjustment method. When we discuss the principal methods in detail we will see just how the AL is determined by them.

It should be pointed out that the concept of an absolute threshold is not without its critics. The classical idea that there is a physiological point where a stimulus suddenly has an effect on the organism is not accepted by many modern workers. Rather than a threshold stimulus being that point where something is "pushed over the brink" and immediate awareness results, modern thinking takes into consideration ongoing processes of the organism and the idea that a threshold is little more than a point in a mathematical-temporal curve. Continuity is especially stressed by contemporary researchers who use such tools as probability theory and detection theory, emphasizing the signal-in-noise nature of threshold measurement. In spite of such criticism, a description of the classical AL and its interpretation is warranted. Just bear in mind that perhaps it should be interpreted as a useful predictive construct and not as some immutable natural limit.

DIFFERENCE THRESHOLD (DL)

The difference threshold is the second measure emphasized by the early workers and described in detail by Fechner. The object of this measure is to determine the smallest change in a stimulus that can be detected by an observer. For convenience, a frequency of 50 percent detection is normally accepted as defining the point of the difference threshold. It might be better to call it the *absolute threshold for a difference*, rather than the difference threshold, because most of what was said concerning the absolute threshold also applies to the determination of the difference threshold. Most of the simpler psychophysical methods can be used for its determination, and the same sort of healthy skepticism of the measure is pointed to by modern theorists.

But, as in the case of the absolute threshold, the concept of a difference threshold has utility as a predictive device, even if it is not based on an absolutely sound theoretical structure. For example, there has been research accomplished by three organizations as diverse as a large liquor distiller, a large soap manufacturer, and the United States Air Force, all of which involved the determination of difference thresholds by conventional techniques. In one the problem was to determine the amount of chance variability in caramel coloring that could be tolerated (not easily detected) in separate batches of whiskey, one was concerned with the amount of perfume to be added to soap, and the third involved the size of disks of light on a vertical display panel.

SENSORY EQUIVALENCE

Sensory equivalence determines how one stimulus must change in order to be equivalent (or equal) to another in some specified attribute. For example, how intense must a pure tone of 100 Hz be for it to sound as loud as a tone of 1,000 Hz? Actually, we can give no simple answer to this question, but must resort to complex and detailed curves that include the actual level of the sounds as well as their differences. For example, if the 1,000-Hz tone has an intensity of a normal voice level, or 70 db (decibels), the 100-Hz tone must be about ten times as intense to result in an equivalent apparent loudness. On the other hand, if the amplitude of the 1,000-Hz tone is quite low, then the 100-Hz tone may have to be 40 db more intense (10,000 times as powerful) to result in equivalent loudness.*

We can, by means of psychophysics, ask many other questions involving sensory equivalence, such as, "How intense must a red light be to appear as bright as a green light?" or "How much pressure is required on the tips of the fingers to be equivalent to a given pressure on the forearm?" Questions such as these are certainly intriguing and often of considerable value in our modern world. As in the case of equivalent sound intensities, however, the results of most sensory equivalence studies give complex, many-faceted relationships, never as simple as Fechner's law would lead us to believe.

RANK ORDER

Several of the psychophysical methods are ideally suited for developing psychological scales of sensory experience—that is, scales of such things as loudness, sweetness, and pain, and, with some reservations, scales of even less concrete experiences such as pleasure or love.

The simplest scale for describing experience-bound data would seem to be a nominal scale wherein experiences are simply given names, and no attempt is made to order or in any way set values to them. Indeed, this was all the ancients thought possible. Today we can go much farther, deriving ordinal, interval, and even ratio scales. In this and the following two sections we will examine briefly the uses of psychophysics that may result in ordinal, interval, and ratio scales.

Often encountered with subject matter that does not easily lend itself to quantification, ordering is a straightforward, uncomplicated procedure: Very simply, given a series of stimuli, what is their correct order according

* The interested reader should not worry too much at this point about the meaning of db or decibel. For the time being it is sufficient to understand that Hz is a measure of frequency and db is a measure of intensity or power. Its meaning and full significance will be considered in detail at a later time.

to some specified attribute? For example, rank the American League short-stops with respect to their worth to their respective teams. An ordinal scale such as this is probably superior to a nominal scale, which would simply have such statements as "good fielder," "fair hitter," "hits in the clutch," and so on. Another example might be to rank ten paintings for their artistic merit. Rank order is probably the simplest of several methods for obtaining numerical data from situations where subjective judgments might appear to be the sole alternative.

SENSORY DISTANCE

A cup of coffee with a teaspoon of sugar is sweeter than one with a half-teaspoon of sugar. A cup with one and one-half teaspoons of sugar is sweeter than one with a single teaspoon. But are the differences in sweetness the same? Several methods lend themselves to the establishment of scales for sense differences, such that defined stimulus values along a continuum result in equal sensory or experiential intervals.

As another example, is the difference in pitch between C and G for different octaves on the piano the same? Certainly the differences in frequency are not the same, but for pitch (the psychological experience of frequency) the two sensory intervals certainly approach in distance the equality they were intended to achieve. On the basis of such data it is possible to construct a scale of pitch that meets the mathematical requirements for an interval scale.

As we will discover later, specialized techniques have been developed to study sensory distance. One noteworthy procedure requires the subject to bisect a sensory distance. For example, what pitch is halfway between C and G? Or how much sugar makes a cup of coffee midway in sweetness between a cup with one-half teaspoon and one with one and a half teaspoons? Although results of such experiments are not always clear-cut and precise, agreement among experimenters and subjects does tend to be rather remarkable, and the existence of interval scales for sensory experience is not beyond reason. Unfortunately, they too are not as simple as Weber and Fechner might have anticipated.

SENSORY RATIOS

The most sophisticated outcome of psychophysics should probably be the development of sensory scales with equal sense ratios. This accomplishment would make possible such statements as "twice as loud," "three times as sweet," and "half as painful." With the development of such scales we would also be able to add and subtract stimuli with predictable results. We might know, for example, when two stimuli could be expected to produce twice the sensory experience of one. This is indeed a difficult area, and only for a few restricted experience modalities do we have anything today approaching satisfactory ratio scales. However, this is one application of psychophysics with a tremendous future. Development in this area is necessary before we can hope to achieve anything approaching a complete understanding of sensory organ–central nervous system functioning.

Let us look at some of the psychophysical methods in more detail. The interested reader is encouraged to obtain additional details from the readings at the end of the chapter. The references by Carterette and Friedman, Guilford, and Scharf are particularly recommended.

Method of Limits

Also called the method of minimal change or serial exploration, as indicated earlier, the method of limits can be used for the determination of thresholds, both absolute and difference. Indeed, this is the primary purpose of the method of limits—to determine thresholds. Let us examine the method in somewhat more detail as it has been utilized for the determination of the two types of thresholds.

ABSOLUTE THRESHOLD (AL OR RL)

The relation between a physical continuum and its corresponding psychological continuum is not as straightforward as, for example, the relation between the position of a needle on a voltmeter and the voltage being fed into the meter. Perhaps there is no such thing as a point where a stimulus "suddenly" has an effect on the organism, like the straw that breaks the camel's back. Rather, there is probably a range wherein experiencing or failing to experience a sensation is largely a function of chance—that is, the result of countless, often indeterminate factors of attention, background noise, physiological processes, and heaven knows what else. Moreover, the criterion of what constitutes a suprathreshold stimulus must also be taken into consideration. As a consequence, the point where a stimulus may be said to evoke a response in an organism must be defined statistically. By convention, the absolute threshold is usually defined as that condition in which the signal is detected 50 percent of the time.

It should also be pointed out that the definition of an AL does not always imply a *detection* threshold. Although we are often interested in determining a threshold for detection, there are other AL's of interest to us. For example, we may have an AL for light detection, but we might also have an absolute threshold for color discrimination, for form recognition (the optometrist's familiar chart), and for even more complex perceptual processes. It should be obvious to the reader that the amount of light necessary to read the optometrist's chart is appreciably greater than that required simply to know that it is there. The AL is a threshold for a psychological experience and is not restricted to a threshold for detection.

Procedure. For the following discussion we will refer to the AL for detection, but the same logic and general procedure could be applied to the other, more sophisticated threshold functions referred to earlier. An AL is determined by presenting to the subject series of stimuli, changing in magnitude by small, discrete steps. For one series of presentations the stimulus is started at a level below the threshold and increased by physically equal increments until the subject provides a positive response. There may or may not be a secondary cue to indicate when the stimulus is presented. In determining the AL for tone perception, there might be a light to indicate when the stimulus is being presented. The subject then indicates by pressing a button, for example, when he hears the tone. To prevent erroneous responses due to suggestion the light cue may be omitted.

Along with the ascending series of presentations, descending series are normally employed. In this case the starting stimulus is suprathreshold and is reduced by small increments until the subject can no longer detect it.

A sample work sheet for a method of limits determination of an absolute threshold is shown in Figure 3–1. In this example an AL for tonal detection was determined with 2-db intensity increments for ten series of presentations. The first presentation (A for ascending) was clearly subthreshold, with a level of 12 db; the second presentation was 14 db, the third 16 db, and so on, until the subject gave a positive response at 28 db. In the second presentation series (D for descending) a clearly audible signal (36 db) was used as the starting point. (In actual practice a short preliminary investigation may be required to locate the approximate AL before setting up the detailed experiment.) Note that in successive runs the subthreshold and suprathresholds starting points are widely varied to discourage guessing and similar unwanted contamination effects.

Difficulties and Limitations. There are several problems and possible sources of error inherent in the method of limits that must be avoided or in some way controlled. One of these is *errors of habituation*. A subject may get into a habit of saying "no . . . no . . . no . . ." for so long that he completely misses the point at which the stimulus is indeed above threshold. In the descending direction, if the subject expects five or six successive suprathresholds signals he may continue reporting them as "yes" when he can in fact detect nothing. A person who is extremely cautious may refuse to change his response until he is sure beyond the shadow of a doubt that a change at threshold level has occurred.

Other subjects commit *errors of anticipation*. They *expect* the signal to change; perhaps they count the number of subthreshold signals and decide that the next one simply *must* be above threshold; perhaps they are just trying too hard to please the experimenter. In any event, errors of anticipation are of serious consequence in the determination of the AL. On the other hand, errors of habituation and anticipation are only exaggerations of normal behavior. All subjects lie somewhere along a continuum of habituation and anticipation.

Both of these errors, habituation and anticipation, can be controlled to a large extent. Probably the most important consideration is adequate motivation and training, along with good instructions. Ideally, all subjects should operate with the same self-instructions and the same criterion for

Direction of Presentation

Stimulus Value, db re .0002 dyne/cm²	A	D	A	D	A	D	A	D	A	D
40						X				
38						X				
36		X				X	X			
34		X		X		X		X		X
32		X		X		X		X		X
30		X		X	X	X		X		X
28	X	X		X	−	X		X		X
26	−	X	X	X	−	−		−	X	−
24	−	−	−	X	−			−		
22	−		−	−	−		X	−		
20	−	−		−	−		−	−		
18	−	−		−	−			−		
16	−			−	−					
14	−			−	−					
12	−			−	−					
	27	25	25	23	29	27	21	27	25	27

Ascending threshold − 25.4 db.
Descending threshold − 25.8 db.
Absolute threshold   − 25.6 db.
Range of uncertainty − 25.4 − 25.8 db = 0.4 db.

Figure 3–1
Sample record sheet for method of limits. Calculation of absolute threshold for 600-Hz tone.

certainty-uncertainty. Considering individual personality differences, such an ideal situation is not likely, but with adequate instructions and training a subject *can* at least establish his own standards and adhere to them.

Several methods are also available to detect subjects highly prone to such errors, and thereby allow for additional instructions and training, or, as a last resort, elimination of the culpable subjects. If we start with a sub-threshold stimulus and keep repeating it without changing its value, a good subject will not make the error of anticipating, that is a "yes" response. Similarly, repeating a suprathreshold stimulus several times without decreasing its value will serve as a check for anticipation in the opposite direction. Habituation can be detected by occasionally slipping in an increment much greater than normal, or by starting a series with a suprathreshold stimulus when the subject expects a stimulus at a level below his threshold. Such "tricks" are never a part of the actual data collection. They are simply thrown in now and then to keep the subject on the ball and to ensure his proper level of performance.

Results. A number of measures are obtainable with the method of limits. We can, for example, locate a threshold for the ascending series of presentations. Note that in Figure 3–1 the value required for detection in the first ascending series was 27 db (halfway between the highest undetected and lowest detected values); the value for the second ascending series was 25 db; and so on, for the five ascending series. The average of these five was 25.4 db, the AL for the ascending series. For the descending series the mean AL is 25.8 db. Note that we seem to have an indication of a slight habituation effect. If there were a true "physiological threshold" and if we had a perfect subject, the AL should be the same for both the ascending and descending series. However, because the ascending and descending series rarely result in the same value for the threshold, the true absolute threshold is usually taken as their arithmetic mean. In Figure 3–1 the AL would be 25.6 db.

The difference between those judgments based on the ascending series and those based on the descending series may be of significance in some cases. Called the range of uncertainty (RU), it is a measure of the difficulty of the task and the performance of the subject. If there were no range of uncertainty (RU = 0) one would suspect that the increments used were too large or that one had a subject with amazing discriminative capability.

Several other measures can, if desired, be obtained from this method. Given enough repetitions (normally more than ten series would be used), one can calculate the variability (standard deviation, standard error of mean, etc.) for the various threshold measures, thus having an index of the subject's consistency or a comparison between subjects.

If the alternated ascending and descending series are presented in sufficient quantity and over a long enough time period, it is possible to show the curve of learning, as indicated by decreasing range of uncertainty and/or increased consistency.

DIFFERENCE THRESHOLD (DL)

The method of limits can also be used to obtain difference thresholds. By definition, the DL is defined as that difference between two stimuli that is detected 50 percent of the time. When used in this way, it is a stimulus difference rather than a stimulus value that is detected, and the method is sometimes called the *method of just noticeable differences.*

Procedure. In this method a standard and a comparison stimulus are presented together and compared for equality. As a function of serial increments (or decrements) to the comparison stimulus the subject indicates whether they are alike or different. In some cases he may be required to indicate which one is larger, brighter, sweeter, and so on. The two stimuli may be spatially separated, as with visual stimuli, or temporally, as with acoustic signals. One advantage of this method for determining DL's is that it does it directly; the subject reports on just noticeable differences (jnd's) or just *not* noticeable differences (jnnd's), depending on the direction of change. If the two stimuli are the same to start with, then the subject discovers a just noticeable difference; if the starting point has two stimuli that are different, then the point to be located represents a just *not* noticeable difference.

An example of a worksheet for this method is shown as Figure 3–2. In this hypothetical experiment a standard weight of 10-g was compared with a variable or comparison weight to determine the DL, or that increment in weight that could be detected 50 percent of the time. We will, of course, get two DL's, one for a comparison stimulus greater than the standard and one for the situation in which the comparison stimulus is the lighter.

In the first ascending series the comparison stimulus first had a weight of 2-g and was called "lighter," a 4-g weight and a 6-g weight were also called "lighter," but both the 8- and 10-g weights were called "equal" to the 10. The 12-g weight was called "heavier" and brought the first series to a conclusion. In the first descending series the comparison stimuli of 20-, 18-, 16-, and 14-g weights were all called "heavier" than the standard 10-g weight. The 12- and 10-g weights were judged to be equal to the standard and the 8-g weight was called "lighter."

As can be seen from Figure 3–2 two separate limen must be determined for each series, Lu and Ll (u and l for upper and lower) and then averages of each must be calculated. Does this mean that our DL is both 2.6 (12.6 − 10) and 1.4 (10 − 8.6)? That would not make much sense, two DL's for a single standard stimulus. Look again; the average value for the comparison called "equal" is really 10.6 g [(12.6 + 8.6)/2] and not 10. In other words, the comparison stimulus, to be judged equal to the 10-g weight had to weigh, on the average, 10.6 g, an error of 0.6 g. In the language of the psychophysicist the PSE (point of subjective equality) is 10.6-g and the constant error is 0.6-g. Such constant errors in the method of just noticeable differences are not at all rare and are due to such procedural influences as time differences, space differences, fatigue, or set. Even when highly balanced designs are employed some constant error is often found; the PSE is rarely identical to the value of the standard stimulus.

The DL then must be the average distance between the PSE and the mean Lu and Ll. In our example the difference threshold, that difference that can be detected 50 percent of the time, is exactly 2 g (12.6 − 10.6 or 10.6 − 8.6). Or, looking at it another way, the DL is one-half the range of uncertainty (Lu − Ll).

Difficulties and Limitations. The method of just noticeable differences is applicable to most situations where a DL is needed. It should be emphasized, however, that a DL determined by a method of limits is frequently

Direction of Presentation

Weight of Comparison Stimulus, grams	A	D	A	D	A	D	A	D	A	D	
20		H				H				H	
18		H		H	H	H		H		H	
16		H		H	H	H	H	H		H	
14		H		H	=	H	H	H	H	H	
12	H	=	H	=	=	=	=	=	H	H	
10	=	=	=	=	L	=	=	=	=	=	
8	=	L	L	L	L	L	L	=	L	=	
6	L		L		L		L	L	L	L	
4	L		L		L		L		L		
2	L				L				L		
Lu	11	13	11	13	15	13	13	13	11	11	(12.6)
Ll	7	9	9	9	11	9	9	7	9	7	(8.6)

Point of subjective equality = 10.6 g.
Range of uncertainty = 8.6 − 12.6 g. = 4.0 g.
Constant error = 10.6 − 10.0 = 0.6 g.
Difference threshold = 2.0 g.

Figure 3–2
Sample record sheet for method of limits. Calculation of difference threshold for lifted weights with 10-g standard.

not the same as one derived by the constant methods (see next section). Both methods provide for a measure called a *difference threshold*), but apparently they are not measuring the same thing—perhaps equality is not the opposite of difference!

We also know that if a subject were to continue after his first report beyond "equal," he might again return to "equal," especially if the increments are exceedingly small and the task difficult: How we can handle such a situation is not clear, so we generally avoid it by stopping as soon as one transition beyond the last equal judgment has been made.

Many of the same difficulties mentioned for AL determination also apply to DL determination. One subject, for instance, would go through an entire series of responses: "low . . . low . . . low . . . low . . . equal . . . high" without the experimenter ever having changed the comparison stimulus! Such subjects, of course, are simply not suited for their tasks, and unless they can be adequately trained they are useless. Indeed, in this case one is making a personality evaluation and not running a psychophysical experiment.

Measures. Although the primary measures obtainable are the DL and the range of uncertainty, the method of just noticeable differences also allows for additional measures. Obviously, a Weber fraction ($\Delta I/I$) can be obtained quite directly. Also, separate DLs for ascending and descending series are obtainable, and indications of habituation and anticipation effects are subject to measurement. The interested reader is encouraged to refer to the readings at the end of the chapter for additional details on methods and applications.

There are several variations to the method of limits that should be mentioned. One possibility involves a continuous change in the stimulus, rather than changes by discrete steps. At least one type of audiometer (an instrument for measuring hearing sensitivity) presents a pure tone below threshold and gradually increases its level until the patient reports he hears it. This, incidentally, is automatic equipment that records the instantaneous sound level at the point indicated by the patient, and then proceeds to repeat the procedure for additional frequencies until an entire audiogram has been plotted.

When the writer was a graduate student he had access to a visual acuity device, a car mounted on a track that moved either directly toward or away from the viewer. By means of an acuity chart (like the one your optometrist uses) mounted on the little car, one could determine the subject's threshold (in distance) for reading the letters on the chart. Distance could then be transposed into the familiar 20/20, 20/40 index of visual acuity. Notice, too, the threshold being measured was a resolution threshold, and not a detection threshold such as we have been considering through most of this chapter.

In addition to continuous and systematic presentations such as these, some experimenters have used a haphazard method and one known as the up-and-down method. Methods derived for computer programing "search" in a predetermined but flexible manner and are highly effective for automatic determination of both absolute and difference thresholds. Some programs "zero in" to determine thresholds quickly and accurately, leaving the experimenter with little to do except read a tape. Variations in the method seem to be limited only by the experimenter's imagination.

The Constant Methods

The constant methods, especially with appropriate modifications, are probably the most frequently used, most flexible, and universally applicable of all the psychophysical methods. Indeed, one often uses one of the other methods to locate parameters approximately, and then adapts one of the constant methods for the experiment proper. Mathematics and procedures for the constant methods have been worked out in almost unlimited detail, and a thorough review would go far beyond the scope of this book. Consequently, we will limit ourselves to highlights only, and the interested reader may go to the original sources.

There are two basic forms of the constant method: the constant-stimulus method and the method of constant-stimulus differences. The unique characteristic of both methods is the calculation of parameters based on percentage of occurrence.

ABSOLUTE THRESHOLD (CONSTANT-STIMULUS METHOD)

In the determination of the absolute threshold, a large number of stimuli are presented to the observer in a randomized order, and he merely indicates whether each stimulus is detected or not. The result is a table of percent detections for the full range of stimuli. These may then be plotted on a curve and the 50 percent point taken as the threshold.

Figure 3–3 is an example of a simple determination of an absolute threshold by the constant-stimulus method. The data in the table at the bottom of this figure have been plotted in the curve. A line of best fit has been drawn through the nine points, each point having been determined by the percentage of times the stimulus at the indicated level was detected. A line drawn from the 50 percent point cuts the curve at an intensity level of 21.6 db, and this is taken at the AL. The distance between the 25 and 75 percent points (the middle 50 percent) defines the range of uncertainty, in this case 19.1 to 23.7 db.

It must be emphasized that there are numerous more sophisticated and probably more precise methods of calculation. There are interpolation methods, median methods, extremely complicated curve-fitting methods, and methods involving the use of tables of mathematical weights aimed at maximizing the influence of those judgments near the limen. Literally hundreds of articles and dozens of often vituperative arguments arose in the past concerning the use of the constant methods. One should not spend undue time on these academic, generally sterile, arguments of philosophical interpretation. For most purposes a simple graphic method such as is shown in Figure 3–3 should be entirely adequate. In some cases it might be desirable to use normal probability paper, in which case the best-fitting straight line could be drawn, rather than the ogive of Figure 3–3.

DIFFERENCE THRESHOLD (CONSTANT-STIMULUS DIFFERENCE METHOD)

The constant-stimulus difference method is the most often used of the psychophysical methods. In this method stimuli are presented in pairs, either simultaneously or sequentially, depending on the sense modality involved and the purposes of the experiment. Unlike the calculation of a DL by the method of limits, in the constant-stmulus difference method, pairs of stimuli are randomized. The subject judges whether the variable stimulus on the right (or on the left, or the second stimulus) is less than, equal to, or greater than the standard. Ideally, such factors as sequence and position are counterbalanced, with the standard stmulus being presented on the left (or first) half of the time, and on the right (or second) half of the time, in some sort of random arrangement. Or the effects of spatial and temporal

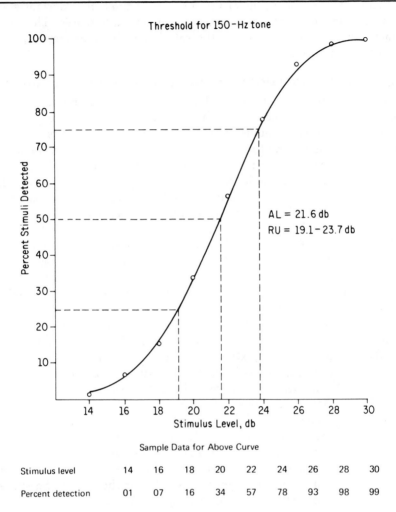

Figure 3-3
Sample graphic determination of an AL by the constant-stimulus method.

arrangement can be retained and teased out in the data analysis if desired. The flexibility of the technique is tremendous, and almost anything of a psychophysical nature can be examined by some modification of the constant-stimulus difference method.

Many of the older, academic discussions referred to earlier also apply to this method. At least one of these arguments should be mentioned. The thinking goes something like this: Any stimulus difference can fit one of three categories: a difference so small that it can never be detected, a difference so large that it can always be detected, and a great gray area where the difference can be detected some of the time. It is this range of uncertainty that presents the problem. What is equal? Is equality a positive attribute or is it negative, the lack of something—this something being, perhaps, the ability to detect a difference. True equality may never exist. With fine enough measuring instruments we might never find two eggs, for example, that weigh precisely the same. Two things are equal only to the extent that we cannot detect a difference.

Some experimenters have argued that three category judgments including "equal" should not be permitted, that a subject must respond with "greater than" or "less than" to all stimulus pairs, even when they are physically alike. Difference thresholds may be smaller when the subject cannot take the easy way out and say "equal" whenever in doubt. Other researchers insist that the perception of equality is a legitimate psychological experience and that omitting it from the acceptable responses of the subject adds intolerably to the artificiality of the situation.

Some additional arguments concern the methodology used to calculate the numerous possible psychophysical measures. What is the significance of a range of uncertainty for two-category judgments as contrasted with a three-category procedure? Considerable argument and a lot of complex mathematics have resulted from the dilemma of two-category versus three-category judgments. The best solution is that, first, each situation must be examined for its own unique requirements and, second, "you pays your money and you takes your choice."

A third category of "equal" or perhaps better defined as "not different" judgments can be included, with the stipulation that subjects should be encouraged to make positive judgments and avoid judgments of "equal" whenever possible. As in all the psychophysical methods, standardized, clear, and forceful instructions to the subjects are very important.

For calculation purposes the "equal" judgments may or may not be included. In the case of DL's they would appear to be useful, if not essential; if a PSE is the objective of the study, then inclusion of equal judgments in the calculations probably adds very little, because they affect only the precision of the measure and not its absolute value.

Sample Problems. Figure 3–4 shows a graphic analysis of data obtained from a constant-stimulus difference experiment based on two-category judgments.* In this experiment a standard auditory tone of 600 Hz was compared with a subsequent variable tone. The second or comparison tone was randomly varied from 592 to 608 Hz in two-cycle intervals. The data collected on a number of individuals over several sessions are summarized in the table beneath the curves. The crossover point for the two psychometric functions indicates the point of subjective equality. In other

---

* Actually, in this experiment "equal" judgments were permitted, but for the purposes of drawing the psychometric functions the equal judgments were divided proportionately. For example, if a particular condition had 80 judgments "high," 20 judgments "low," and 10 judgments "equal," the latter would have been divided eight "low" and two "high."

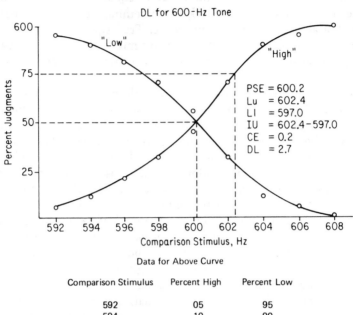

Figure 3-4
Method of constant-stimulus differences; two-category judgments. Subjects judged whether a comparison stimulus was "higher" or "lower" in pitch than a 600-Hz tone.

words, the second of two stimuli, on the average, had to have a frequency of about 600.2 Hz to sound equal in pitch to a preceding 600-Hz standard.

This chart also shows one method for calculating the difference threshold, utilizing the 75 percent points for both judgments "low" and "high." Again called Ll and Lu, these values are about 597.0 and 602.4 for an uncertainty interval of 5.4. The DL is then one-half the interval of uncertainty, or 2.7. That is, a difference as great as 2.7 Hz can be detected 50 percent of the time.

In this example a method for determining the DL similar to that used for the method of limits was employed. Actually there are many methods for calculating a difference threshold, and experimenters in the field are far from being in agreement as to which method is best. However, as long as we define it adequately, we may use any legitimate method we choose, bearing in mind that had we used some other, perhaps more sophisticated method, the results would not have been precisely the same.

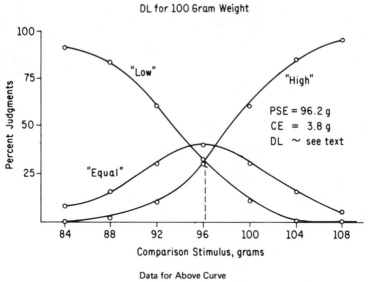

DL for 100 Gram Weight

PSE = 96.2 g
CE = 3.8 g
DL ~ see text

Comparison Stimulus, grams

Data for Above Curve

Comparison Stimulas	Percent High	Percent Equal	Percent Low
84	00	08	92
88	02	15	83
92	10	30	60
96	30	38	32
100	60	30	10
104	85	15	00
108	95	05	00

Figure 3-5
Method of constant-stimulus differences; three-category judgments. Subjects judged whether a comparison weight was heavier (high), lighter (low), or equal to a 100-g standard weight.

In Figure 3–5 an example of three-category data has been plotted. In this case a standard weight of 100 g was compared with a variable ranging from 84 to 108 g in 4-g steps. Note the rather large constant error (3.8 g), probably a time error, since one weight was hefted subsequent to the other, and no counterbalancing was used.

An even greater variety of techniques for determining a wide range of measures is available when "equal" judgments are included in the calculations. And even more differences of opinion are found than was true for the method of limits. Consequently, a DL is not present for this example. If we use half the distance between the 50 or 75 percent points as we did before, we would be omitting, perhaps wasting, the "equal" category entirely. Some of the techniques do indeed include the "equal" judgments, but their complexity and their disputed status militate against their inclusion in a book of this depth.

Regardless of what technique is used, the three-category presentation does have an advantage in facilitating comparisons of one condition with another. Comparing different curves with their distributions of "equals," for example, can be enlightening to the extent that "uncertainty" can be observed directly rather than by inference. Once more the reader is encouraged to consult the references if he is interested in the nitty-gritty of the numerous methods of calculations and the arguments of the numerous proponents of one method or another.

Method of Average Error

With this method we obtain a true PSE. Also called the *reproduction* or *adjustment method,* this technique circumvents the need to infer a PSE as in the other methods, because the subject himself makes the adjustment on one of the two stimuli until he reaches a point where he can say "Voilà, they are equal!" A practical application of the method can be found in some modern exposure meters, where the photographer adjusts a small spot of light until it is the same brightness as its surround.

In many respects the method is similar to the method of limits. The variable stimulus may originate either above or below the standard, and calculations, for the most part, are similar. The principal differences are that the subject makes the adjustment and a continuous movement rather than discrete steps are generally utilized. In some cases, unlike the method of limits, "bracketing" is permitted. That is, the subject can go slightly beyond the PSE and zero in on it with successive small adjustments until he is satisfied with his match.

The same general advantages and disadvantages mentioned for the method of limits tend to apply to this method. In addition, we must bear in mind that we are not evaluating a sensory-perceptual experience independent of a motor response. In some cases, the error may be confounded by the subject's motor limitations.

There are numerous variations and possible modifications to the method. It can be used for AL determination when employed with a single stimulus. As another variation, discrete step changes rather than continuous changes may be employed. In this case the only difference between an adjustment method and a method of limits would be the identification of *who* makes the change in the variable stimulus.

Summary

In this chapter we looked briefly into the historical background of the psychophysical methods, including the primary contributions of the two pioneers Weber and Fechner. In addition, we identified six broad uses for psychophysics: the determination of absolute thresholds, difference thresholds, sensory equivalence, rank order, sensory distance, and sensory ratios. Finally, we examined briefly the three primary psychophysical methods:

the method of limits, the constant methods, and the method of average error. In the following chapter we examine additional techniques designed to evaluate more complex sensory-experiential relations.

Suggested Readings

1. S. S. Stevens. "Mathematics, Measurement, and Psychophysics," chap. 1, in S. S. Stevens (ed.), *Handbook of Experimental Psychology*. New York: Wiley, 1954. These 49 pages contain a wealth of background information on measurement in general. Number systems, scales of measurement, and a general approach to psychophysics makes this a valuable background source.
2. From J. P. Guilford. *Psychometric Methods*, 2d ed. New York: McGraw-Hill, 1954. I suggest chap. 1 for a short (19 pages) introduction to psychological measurement. Although all of this book is of great significance to experimental psychologists, chaps. 4 to 6 (70 pages) might be considered the "bible" for psychophysical methods. Chapters 7 to 12 (190 pages) have similar importance for scaling techniques (to be considered in the next chapter). Although even the serious student might not sit down and read this book from cover to cover, it should be available for reference when needed.
3. From R. S. Woodworth and H. Schlossberg. *Experimental Psychology*, rev. ed. New York: Holt, Rinehart and Winston, 1954. Chapters 8 and 9 of this excellent text summarize threshold determinations and scaling methods, respectively, in a total of about 75 pages. Although not nearly as complete as the previous reference, these two chapters should be familiar to the serious student of psychophysics and experimental method.
4. From J. F. Corso. *The Experimental Psychology of Sensory Behavior*. New York: Holt, Rinehart and Winston, 1967. Chapter 7 is a shorter (40 page) up-to-date summary of psychophysical methods with a somewhat different approach, and including descriptions of scaling. It is suggested for its somewhat broader coverage with less depth, as contrasted with the preceding references.
5. L. L. Thurstone. "Psychophysical Methods," in T. G. Andrews (ed.), *Methods of Psychology*. New York: Wiley, 1948. These 34 pages, comprising chap. 5, provide an excellent coverage of the area of psychophysics. It is written in an easy, readable manner and is highly recommended.
6. From Edward C. Carterette and Morton P. Friedman (eds.). *Handbook of Perception, vols. I and II*. New York: Academic Press, 1974. Both of these two previously mentioned volumes contain material relevant to the application of the psychophysical methods. See, in particular, chap. 1 of vol. II, "History of Psychophysics and Judgment" by F. Nowell Jones.
7. From Bertram Scharf (ed.). *Experimental Sensory Psychology*. Glenview, Ill.: Scott, Foresman, 1975. In addition to a fine introductory chapter by Professor Scharf, "Psychophysics," chap. 2, by Joan Gay Snodgrass is well worth reading. These 67 pages contain a wealth of information as well as a very fine bibliography. The serious student would do well to read these two chapters.

4 / methods for studying the senses—II

The early psychophysical techniques discussed in the preceding chapter were primarily concerned with determining thresholds and similar physiologically (so the early workers believed) limited constraints on sense organ performance. Only incidentally did they aspire to the development of interval or ratio scales of sensory functioning. Although such operationally observed constructs as difference thresholds and just noticeable differences did indeed foretell the development of true phenomenal experience scales, the final development of such scales remained for the future, with more "tools of the trade" being designed specifically for their determination.

In this chapter we examine some of those methods in a somewhat logical sequence, reflecting both historial and procedural perspective. These approaches are both simpler in concept and, in some cases, more sophisticated than the three psychophysical methods considered in the previous chapter.

We conclude this chapter with a brief look at three modern approaches to determining the relation between the external world and the world of experience. Although these three approaches are probably too broad to be categorized as psychophysical methods, their inclusion in a book of this type is imperative. They reflect the direction of the future and should be familiar to the contemporary sensory-perceptual psychologist.

Method of Rank Order

An order-of-merit technique, because of its simplicity and apparent validity, has much to recommend it. Many evaluations do not lend themselves to quantification, and a rank ordering is the best that can be hoped for. Ordering may be be done directly, with no (or little) reliance on objective measures, such as: "rank seven different odors on a scale of pleasantness-unpleasantness." In this procedure no attempt is made to equate differences within the scale; that is, no assumption is made that the interval between the fifth and sixth odors is in any way comparable to the difference between the first and second. Although this lack of an interval scale may appear to be a drawback, in many cases the absence of scores or other quantitative data make any other approach impossible.

Several other examples might be mentioned. Many colleges provide a rank order of their graduates as well as the individual cumulative grade average. In this case rank order, even when a more sophisticated rating is available, is used for purposes of ease of interpretation and comparison.

Determination of automobile-racing champions is based on a form of ranking wherein points are awarded for finishing first, second, and third for each race and then accumulated throughout the season. At the end of the season the driver with the most points is the champion. At our local track the winner of each race receives 50 points, the second place finisher 48, and on down to 2 points for finishing last. Unfortunately, when one driver consistently finishes a half-lap ahead of the bunched second, third, and fourth cars, the point spread for an individual race is incapable of showing this marked supremacy. The winner gets only 2 points more than the second-place finisher whether he wins by a full lap or by 6 in. When applied to psychological problems the same lack of direct quantification must be recognized.

There are, however, a number of approaches that, by means of pooling several rankings, attempt to arrive at scales that *do* show relative position within the rankings, at least when totaled over an entire season or a group of several races. Simply averaging the rank of each individual over all the rankings is an obvious step in that direction. In our racing example, over many races the man who always wins would have an average rank of one; the more evenly matched second-, third-, and fourth-place cars would vary in their finishing orders from race to race so that their average rank would be greater than two, thereby resulting in a significant numerical advantage for the consistent winner. The accumulation of points from race to race would accomplish the same thing.

A number of additional, more sophisticated approaches for deriving scales from rank-order data have been advanced at various times. Each of these methods attempts to meet the problem of interpreting pooled results. The characteristic being rated may be distributed normally in the population, distributed rectangularly, or distributed in a markedly skewed fashion. A pooling technique satisfactory for one form of distribution may be quite misleading for another.

One such method, although not precisely ranking, does facilitate the interpretation of large numbers of data. Ranking 100 values would be exceedingly difficult, and in the long run probably meaningless. This approach provides for a limited number of slots, ten, for example, and the rater places the data in them according to some a priori instructions. He may approximate a rectangular distribution by apportioning the data equally among the various slots, or he may approximate a normal distribution if so instructed. As in all examples of rating-scale formation, instructions to the rater, whether implicit or externally induced, are of extreme importance.

Guilford (1954) suggests five or six methods for deriving scales from rank-order data and the interested reader is referred to this source for detailed procedures. One of the methods entails the comparison of each rank with every other rank on a paried comparison basis. This is an indirect application of the following basic procedure.

Method of Paired Comparisons

A second technique, the method of paired comparisons, is useful when the stimulus cannot be measured in objective terms. It has probably been used most often for evaluating aesthetic judgment. As the name would imply, the procedure for this method is to compare each stimulus with every other stimulus on some basis such as beauty, artistic merit, and so on. Because a total of $N(N-1)/2$ different pairs can be made from any series of stimuli, the evaluation of ten stimuli would require 45 separate judgments. It is clear that when the number of stimuli becomes large the method becomes time-consuming and unwieldy. (For 100 stimuli a total of 4,950 individual judgments would have to be made by each rater.)

A sample work sheet and summary table for the method is shown as Figures 4–1 and 4–2. In Figure 4–1 the result of ten stimuli being examined with a paired-comparison technique by a single rater is shown. The sample numbered 6 appears to be the choice of this rater, who selected it over every other sample except for the 5. Actually, a rating based on one observer and resulting from just 45 comparisons would be highly subject to chance variability and not very meaningful.

The presentation in Figure 4–2 provides a more meaningful analysis, based on a large number of comparisons by several raters. This was an experiment performed for a large soap manufacturer and the stimuli were ten bars of soap varying in the amount of perfume they contained. The question asked was something like this: "How much perfume should be put in a new brand of soap? If too much sweet perfume is used the soap may be rejected by potential male users; if too little perfume is used and the final product smells like soap, women may refuse to buy it. But is there a happy middle ground where both men and women may like the smell of the soap? Or must separate 'his' and 'hers' soaps be manufactured, differing primarily in their perfume content?" This was the problem we attempted to solve by a paired-comparison technique, with subjects choosing between all possible pairings of the ten samples. Figure 4–2 presents part

	Standard								
Comparison	10	9	8	7	6	5	4	3	2
10									
9	9								
8	10	8							
7	7	7	7						
6	6	6	6	6					
5	5	5	5	5	5				
4	4	9	4	4	6	5			
3	3	9	8	3	6	3	4		
2	10	9	2	7	6	2	2	2	
1	10	1	8	7	6	5	1	1	2

Summary for Single Rater

Soap	10	9	8	7	6	5	4	3	2	1
Preference	3	4	3	5	8	7	4	3	5	3

Figure 4–1
Method of paired comparisons (sample work sheet for one rater). Ten bars of soap, varying in perfume content, were presented to a single subject in all possible two-bar combinations. The subject made 45 judgments as to which of the paired bars were the more pleasant to smell.

of the data, but does not indicate whether the data were for the males, the females, or the combined results. Although these data are not extremely revealing, they do indicate that samples 5 and 6 were preferred almost three-fourths of the time and, except in comparison to each other, were clearly preferred over all the other samples. It would appear, too, that there is not much to choose between these two.

This last statement hints at another use for the paired-comparison technique. We once did an experiment for a distillery in which the problem concerned the necessary amount of quality control in coloring the final product. When a bartender pours a drink for a customer at the bar from a newly opened bottle, it won't do for the customer to notice a difference in the color of his drink, as compared with his neighbor's that came from the just-emptied bottle. The customer is likely to exclaim, "Who watered my drink?" It therefore behooves the distiller to ensure that all batches of the same spirits have the same color, at least within the normal discriminatory limits of the sober customer. This was the problem we attacked. Subjects matched samples for coloring (which of each pair is darker?) and the result was something like a difference threshold for caramel coloring, but de-

Code Numbers of Soap

	10	9	8	7	6	5	4	3	2	1
10		.52	.55	.60	.85	.83	.80	.75	.70	.60
9	.48		.51	.63	.80	.78	.55	.55	.50	.49
8	.45	.49		.65	.70	.70	.50	.55	.40	.35
7	.40	.37	.35		.65	.60	.48	.35	.30	.20
6	.15	.20	.30	.35		.48	.32	.18	.10	.02
5	.17	.22	.30	.40	.52		.40	.22	.20	.15
4	.20	.45	.50	.52	.68	.60		.54	.40	.30
3	.25	.45	.45	.65	.82	.78	.46		.55	.32
2	.30	.50	.60	.70	.90	.80	.60	.45		.40
1	.40	.51	.65	.80	.98	.85	.70	.68	.60	
Means	.31	.41	.47	.59	.78	.71	.53	.47	.42	.31

Figure 4–2
Sample summary table for method of paired comparisons (proportion of time soap numbered on top was preferred to number listed on side). This table presents the summary results of a large number of subjects such as the one illustrated in Figure 4–1.

termined by a paired-comparison technique. The smaller the DL, the greater would be the amount of precision required on the part of the distiller.

The careful reader may have already noted the similarity between the constant-stimulus difference method and the method of paired comparisons. In the former, each stimulus is compared with a standard; in the latter, each stimulus is compared with every other stimulus. In an experiment such as the soap-smelling one, the rater probably would not even know which method was being used. Many of the sophisticated data analysis techniques for the constant-stimulus difference method can (with necessary modification) also be applied to the method of paired comparisons. As before, their complexity, controversiality, and specialized nature militate against their inclusion in a book of this broad coverage and limited psychophysical emphasis.

Scaling Methods

The idea of scaling things is not new. Industrial psychologists, military commanders, and others have for many years used scales to aid in the evaluation of the competence and, in some cases, personality, of their charges. Generally referred to as *rating scales,* those developed are purely nominal, ordinal, or numerical scales. Considerable effort has been expended on developing such scales and some have been highly successful. But such scales as those found in the military's Officer's Evaluation Report, as an example, differ in a fundamental way from the scaling procedures we will discuss in this section. Such scales merely locate an individual along some continuum, perhaps psychological; they do not attempt to relate this position to some other physical, measurable continuum in a quantitative manner. The purpose of scaling as considered in this section is to relate a continuum of behavior (experience) to a continuum of some physical event in a meaningful, quantitative way.

INDIRECT METHOD

When Fechner suggested that just noticeable differences were equal unless always or never recognized, he was stating the basic premise of the indirect method of constructing a sensory-physical scale. If we could accept the formula of Fechner for a sensory experience, we should be able to plot a curve such as shown in Figure 4–3. If Fechner's $S = k \log I$ were perfectly valid this curve would, if the stimulus values were expressed in log units, be a straight line. The curve of Figure 4–3 is indeed a hypothetical function, for, as we indicated earlier, Fechner's law does not hold throughout the range of most sensory experiences.

To derive a scale such as this that would be valid, it would be necessary to calculate a number of jnd's (DL's) and fit a curve to these points. We would not need to measure all the possible jnd's, but with a sampling of 10 or 15 the best-fitting curve would be a good indication of the relation of the experience and the physical event.

The result would be an interval scale of sensory experience. It would not be a ratio scale unless we took the liberty of calling absolute threshold "zero," and this would be a presumption open to serious question.

As we indicated earlier, the magnitude of a jnd, like other psychometric values, is not entirely independent of the manner by which it is determined. The DL obtained by a constant-difference method is not necessarily the same as a jnd arrived at by a more direct method. Consequently, the meaning of a scale derived by such indirect means is problematical.

The Law of Comparative Judgment. Modern work on indirect scaling owes much to the efforts of L. L. Thurstone, who advanced his Law of Comparative Judgment in 1927. Thurstone's idea was that a stimulus gives rise to a discriminal process within the subject that, rather obviously, varies from presentation to presentation. If enough repeated measures are taken and the amount and shape of the dispersion of the data are known, measures of psychological distance can be calculated. The method has been frequently employed with data of a more "psychological" than "psychophysical" nature. Thurstone's methods have been utilized in scaling various social and personality attributes with some degree of success.

It should be pointed out that Thurstone's method does not dictate a

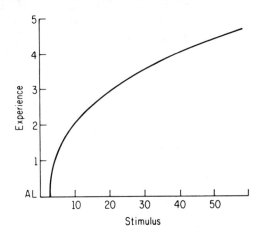

Figure 4-3
Hypothetical function relating magnitude of the sensory experience to the magnitude of the stimulus.

specific method of data collection. Various conventional methods for collecting data are available and have been used. Paired comparisons suggests itself as an obvious method; Rank order methods have likewise been utilized, with statistical transcriptions in accordance with methods suggested by Guilford (1954, Chap. 8).

The interested student is encouraged to read the original work of Thurstone (1959) to gain a thorough understanding of the technique.

DIRECT METHODS

Modern proponents of scaling techniques often lean to the use of more direct methods in lieu of the older, indirect psychophysical method. Such approaches, although admittedly somewhat subjective, do tend to eliminate or greatly reduce the effects due to different methods referred to earlier. In addition, better handling of the sticky "zero" problem is possible when direct methods are employed.

Several related approaches for application of the direct methods are available. We will describe, briefly, only two.

Fractionation Method. A method to determine sense ratios was used by Merkel around 1890, in which he attempted to derive a sensory magnitude scale by means of doubling a sensory experience (Woodworth, 1954). The method was forgotten until revived in the 1930s by S. S. Stevens, who pointed out its value as a tool for developing a scale for loudness. Stevens, however, achieved his greatest success by a process of halving the experience, rather than doubling it—hence the term *fractionation*.

It would appear that the most direct way to obtain a ratio scale is appropriate application of a fractionation method. It is perhaps the only method that can be said to provide a true ratio scale. The underlying assumption, of course, is that people can recognize equal sense ratios— that is, equal relative distances on a psychological continuum—and that they can make appropriate ratio responses, not merely matches as in conventional psychophysics. As a matter of record, the success with which observers *can* produce ratio scales would probably astonish the Webers and Fechners were they to observe research in a modern psychophysical laboratory.

A typical fractionation experiment goes something like this. Utilizing a scalable standard stimulus, the observer either adjusts or selects an appropriate variable stimulus that stands in some specified ratio to the standard. The subject might, for example, adjust a variable stimulus to a point where it is one-half as loud as the standard, or twice as bright, or one-half as sour. To be sure, many judgments must be averaged to reduce chance variability, and if the scale is to be representative of more than one person, many subjects must be used.

Combining of a large number of subjects does not always result in a practical scale. There is always the possibility that a scale based on the average of a large number of subjects may be representative of none of them. Most of us are aware of how multiple plateaus in each individual learning curve may disappear when curves for several persons are combined. The whole may obscure the nature of the parts. In spite of such negative instances, however, the remarkable success achieved by such workers as Stevens *does* seem to indicate a bright future for the development of true ratio scales of sensory experience.

There are many modifications and variations in the procedure. One approach involves an adjustment in which the subject halves a difference between two stimuli—that is, he locates the midpoint between two sensory experiences. Such a bisecting procedure has been used by Stevens to verify results obtained by the simpler fractionation method. It is also theoretically possible, although difficult in practice, to fractionate in thirds, quarters, or any simple fraction. Such complications make the task of the subject more difficult, but are not impossible.

There are also several different ways in which a scale may be derived from fractionation data. In general, these methods are relatively simple, relying on commonly used measures of central tendency and simple arithmetic. For the person interested in deriving scales by fractionation techniques the suggested readings by S. S. Stevens at the end of the chapter are particularly recommended. Certainly anyone wishing to use any of the methods in research of his own should be familiar with these readings.

Single-Stimulus or Direct-Magnitude Estimation. We learned that in the constant-stimulus method, a stimulus is presented in a pseudorandom fashion and the observer reports its presence or absence. In the scaling technique of Direct-Magnitude Estimation a single stimulus is again used, but now all stimuli are above threshold and the subject simply assigns some value to each. In normal practice the experimenter gives a standard signal to the subject to serve as an anchoring point and informs him of its assigned value, such as five, ten, and so on. The subject then proceeds to assign values to each of the entire series of stimuli, based on his impression of their relationship to the standard and—and this is very important—to the instructions provided by the experimenter. In some cases, the standard signal may be given before each variable, thus approximating somewhat more closely the method of constant-stimulus differences. In other applications the standard may vary, being, as an example, the preceding variable stimulus. The important consideration, however, is that the subject *assigns* values to each sensory experience.

Relating the assigned numbers to the stimulus values is then a relatively straightforward procedure, generally followed by curve fitting and the derivation of the physical-sensory scale.

For a technique as subjective as this, the importance of the instructions given the subject cannot be overemphasized. Procedures too are of extreme importance if results are to be repeatable and generalizable. Stevens outlines in great detail some of his musts, such as the following: Use a standard of intermediate value, keep sessions short (10 minutes), use a simple number such as 10 for the standard, use one standard only for a given session, let the subject present the stimuli to himself, do not suggest what values should be assigned (except for the standard) (Stevens, 1956). It should be clear to the reader that any departure from these suggestions, such as utilizing the weakest or lowest stimulus as the anchoring point, would influence the final results.

Stevens's Power Function. No account of scaling could be complete without reference to the life-long work of the late S. S. Stevens. In addition to his numerous contributions mentioned in the preceding paragraphs, and many more to be cited in later chapters of this book, Stevens advanced the hypothesis of a power function to relate a stimulus to an experience, in contradistinction to Fechner's logarithmic ($S = k \log I$) relationship. He worked out numerous exponents for various functions, demonstrating that a sensation grows in proportion to a stimulas raised to some power. These exponents were worked out for a vast variety (more than 20) of stimulus-sensation relations, such as loudness, brightness, smell, taste (sweet and salt), vibration, visual area, angular acceleration, vocal effort, and temperature (cold and warm) (1970). See Figure 4–4 for an example of several power functions based on cross-modality matches. In this experiment subjects adjusted the values on each continuum to match the brightness of a circular luminous target viewed in a dark room. The existence of a power function is, of course, demonstrated by the straightness of the lines connecting the points.

In spite of its relatively wide acceptance, the power function approach of Stevens does have its critics. The failure of Stevens's "Neural Quantum" approach to encompass absolute thresholds is emphasized by Corso (1973), as well as several other weaknesses. The interested student should read

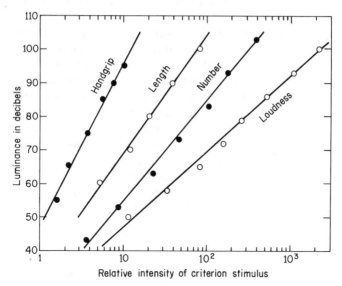

Figure 4–4
Equal-sensation functions determined by cross-modality matches between brightness
and four other continua. (From S. S. Stevens, *Science*, 170 (1970): 1044. Copyright
1970 by the American Association for the Advancement of Science.)

the Corso-Norman note exchange listed in the readings at the end of the
chapter.

Signal Detection Theory

Signal detection theory, the most recent approach to the study of sensory
experience, should be familiar, at least in principle, to all students of
sensory-perceptual relations. Because it entails some complex thinking, no
attempt is made here to provide enough information for successful application of the method. If however this section gets across the general idea
and significance of the approach, it will have achieved its purpose.

BACKGROUND

Some years ago the principles of statistical decision theory were translated into a theory of signal detection, primarily for use in the description
and ultimate prediction of radar signal reception (see Peterson et al., 1954).
It was recognized that radar signals are specialized conditions in a background of noise, and their reception or nonreception does not follow any
simple threshold analogue, but rather some function that should include
a statement of probability. The theory of signal detection accepted the
principles of decision theory, in that general hypothesis acceptance or rejection was not considered to be adequately descriptive. On the contrary,
in a general decision procedure, statistical hypotheses rather than general

hypotheses are evaluated. For those not familiar with the terminology, a general hypothesis is a deductive logic statement such as "all birds have wings." If we find one bird without wings, then we can reject the hypothesis. A statistical hypothesis, on the other hand, requires special rules for rejection and can be rejected only at some probability level.

Several years after the adoption of the theory for radar signal detection, the theory came to the attention of several workers at the Massachusetts Institute of Technology, who recognized the generality of the theory and its possible applicability to problems of human signal detection (Tanner and Swets, 1954; Swets, 1961). Indeed, to these workers the theory appeared to provide a framework for describing the behavior of the human observer in a large variety of detection and perceptual tasks. Swets and others then proceeded to adapt the theory to the human, the result being signal detection theory applied to human observers.

SENSORY THRESHOLDS

One of the key aspects of signal detection theory is its rejection of the concept of a sensory threshold. In classical psychophysics a sensory threshold was considered an immutable attribute of the sense organ and its associated structures. It was presumed that there was a definite point in a physical continuum beyond which a sense organ would invariably respond. Variability as observed in a psychophysical experiment was due to chance factors and should be eliminated to the extent possible. If this chance variability could be eliminated then, Eureka! the threshold would be there, standing out clearly for all to see.

Although not entirely rejecting the all-or-none law in the case of extremely simple structures such as muscle fibers or individual neurons, the proponents of sensory detection theory took a different tack. Even if it were true that there is a point where a single straw will break the camel's back, we are not going to find this point. An analogue to noise in an electrical system will prevent our identifying this point with anything approaching optimum precision. Furthermore, why should we wish to find this magical point anyway? The aim of science is prediction, and we can only predict accurately if we include *all* the influences involved. To the modern detection theorist, a threshold is a statistical concept, a probability of detection based on factors probably too numerous to enumerate. The emphasis is not that a true threshold does not exist, rather it is more like "Who needs a threshold concept? We can predict behavior better if we use the constructs of sensory detection theory and include the influences of noise, the operating characteristics of the receiver (organism), and general probability considerations."

DESCRIPTION

In the basic experiment utilizing detection theory an observer must decide whether an experienced event is caused by noise (random influences) alone or is due to the presence of a signal in the noise. A signal is pre-

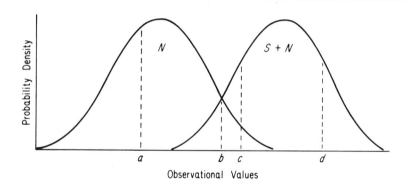

Figure 4–5
Hypothetical density function of noise and signal plus noise.

sumed to shift the overall distribution (noise plus signal) and the degree of shift should, it is clear, indicate the strength of the signal. Although this is basically what is done in all psychophysical methods (although perhaps not recognized as such), the unique feature of detection theory is its approach to the data analysis and interpretation.

One aspect of experiments using this technique is the concept of a probability density function such as exemplified by Figure 4–5. This curve is based on the assumption that any observation may arise either from noise alone or from noise plus a signal.

In Figure 4–5 the probability density functions have been plotted for noise alone and for the condition combining noise and a signal. The distribution labeled N represents the probability density function for a positive response under a condition of noise alone; the distribution labeled $S + N$ is the probability of a positive response when the signal and noise are combined (as in most instances). Because the observations will be of a greater magnitude under the $S + N$ condition, the average for this distribution will be higher than the average for the N distribution. Note too that when the observation has a value of a, the probability of detection of (experiencing) the combined event is simply the probability of experiencing the noise. As signal strength is increased through b (equal probability) to d, the likelihood of an error in which noise is identified as signal approaches zero.

This last statement points to another advantage of the detection theory model. Levels of confidence in accepting or rejecting various hypotheses concerning the presence of a signal can be manipulated with extreme facility. Statements concerning the probability of rejecting the hypothesis that a signal does not exist when it does indeed exist, and conversely, that a signal exists when only noise is present can be made with ease and precision.

There are numerous other concepts developed for the application of sensory detection theory, too involved to consider in this section. The concept of an ROC (receiver-operating-characteristic) is useful in describing the sensory process. It is possible also to control the criterion and to manipulate such aspects as payoff for correct versus incorrect decisions. In summary, the technique, although difficult in its conceptual framework, holds great promise for an ultimate understanding of sensory-perceptual phenomena.

Information Theory

Still another approach, borrowed from a discipline other than sensory psychology but useful in many instances, is that involving information theory. It is generally more applicable to such areas as linguistics or decision making, but information theory can be helpful as a framework for understanding sensory-perceptual phenomena.

As described by its proponents, one unit of information is that amount of information that will reduce uncertainty by one-half. If you have a deck of 64 cards, half red and half black, and divided equally according to suits, and I ask you to identify the one card I am thinking of, your uncertainty encompasses the entire pack; the one I am thinking of could be any one of the 64 cards. But if I give you one piece of information, "I am thinking of a red card," now your uncertainty only involves 32 cards, the red ones. If I then tell you that the card I have in mind is a heart, your uncertainty is again reduced by one-half, because only 16 of 32 red cards are hearts. In the language of information theory, I have given you two *bits* (short for *binary digits*) of information, each of which enabled you to reduce your uncertainty by one-half. It should be apparent, if you continue the subdivision to the end, that I would have to give you 6 bits of information to assure your identifying the card I am thinking of with no possibility of error and no guessing. There are, then, 6 bits of information in a sample of 64 items. If the deck had contained 128 cards, 7 bits of information would be represented, and so on, in powers of 2. This is the key—powers of 2—and the amount of information in any symbol or statement is measured by the amount of uncertainty reduction according to a power-of-2 law. Notice that $2^4 = 16$, $2^5 = 32$, $2^6 = 64$, $2^7 = 128$, and so on.

Usually the numbers do not come out as even as in the example. In identifying a letter at random from the alphabet we would need 4 bits of information to identify a letter from a 16-letter alphabet, and 5 bits of information to identify a letter from a 32-letter alphabet. To identify a specific letter in a 26-letter alphabet we would need between 4 and 5 bits of information. We would, of course, settle on 5 bits to be certain of never missing the desired letter. For precise calculation, the number of bits in a 26-letter alphabet would be found as $2^b = 26$ (the power that 2 would have to be raised to for it to equal 26). Actually, it would be something like 4.6 bits of information.

The information theory approach, it should be noted, is related to the detection theory model, and the two can be combined profitably for statistical analysis purposes. Many of the conventional psychophysical approaches can be used, with design and interpretation in terms of information theory concepts and the broad conceptual background of communications. Psychophysical experiments in the broad area of learning and learning theory are particularly amenable to the information theory approach.

Adaptation Level

Another interesting approach involves the theory of *adaptation level*. Extensively developed by Harry Helson (1943, 1964), this approach examines the fact that judgments tend to move in directions away from some middle point, that is, toward an "adaptation level." The theory arose from experiments by Helson on induced color. For example, if one observes a series of surfaces of different reflectances ranging perhaps from very dark gray to near white (illuminated by monochromatic light) surfaces of intermediate reflectance appear gray, surfaces of greater reflectance are the color of the illuminant, and surfaces of lower reflectance take on the complementary color of the illuminant.

In addition to its recent application to nonsensory psychological phenomena, extensive work has been accomplished by other investigators with respect to sensory judgments. Among the most precise testing of the predictive value of the hypothesis is the work of Parducci (1971) and his co-workers. The interested reader should begin by becoming familiar with the definitive articles by Helson.

Use of Computers

This section does not discuss actual methods for psychological research. Its emphasis is on the importance of the modern digital computer as a tool for research. An analogue computer may be ideally suited to some special instances, but for general-purpose use and overall flexibility the digital computer is unequaled.

A psychophysicist (or almost any psychologist, for that matter) who, 15 years from now, does not have a basic understanding of computer technology will be as hard to find as a pop singer without a guitar. The age of the computer is with us and the serious student must keep up with the times.

DATA REDUCTION

What can computers do for us? First of all, the once laborious task of manually processing data collected in a psychological experiment can be all but eliminated by the rapid and accurate calculations of the modern digital computer. I once, for example, had a very simple program for processing grades of my students, using a time-sharing system with a

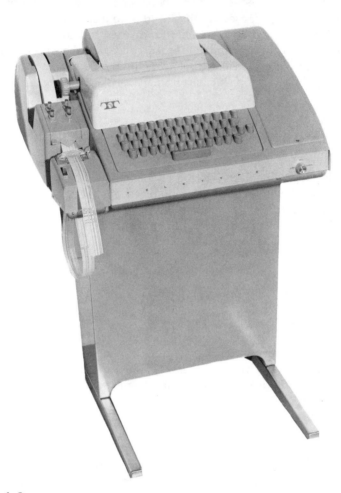

Figure 4-6
Teletype® Model 33 data terminal. (Photograph courtesy of Teletype Corporation, Skokie, Illinois.)

Flexowriter (see Figure 4-6). A sample printout from this program is shown as Figure 4-7. Note that when the computer says "READY," merely enter the grades in any order by typing, for instance, 76, 62, 66, 78, and so on, and then the order for the computer to do its job, in this case BASIC. The computer then gives the date and the time of day. It counts the number of entries and prints out the result as SAMPLE SIZE; in the example of Figure 4-7 the number of students taking the quiz was 28. The next step is the calculation and printout of the mean, the median, and the standard deviation. Then the computer proceeds to rank the grades, printing out each grade in order with its rank, its deviation from the mean, its

```
READY
00001   DATA   76, 62, 66, 78, 70, 24, 60, 90, 78, 80, 66, 86, 82, 86, 82, 74
00002   DATA   78, 60, 72, 84, 58, 90, 88, 78, 86, 72, 60, 36
$BASIC
```

	03/09/78		12:51	

SAMPLE SIZE	28	
MEAN	72.21	
MEDIAN	77	
STANDARD DEVIATION	15.197	

	SUBJECT	SCORE	DEVIATION	STAND SCORE	CENTILE
A	1	90	17.79	1.17	87.9
	2	90	17.79	1.17	87.9
	3	88	15.79	1.04	85
	4	86	13.79	0.91	81.7
	5	86	13.79	0.91	81.7
B	6	86	13.79	0.91	81.7
	7	84	11.79	0.78	78
	8	82	9.786	0.64	74
	9	82	9.786	0.64	74
	10	80	7.786	0.51	69.5
	11	78	5.786	0.38	64.8
	12	78	5.786	0.38	64.8
	13	78	5.786	0.38	64.8
	14	78	5.786	0.38	64.8
C	15	76	3.786	0.25	59.8
	16	74	1.786	0.12	54.6
	17	72	$-.2143$	-0.02	49.4
	18	72	$-.2143$	-0.02	49.4
	19	70	-2.214	-0.15	44.2
	20	66	-6.214	-0.41	34.1
	21	66	-6.214	-0.41	34.1
D	22	62	-10.21	-0.67	25
	23	60	-12.21	-0.80	21
	24	60	-12.21	-0.80	21
	25	60	-12.21	-0.80	21
	26	58	-14.21	-0.94	17.4
E	27	36	-36.21	-2.38	0.8
	28	24	-48.21	-3.17	0.0

Figure 4–7
Sample printout from computer terminal. This is a sample from a quiz given to a
statistics class. A printout such as this hanging on a bulletin board enables students
to see how well they did in comparison to other students.

standard score, and its percentile rank. The instructor can also get a histogram of the distribution, all in a form ideal for posting on the classroom walls. The total job takes perhaps five minutes, almost all occupied by the slow printout of the mechanical typewriter. Today, of course, modern high-speed printers can supply the complete printout in considerably less than five minutes. Just imagine how long it would take me to calculate manually these standard scores and percentiles.

The degree of precision, the alignment and neatness of the presentation, and so on, are all at the discretion of the person doing the programming. If desired, I could have carried out my calculations to several more decimal places and I could have presented normalized centile values, rather than those based simply on the area under the normal curve. There is almost no limit to what can be done by an individual with a little ingenuity and a basic knowledge of programming.*

Experiments can be designed to capitalize on the capabilities of the computer as a calculating tool. Data can be collected automatically on punched cards or magnetic tape. In some cases the processing of the data and the final statistical analysis may be completed before the subject leaves the laboratory.

ON-LINE COMPUTER CAPABILITY

Computers can be programmed to run experiments. Not only can they process the final data, but they can also generate and present the stimuli in a preplanned (or random) fashion, and make necessary changes as a function of the subjects' responses. Completely automatic experiments can, conceivably, be designed. It is not uncommon for many animal studies, for example with rats or pigeons, to rely heavily on computers to program the stimuli, provide the rewards, and simultaneously record the subjects' responses, all with a minimum of intervention by the experimenter. To be sure, the latter must program the computer so that it "knows" what to do.

I once employed a simple program to generate a multihued information display that simulated certain military status boards. It was possible to obtain random location and identity of known and unknown aircraft, entirely simulated, and suitable for experimentation with human subjects.

Computers, under the control of qualified experts, can be used to simulate—that is, model—many human functions for concentrated study. Models of neural activity, pattern recognition, and signal detection have all been achieved with some degree of success.

ADDITIONAL USES FOR COMPUTERS

Another use for the computer is to store and retrieve information. Although it may not be one of the more important uses for the psycho-

---

* The program demonstrated by Figure 4–7 was accomplished with BASIC Language. Modern forms of Fortran, for example, are more likely to be encountered by the beginning student.

physicist, the capability of storing vast amounts of information in a small space and retrieving all or part of it on demand is an important capability of the modern computer.

Of course, not every psychologist interested in sensory-perceptual phenomena requires such a complete knowledge of computer technology as to be able to write extremely complex programs. To do this well requires a thorough knowledge of computer programming in the language of the computer. When complex programming in computer language is required, the average psychologist might better obtain the expert assistance of an interested and cooperative professional programmer. In addition, computers with the size and complexity to handle lengthy and complex programs are relatively expensive and not always available to the average psychologist.

For routine work, however, the qualified sensory psychologist should have a basic understanding of how a computer works. He should be familiar with its parts, its input and output capabilities, and what it can do for him. He should understand elementary programming. Time-sharing systems with limited capabilities are becoming readily available at nominal cost. Modern time-sharing systems frequently have executive programs that permit the scientist to use simple programming language such as BASIC, FORTRAN, or APL. The sensory-perceptual psychologist should be able to write his own program in such simple language and should be able to use simple time-sharing systems such as exemplified by the console shown in Figure 4–6.

Summary

In this chapter we have presented additional methods of a more recent and, in several cases, more sophisticated nature, for the investigation of psychophysical problems. We examined the older methods of rank order and paired comparisons. More recent and more sophisticated scaling methods were discussed briefly, and their importance for future, highly definitive research was indicated. A brief look was directed at the application of signal detection theory to psychological problems, and the significance of this trend was noted. The application of information theory to psychological problems was mentioned, and the importance of the computer as a tool in modern research was stressed.

Suggested Readings

1. G. A. Miller. "The Magical Number Seven, Plus or Minus Two: Some Limits on Our Capacity for Processing Information," *Psychol. Rev.* 63 (1956), 81–97. This is a classic article on the human's limitations in making absolute sensory judgments. Limitations in the number of absolute steps in psychological continua are discussed in terms of units of information theory called "bits,"

and the manner in which people mitigate this problem by utilizing linguistic coding is considered. This is a thought-provoking article, one requiring a little effort to read and understand, but well worth the trouble.

2. J. P. Guilford. *Psychometric Methods*, 2d ed. New York: McGraw-Hill, 1954. As suggested earlier, this reading is from the "bible" of psychophysical methods. Chapters 7 and 8 (142 pages), dealing with the method of paired comparisons and the method of rank order, are particularly useful for the serious student and are quite complete. Chapters 9 to 11 elaborate on scaling and rating techniques; these 102 pages do for scaling what the earlier chapters do for the more basic psychophysical methods. Recommended for the serious student.

3. S. S. Stevens. "The Direct Estimate of Sensory Magnitudes: Loudness," *Amer. J. Psychol.*, 79 (1956), 1–25. This is a highly recommended reading describing a scaling technique in considerable detail as employed in the scaling of loudness. This article also provides the "suggestions" emphasized by Stevens to ensure validity of a scaling procedure.

4. J. A. Swets. "Is There a Sensory Threshold?" *Science*, 134 (1961), 168–177. This article is recommended for the student with an interest in the detection theory approach to psychological research. Although its title sounds as though it was aimed purely at the question of thresholds, the coverage of the article is broader and presents a brief description of the entire approach. It is one of the shortest descriptions of the method, although it is not especially easy to read and understand.

5. J. A. Swets, W. P. Tanner, Jr., and T. G. Birdsall, "Decision Processes in Perception," *Psychol. Rev.* 68 (1961), 301–340. This article of some 39 pages is quite complete. In addition to explaining the approach, the authors include five sample experiments utilizing the signal detection method. It is recommended for the serious student with the necessary background.

6. F. Attneave, *Application of Information Theory to Psychology.* New York: Holt, Rinehart and Winston, 1959. This is an excellent short description (88 pages plus a short appendix) of the application of information theory to psychological problems. It starts out at an elementary level, using the game of "Twenty Questions" as an example of information theory application, and proceeds in orderly steps to establish a basic understanding of the technique. It is highly readable and a must for the student interested in learning about information theory as applied to psychological problems.

7. S. S. Stevens. "Perceptual Magnitude and Its Measurement," in Edward C. Carterette and Morton P. Friedman, *Handbook of Perception, vol. II, Psychophysical Judgment and Measurement.* New York: Academic Press, 1974. This is one of the last, and possibly best, summaries by the late S. S. Stevens. It is absolutely essential reading for any student seriously interested in scaling. The chapter begins with a description of Fechner's law and progresses systematically through the gamut of scaling as expounded by Stevens. It also has an extensive bibliography.

8. L. L. Thurstone. *The Measurement of Values.* Chicago: University of Chicago Press, 1959. This reading is recommended for the serious student interested in learning of the work of Thurstone at first hand. A collection of his writ-

ings, it is not a simple secondary reference, but goes to the original source for more basic and detailed background information.

9. John F. Corso and Donald A. Norman. "Neural Quantum Controversy in Sensory Psychology," *Science* 181 (1973):467–469. This reading consists of two letters. One, by Corso, offers criticism of the Stevens' power function theory and an answer by Donald A. Norman. It is a good article, if for no other reason than to demonstrate the existence of fundamental disagreements between workers in the field.

10. Joan Gay Snodgrass. "Psychophysics," chap. 2, from Bertram Scharf (ed.), *Experimental Sensory Psychology.* (Glenview, Ill.: Scott, Foresman, 1975). Pages 30 to 65 of this previously cited reference are particularly pertinent to the material covered in this chapter. Both signal detection theory and scaling techniques are covered in considerable detail and in a highly understandable manner.

11. John A. Swets. "The Relative Operating Characteristic in Psychology," *Science* 182 (1973):990–1000. This is a fine article, of a technical nature, suitable for the advanced student interested in the application of signal detection theory to psychology.

5 / nature of light and development of vision

Introduction

You may be surprised to learn that the brilliant Plato thought vision was produced by particles being squirted out of the eye and falling on an external object. Today Superman has a similar talent that would have thrilled (and vindicated) Plato—a capability of emitting rays from his eyes to destroy the enemies of society who challenge the peaceful existence of Clark Kent and his friends.

But less than fifty years after the death of Plato the Greek mathematician Euclid was to recognize that the eye is indeed sensitive to some substance arising from the outside. To be sure, the theories of Euclid, Galen, and others were not entirely adequate in that they failed to recognize the cameralike nature of the eye, believing that a cone of rays emanates from the external object and is perceived by means of the lens, then thought to be the sensitive element of the eye.

Other, later individuals, such as the Arab philosopher Alhazen and Leonardo da Vinci, approached an understanding of the basic functioning of the eye, but it remained for Johannes Kepler in 1604 to describe the eye as we know it today. Except for detailed functioning, his description of the eye as similar to the camera obscura, a device for projecting an inverted image on a screen, was complete and accurate. With elaborations by Christopher Scheiner, René Descartes, Christian Huygens, and Sir Isaac Newton, our knowledge of the gross anatomy of the eye has needed little modern refinement. (See Begbie, 1973, for a highly readable introduction to the history of vision.)

Nature of Light

But what is the nature of the substance that emanates (or is reflected) from objects in the external world? Since we first became aware of the general functioning of the eye, our understanding of the visual stimulus has taken two distinct approaches. One theory, advanced by Newton, held that light is made up of particles, or corpuscles; another theory, advanced by Christiaan Huygens, supported the existence of waves or pulses in a universal medium (ether). The argument is not completely settled today. Indeed, modern thinking tends to support both protagonists (see, for example, Bouman, 1962).

Light behaves much like Huygens' theory would predict, traveling at different speeds in media of different density in accordance with Descartes' law of refraction, which developed the concept of a refractive index for light-transmissive materials. The apparent bending or refraction of light as it passes from one medium to another (air to glass, for example) is strong evidence for the wave theory of light, thus supporting Huygens' theory.

Moreover, light of different wavelengths is bent at different angles. When Newton passed white light through a prism, breaking it down into the spectral colors, he was probably not aware of the evidence he was amassing in support of his rival's theory. Although Newton did not understand it, we now know that each of the spectral hues he obtained is of a different frequency and wavelength and that the visible spectrum is just one small part of a very great range of electromagnetic radiation.

These electromagnetic waves (see Figure 1–1), ranging from 10^{-14} to 10^6 m in wavelength for the known spectrum, travel, in a vacuum, at a velocity of 3×10^{10} cm/sec, or about 186,000 miles per second. As mentioned in Chapter 2, visible light represents only an exceedingly small portion of this total spectrum—slightly less than the equivalent of one octave from the seventy required to represent the entire spectrum.

As Newton first demonstrated, visible light can be broken down further, as was shown in Figure 1–1. Violet light has a wavelength of about 400 nm (about 1/70,000 inch), whereas red light has a wavelength on the order of 700 nm (about 1/40,000 inch). Other spectral hues lie in between these two extremes.

Although it is difficult to measure in terms of frequency, light can be described in this way if we so desire. Using the formula $f = s/\lambda$, where s is the speed of transmission and λ is the wavelength, we can calculate the frequency for any point on the electromagnetic spectrum. Note from Figure 1–1 that a radio wave with a wavelength of about 300 m has a frequency of 1,000 kc (10^6 Hz). Radio station KDKA in Pittsburgh puts out a radio signal with a wavelength of 300 m. Contrast this with a visual wavelength of 500 mμ (green light), which has a frequency of between 10^{14} and 10^{15} Hz, or 10^{11} and 10^{12} kc.

But light also behaves as if it consists of small packets of energy called *quanta.* The response in the retina of the eye is such that it can be understood only in terms of a quantum theory. It would appear that the chemical reaction in a single element (rod or cone) requires a minimum of one quantum of energy in order to take place. To be sure, we cannot see a single quantum of visible energy, largely because absorption and reflection in the less than perfect transmission portions of the eye permit only about 10 percent of the energy actually to reach the sensitive elements in the retina. A total of five to eight quanta *are* sufficient to elicit the experience of a flash of light. This is still a remarkable sensitivity; the eye, under optimal conditions, can detect a candle at a distance of more than 15 miles!

Much of our knowledge of the quantal behavior of the eye is due to the pioneering work of Selig Hecht and his associates at Columbia University (Hecht et al., 1942). Starting out with an assumption of maximum sensitivity of the retinal elements, these researchers demonstrated the sensitivity of individual photoreceptors on a statistical-probability basis.

A quantal theory of light is also useful in understanding the relation of intensity and time factors in vision. It has long been known that there is a reciprocal relation between the intensity and the duration of a visual stimulus. The eye integrates energy over time (on the order of one-tenth second), and a weak stimulus presumably requires more time for the chemical reaction to take place. For a sufficiently intense stimulus, time is of less significance, but for stimuli near threshold a finite amount of time is required for the chemical integrative process to run its course. A pure wave theory of light could not adequately foresee such a relationship.

Evolution of Vision

As indicated before, sensitivity or irritability to some portion of the electromagnetic spectrum appears to be a universal characteristic of protoplasm. Note again Thomas Moore's beautiful recognition of a positive phototropism: ". . . as the sunflower turns on her god, when he sets, the same look which she turn'd when he rose." Most organisms, both animal and vegetable, demonstrate some sensitivity to radiation in the general range we refer to as light. It would appear that even animals possessing highly specialized light-sensing organs may still retain a "general" sensitivity to light. It has been demonstrated that animals as high in evolution as the sparrow are able, in some unknown manner, to sense the presence of light without the use of the normal visual mechanism. Several workers, including Underwood and Menaker (1970, 1971), have showed that blinded sparrows evidence testicular response to variations in light and dark periods (simulating day-night relationships) even when the eyes are totally blinded and the retina is nonfunctional. Wetterberg et al. (1970) suggest that the Harderian gland, located near the eye, may serve, at least for neonatal rats, as a primitive sort of light receptor. Removal of this gland is said to abolish response to light in blinded animals. Harth and Heaton (1973), on the other hand, consider dermal sensitivity to be the key to visual sensitivity in newly hatched pigeons.

There are several cases on record of individuals in Russia, mostly women, who could literally "read" with their skin. They were able to identify printed characters, both in shape and color, simply by running their fingertips over them. Even when a thin sheet of glass was interposed between the fingertips and the printed matter, some of the subjects could still identify the printed characters, apparently as a result of their radiations in the infrared region (Novomeiskii, 1965). One such subject was tested in detail by four investigators (Zawala, 1967). The positive results they obtained were attributed to differential cooling of the skin by the differently colored stimuli.

The well-developed visual organs of higher animals have come a long way from the general sensitivity of the sunflower, the phototropism of the single-cell animal, or the testicular response of the sparrow.

Just as specialized cells and groups of cells developed to facilitate reproduction and assimilation, so did specialized cells develop to enhance the irritability function. Probably the earliest "sensory" cells for electromagnetic radiation were little more than ordinary cells with an increased amount of dark pigment, thus producing a reduction in reflection and an increase in absorption of the impinging energy. A further refinement such that these pigmented areas were able to react to the absorbed light energy in a differential manner was a much later development and was essential for the ultimate genesis of color discrimination.

PIGMENTED PATCHES, EYESPOTS

The very simple protozoan *Euglena* provides us with an example of a very early stage in the development of light sensitivity. As seen in Figure 5–1, *Euglena* is quite a simple, single-celled animal. At the anterior end of its body, near the base of the flagellum, however, it has an "eyespot," a small patch of reddish pigment sensitive to light. The action of the flagellum, which propels the small creature, is dependent on the illumination falling on the "eyespot," thus determining whether *Euglena* will swim into or out of an area of brighter or dimmer illumination (Maier and Schneirla, 1935). To be sure, the situation with respect to the *Euglena* is not quite this simple and straightforward. As Diehn (1973) points out, only organisms with the eyespot or stigma exhibit positive orientation with respect toward the light source. Mutants lacking the eyespot may react to light, but not in a predictable phototaxic manner.

In more complex, multicellular animals light sensitivity is often mediated by pigmented cells scattered over the skin, as in the earthworm. Although basically an inhabitant of darkness, because of factors such as humidity and temperature, the behavior of the earthworm is not nearly as simple as pure negative phototropism might predict. Under proper conditions the worm may go toward an area of brighter illumination, ap-

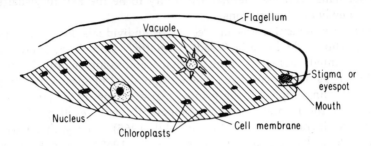

Figure 5–1

The protozoan *Euglena*. This simple creature is one of the earliest organisms to possess a light-sensitive organ, the eyespot. Note, however, that the presence of chloroplasts gives credence to the argument of some biologists that it is really a plant, rather than an animal. (Modified from *Principles of Animal Psychology* by N. R. F. Maier and T. C. Schneirla. Copyright 1935. Used with permission of McGraw-Hill Book Company.)

parently as a result of the interaction of such factors as the humidity and temperature of its environment.

Most organisms have their patches of pigment concentrated in such a manner that they appear to provide the animal with a crude indication of direction. Some planaria, or flatworms, for example, have paired clusters of pigmented cells, known as *ocelli*, at the anterior end; and some marine worms are blessed with several pairs of ocelli sensitive to light. Sea urchins, on the other hand, have numerous pigmented spots scattered about on their bodies.

Even when the species has well-developed, specialized light receptors, some still retain the capability for generalized phototropic sensitivity. As an example, the crayfish, in addition to its typical compound eyes, also has photosensitive nerve fibers near the undersurface of its segmented abdomen (Kennedy, 1963).

VISUAL PITS AND SIMPLE EYES

The next evolutionary stage in the phylogeny of the eye appears to be the development of pits or indentations that include the sensitive pigments. These would appear to serve several purposes for survival: for one thing, some mechanical protection of the sensitive pigments from the outside elements would be expected to result from their being located at the bottom of indentations in the animal's surface. In addition, if the pits have any appreciable depth, shadowing could serve as an indication of the direction of the light source.*

---

* In many lower animals (fish, snakes) sensory cells for stimuli other than light are frequently found in pits in the skin. These may serve as chemical receptors, or in some cases as receptors for acoustic or vibratory stimulation, as well as for temperature. The temperature-sensitive pits in some snakes are a good example, known to almost everyone.

The limpet, a marine shellfish, has a relatively simple visual pit. For his quiescent existence, hanging on a rock by his single "foot," the limpet probably needs little more than simple sensitivity to light, and perhaps moving shadows. In the limpet the designation of sensitive pigment might be an oversimplification. It would appear that the limpet has something like a primitive retina, a layer of tissue made up of many individual cells with neural fibers proceeding to the central nervous system.

Oliver Wendell Holmes was probably not aware of its unique visual capability when he wrote of "the ship of pearl, which, poets feign, sails the unshadowed main. . . ." The nautilus, a cephalopod mollusk related to the squid and octopus, is indeed a remarkable animal, apparently achieving an astounding level of visual functioning, all without the benefit of any lens or focusing device. The eye of the nautilus is like a pinhole camera, the Camera lucida of the ancients (see Figure 5–2). Thus a primitive focusing effect is obtained and the animal is said to be able to respond to the slightest movement of its anticipated dinner. The simple structure of the eye hardly provides the nautilus with much detailed pattern vision, and surely the amount of light admitted to the eye must be quite limited. But the pinhole camera apparently provides a primitive form of vision that is adequate for the needs of the creature.

In anticipation of later developments, we can see that improvement would result from the formation of a transparent membrane to cover and protect the visual mechanism inside. And a still later stage in evolution would see the formation of a simple lens, either from the primitive corneal layer or immediately behind it.

Although the visual mechanisms we are describing seem to portray an increasing complexity in phylogenetic development, they do not in fact portray a simple phylogenetic series. Actually, to trace any specific complex eye of higher-order animals back to its primitive ancestors is a difficult if not impossible task. In the process of evolution many directions were taken before the present levels were reached. Some of these directions were unsatisfactory and the species became extinct. Many other developments led to blind ends—that is, species that were served adequately by their unique organs but from which no important or significant developments evolved. Some primitive eyes evolved into the mammalian eye, and parallel development resulted in the compound eye of the arthropods, each satisfactory for its bearer, but neither evolving from the other.

One of the most fascinating examples of an animal appearing to take the wrong turn and ending up in a dead end is that of *Copilia*, a tiny arthropod about the size of a pinhead (see Figure 5–3). The eye of this creature has a well-developed primary or objective lens mounted on the end of a stalk, but only a single receptor with its own smaller lens. The receptor is attached to a small muscle and it is believed that this muscle moves the receptor back and forth in the focal plane of the lens, thus scanning the image much like some modern electronic devices built by man.

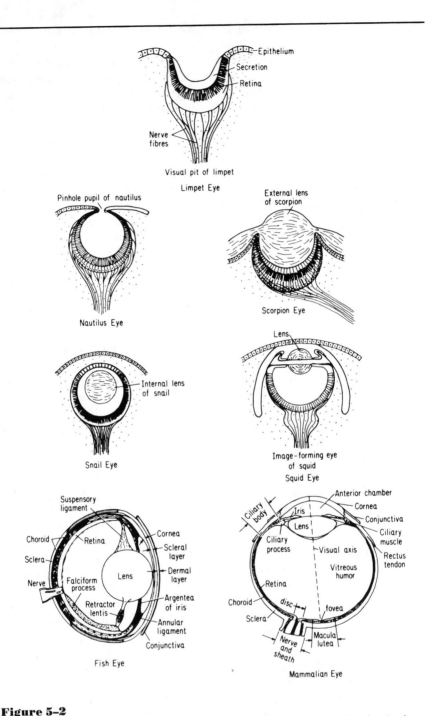

Figure 5–2

Schematic drawing of representative eyes. Note the progression from the simple pit of the limpet to the drawing depicting the mammalian eye. Notice too the nearly spherical shape of the fish's lens, presumably designed to move back and forth, rather than to change shape, in the action of accommodation. (Above figures from G. L. Walls, *The Vertebrate Eye,* 1942, courtesy of the Cranbrook Institute of Science; the first five figures are from a modification by R. L. Gregory, *Eye and Brain,* 1966, courtesy of George Weidenfield & Nicholson Ltd.)

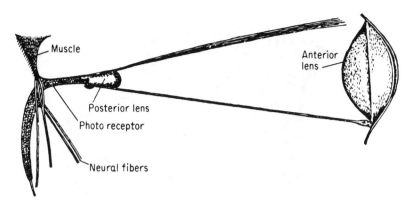

Figure 5–3
Scanning eye of Copilia. The eye of this minute arthropod appears to have a pair of lenses and a single receptor element. It would appear that the muscle attached to the receptor causes the latter to move back and forth, thus providing a scanning effect. (From "Eye and Camera" by George Wald, 1950, © Scientific American, Inc. All rights reserved.)

COMPOUND EYES

A direction of evolutionary development that apparently proved to be quite successful resulted in the existence of so-called *compound eyes*. Probably more creatures today have compound eyes than any other type of visual apparatus, and the situation in the past was probably not much different. The earliest known eyes, from the trilobites of the Cambrian period 500 million years ago, appear to have been compound.

Although many still retain some simple ocelli, most arthropods have compound eyes that are ideally suited for detecting movement (see Figure 5–4). Compound eyes consist of numerous (1 to 30,000) units, or *ommatidia,* each of which is a separate receptor, many having relatively simple, direct connections to the central nervous system. Such a proliferation of individual "eyes" makes for rapid visual processes and the ability to detect shadows or contours moving across the surface of the organ with a minimum of delay. Usually it is sufficient to move a shadow over a housefly only once before it flies away.

Although each ommatidium is indeed a single receptor structure, it is a disarmingly complex and sophisticated entity. At one end, each ommatidium has a simple lens facet and a secondary lens cylinder. The wave-guide nature and high directivity of each ommatidium should be obvious; only light traveling in a direction parallel to the optical path of the element is likely to activate it. If light is coming from the proper direction it will pass through the transparent tissues to a light-sensitive element, consisting of several cells in a flowerlike cluster. By the facilitation, not yet

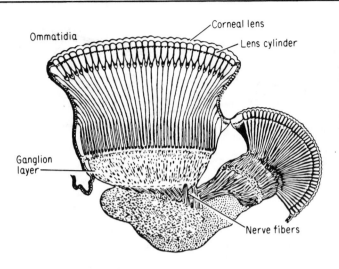

Figure 5–4

A compound eye. The eye of the mayfly, *Chloeon*, is unique in that it has a double-segmented compound eye. The larger component presumably provides detailed vision, while the smaller part to the right permits coarser, wide-angled vision. (From "Eye and Camera" by George Wald, 1950, © Scientific American, Inc. All rights reserved.)

well understood, of another cell known as the *eccentric cell,* a nerve impulse is evoked in a fiber leading from the receptor.

Form vision with the compound eyes of the arthropods must be quite rudimentary. But for the high-speed movements and simple behavior of insects, the compound eye is an ideal arrangement.

The development of the compound eye has had a fortunate side effect. The relatively large size of the ommatidia (in some species) and their direct linkage with afferent neural fibers make them an ideal subject for laboratory research. Much of what we know about the neural and chemical activity in light-sensitive organs was gleaned from research on compound eyes. For this purpose the eye of *Limulus* (horseshoe crab) has been found to be of particular value.

COMPLEX EYES

With the exception of a few oddballs like *Copilia*, those higher animals that did not perfect compound eyes moved in a direction of increased complexity of the simple eye. The compound eye of the arthropods did not work too well except for such short distances as concern these small creatures, and it did not provide much pattern or form vision. The simple pinhole device, on the other hand, did not provide adequate sensitivity to dim light nor adequate image formation. Moreover, such primitive eyes did not permit much in the way of accommodation for varying distances.

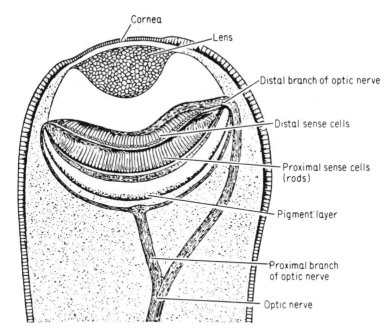

Figure 5–5
Detail of scallop eye. Note the double-layer retina. The layer farthest from the lens is made up of cells not-unlike conventional rods, while the layer closer to the lens is made up of cells which fire at the cessation of a stimulus. (From "Inhibition in Visual Systems" by Donald Kennedy, 1963, © Scientific American, Inc. All rights reserved.)

Through evolution, the principle of the nautilus's simple pinhole eye was adopted, and with the further development of such refinements as protective coverings, lenses, focusing systems, and multilayered retinas, progress was rather straightforward. An ultimate in sophisticated visual mechanisms (up to now, at least) was the result, culminating eventually in the paired visual organs of the vertebrates.

Several "stages" in this development can be seen in Figure 5–2. The scorpion, as an example, developed a fixed "lens," apparently in contact with its sensitive retinal layer. The snail, on the other hand, developed an internal lens (probably also fixed focus) bathed in its own intraocular fluid, probably not greatly unlike the aqueous fluid in our own eyes (and, incidentally, not dissimilar to the saline solution of the seawater that originally bathed the visual organs of all animals). Many other organisms developed similar, perhaps more highly specialized structures, often permitting a primitive form of accommodation.

The scallop, a bivalve mollusk (see Figure 5–5), sports a row of bright blue eyes along the edge of its shell. Did you ever think when you ate a platter of French-fried scallops that the tasty little creatures had pretty blue eyes? Each of these eyes has a simple cornea and what appears to be a fixed-focus lens. Curiously, the scallop has a double-layer retina, one layer responding to the onset of a visual stimulus, the other discharging when the light is terminated (Hartline 1938, Gorman 1969). Many higher-order animals, including man, appear to have both "on" and "off" receptors, but few are as clearly delineated structurally as in the scallop. We will in a later chapter consider in more detail man's visual receptors that indicate the onset and the termination of a signal.

Although most higher-order animals adjust their eyes (accommodate) for distance by changing the shape of their crystalline lenses, the octopus appears to have a more primitive approach. His hard, crystalline lens moves back and forth like the lens of a camera, adjusting according to the distance of his prey. Although the octopus does have a rather large eye and a very well-developed retinal structure, the limited range of its accommodative capacity is probably an important factor in restricting the size of the creature's dinner table. Normally it seizes its prey at a distance of 2 to 3 m, presumably the accommodative range of its eye. At other, shorter distances the octopus must rely on chemically sensitive disks in its long tentacles.

THE VERTEBRATE EYE

If there was ever a "wonder of science" the vertebrate eye is surely it. The eye is truly a magnificently designed and almost perfectly conceived instrument. Its range of sensitivity is greater than any camera-film combination, its absolute sensitivity approaches that of the finest man-made instrument, and its ability to resolve fine detail is almost unbelievable. As an example of its excellence of design, most organs of the body have capillaries coursing through them, supplying nutrients and removing waste products. But a cornea with blood vessels in it would not be very transparent. So the cornea is serviced directly by the aqueous fluid behind it, rather than by intrinsic, semiopaque blood vessels. Furthermore, this aqueous fluid is completely renewed every four hours to ensure adequate conditions for survival of the tissue it supplies. It is obviously important too that the lens of the eye be transparent. Early in life, even the pigmented cell bodies disappear from this structure, and barring metabolic problems later in life, it maintains a remarkable degree of transparency.

The great variety of specialized development for various species is noteworthy. A hawk soaring hundreds of feet in the air can distinguish a small rodent scurrying along the ground. Some animals not only can detect and utilize light, but also can discriminate different wavelengths within the visible spectrum. We take this color vision for granted, but it is indeed a remarkable evolutionary development. Still other animals survive with a minimal dependency on their visual abilities, substituting the sense of smell or an acute sense of hearing. Most rodents, bats, and similar animals that live in burrows in the ground, dark caves, and the like utilize senses other than vision for most of their survival functions. Owls have apparently developed such a sensitivity to light that their vision in daylight is severely impaired, and dogs' distance vision is notoriously poor. Although man is one of few mammals with true color vision, some lower animals (e.g., birds) are said to have excellent color vision.

When we do find a remarkable visual capability or limitation for a particular species, we should not necessarily attribute it to the eye itself, at least not to that part of the eye that we can see and generally refer to as the eyeball. It is the magnificence of the computer behind it that gives the eye much of its advantage over man-made optical instruments. The eye actually has many optical defects if examined by itself. It is often somewhat misshaped, its range of focusing is not always adequate, and the medium through which the light must pass is not always very transparent, frequently containing loose cell bodies, scaled epithelial cells, and various debris floating around in it. But as an extension of that amazing neural computer known as the brain, the eye can perform unbelievable feats.

Development of the Mammalian Eye

Let us look briefly at the development of an individual eye, which in a limited sense tends to recapitulate some of the general phylogenetic development of all mammalian eyes. The old schoolboy tongue-twister "ontogeny recapitulates phylogeny" has long been demonstrated to be of limited truth. As a result, those instances where it *does* seem to apply, and the development of human sense organs seems to be one, take on added interest.

THE RETINA

The *retina*, or light-sensitive surface of the eye, develops from the very early, poorly differentiated, and still hollow forebrain of the embryo, and the first evidence of this development heralds the overall development of the eye. Indeed, a thickening of the forebrain wall, called a *placode*, identifies the eventual location of the retina and can be observed in an embryo of less than 4 mm. Early in development the paired placodes begin to migrate laterally; at the same time, an outward bulging of that part of the brain wall including the placode results in the formation of the *primary optic vesicle* (see Figure 5–6). At such an early stage this simple vesicle is little more than a hollow swelling in the wall of the forebrain. Concurrent with the development of the optic vesicle, the ectoderm layer in front of it thickens, forming a lens placode that will eventually develop into the lens of the eye.

As the optic vesicle develops further, it undergoes a complex invagination process: The base of the vesicle constricts so that the primary optic vesicle takes on the form of a hollow ball on the end of a hollow tube (see bottom drawing of Figure 5–6). Simultaneously, as can be seen from this figure, the forward wall of the vesicle invaginates so that the result is a double-walled structure, known rather appropriately as the *optic cup*. This

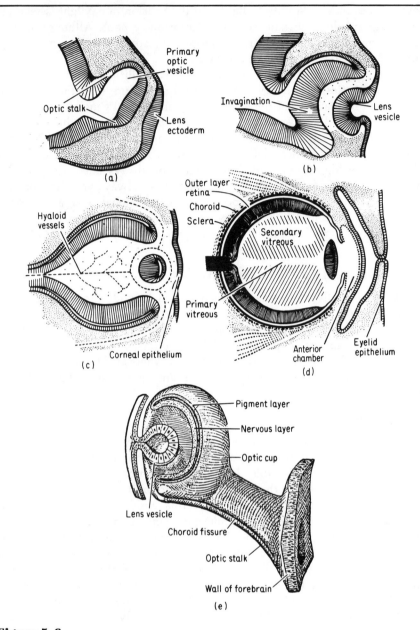

Figure 5–6
Development of the mammalian eye. Drawings (a) through (d) show the orderly progression from the original "bulge" to the nearly developed eye. Drawing (e) presents an interesting cross-sectional view of a stage between (b) and (c). [(a)–(d) from A. W. Ham, *Histology,* 6th ed., 1969, by permission of J. B. Lippincott Company; (e) from I. C. Mann, *The Development of the Human Eye,* 1928, by permission of Cambridge University Press.]

double-walled entity is destined to become the retina; the optic nerve will arise from it and proceed by way of the stalk to the brain, and the *hyaloid artery* will enter the eye through the same stalk to nourish the developing retina and its associated structures. Although the hyaloid artery will eventually atrophy and fade away, other blood vessels will continue to service the inside layers of the adult eye. These vessels pass through a narrow slit in the cup known as the *choroid fissure* that eventually closes up, enveloping itself around them.

At an early stage the sides and rear of the optic cup are made up of two layers with a space between them. The inner of these two layers develops into several layers of cells and becomes the retina proper (sensory area); the outer layer develops a pigment, *fuscin*, and becomes the black-pigmented layer. These two layers merge together as the space between them disappears, and the combination becomes the retina as we know it.

Before the choroid fissure has closed completely, the nervous layers of the retina undergo considerable development. The outermost layer of cells differentiates (in man, at least) into the sensory neuroepithelial *rods* and *cones*, the second layer of cells proliferates into *bipolar cells*, and a third layer is made up largely of *ganglion cells*. These latter send out fibers that converge from all parts of the retina, leaving the eye by way of the still open choroid fissure and proceeding to the brain. Note that this development results in a retina that is "backward," in that light must pass through the nerve fibers and the nonsensitive cell layer in order ultimately to arrive at the sensitive rods and cones.

THE LENS

Meanwhile, back in the embryo, the lens plate or lens placode has not been sitting idly by watching the remainder of the eye develop. Arising from the ectoderm layer of the embryo, a thickened placode develops into an indentation (lens pit) and subsequent invagination not entirely unlike that of the optic vesicle. Known as the *lens vesicle*, this hollow chamber, or bulge into the main cavity of the eye [see (b) and (c) of Figure 5–6], pinches off from the primary ectoderm layer. Subsequently, the walls of the cup come together, forming a sac with a thick wall on the side facing the retina and a thin wall on the other side. At a sufficiently early stage the large primary optic vesicle is almost filled by the smaller lens vesicle. The thin wall of the lens vesicle develops into the lens epithelium, and long cells in the thick wall continue to grow, so that by about the seventh week of development the entire cavity has been obliterated. The elongated cells lose their relatively opaque nuclei and become the lens fibers. With the formation of a lens capsule from the epithelium, the lens is essentially complete.

The tissue of the lens proper is entirely nonvascular. During its early development, however, blood vessels from the hyaloid artery spread over its rear surface. Along with additional vessels on the front surface, the gross structure is known as the *vascular tunic* of the lens. It flourishes during the period of rapid development, and at birth has usually disappeared along with the hyaloid artery, leaving a structure of remarkable transparency and flexibility.

ADDITIONAL STRUCTURES

The remaining structures of the eye, of course, develop along with the retina and lens. The chamber between the lens and the retina becomes filled during the second month with a fibrillar jelly, known as the *vitreous body*, presumably a "secretion" from the inner surface of the eye. Other fiberlike growths attach themselves to the lens and become the *suspensory ligaments* for later growth and attachment to the *ciliary muscle*.

During the seventh week tissue surrounding the optic cup begins to differentiate and specialize into two accessory coats. The outer coat is more dense and becomes the white fibrous tissue known as the *sclera* or *sclerotic coat*. Actually, this coating corresponds to the *dura mater* of the brain, with which it is continuous by way of the optic nerve. In the front of the eyeball, the sclerotic coat is quite transparent and we recognize it as the *cornea*.

The inner of the two coats covering the optic cup is called the *choroid*. Located between the sclera and the pigmented layer of the optic cup, this later acquires a high vascularity and corresponds to the *pia mater* of the brain. Even in embryos as young as six weeks the choroid plays an important role in the blood supply to the retinal surface.

Although we could examine the development of countless other structures of the eye, we will not do so at this time. Suffice it to say that their developments are orderly and can very often be understood in the light of the phylogenetic scale. We will examine additional structures in the following chapter, where we consider the anatomy and physiology of the adult eye. For the student interested in the embryological development of such parts of the eye as the iris, the ciliary body, or the eyelids, numerous excellent embryology texts are available.

The thoughtful reader should have noticed the close relationship of the eye and the brain: the extension of the forebrain to form the retina, the relation of the choroid and the pia mater of the brain, and the common origin of the sclera and the dura mater. This was the principal reason we spent so much time on the embryological development of the eye and introduced so many new terms. A student of the eye must realize that it is a remarkable instrument, not just because of its optical qualities, but, of even greater importance, because of its profound data-processing capabilities.

Summary

In this chapter we have tried to present some of the background of vision and the development of the visual organs. We examined first the nature of light, its location on the broad electromagnetic spectrum, and its characteristics as both a wave and a particle phenomenon. As a second step we traced the phylogenetic development of vision, beginning with highly primitive light sensitivity, progressing through the formation of pigmented patches, simple visual pits, and culminating finally in the evolution of compound and complex eyes. The last part of the chapter traced the ontogenetic development of several structures of the human eye, to show some comparability of ontogenetic and phylogenetic development, and the remarkable nature of the eye as an extension of the brain.

Suggested Readings

1. From N. R. F. Maier and T. C. Schneirla. *Principles of Animal Psychology.* New York: McGraw-Hill, 1935. While I recommended this entire reference for Chapter 1 as general reading, some parts are of particular significance to the development of visual systems. The first 266 pages are replete with illustrations and descriptions of visual mechanisms of lower organisms. The interested reader can obtain a great deal of valuable information by scanning all these pages and then reading those of specific interest.

2. Lawrence Kruger and Barry E. Stein. "Primordial Sense Organs and the Evolution of Sensory Systems," from Edward C. Carterette and Morton P. Friedman (eds.), *Handbook of Perception, vol. III, Biology of Perceptual Systems.* New York: Academic Press, 1973. Although the title of this article does not so indicate, its primary topic is the development of visual systems. In some respects this reading is a more accessible, much condensed presentation of material included in the preceding reference. If you are interested in the development of the human eye this is a good place to start.

3. G. Hugh Begbie. *Seeing and the Eye.* Garden City, N.Y.: Doubleday, 1973. The first chapters of this little book are of particular value because they present a brief, easy to understand history of visual study and knowledge. Later chapters present much of the same information to be found later in the book you are now reading

4. G. Wald. "Eye and Camera," *Scientific American,* August 1950. This is an interesting, well-written, and relatively short description of the eye. Background history is provided, and although considerable detail about visual functioning is omitted, the analogy between the eye and the camera is carried all the way through the nature of the sensitive emulsion. These 10 pages are interesting and quite easy to read.

5. From H. R. Schiffman. *Sensation and Perception: An Integrated Approach.* New York: Wiley, 1976. Chapter 11 of this recent book presents a lucid and highly readable description of the visual system. As supplementary reading it is highly recommended.

6. M. A. Bouman. "History and Present Status of Quantum Theory in Vision," in W. A. Rosenblith (ed.), *Sensory Communication.* New York: Wiley, 1962. This is a fine summary of the quantum theory of vision as of the publication date. It is recommended for the serious student, who should not find it unduly difficult.

7. From R. M. Evans. *An Introduction to Color.* New York: Wiley, 1948. Chapter II of this excellent book, titled "The Physical Nature of Light," does

what it is supposed to do in a very acceptable manner. These 14 pages go into the matter in more detail than is required at this point in the consideration of sensory-perceptual processes. However, the material is highly readable, and the inclusion of several pages on such topics as general receptors and photometry will help prepare the reader for more specific visual problems to be considered later.

8. From M. Wilson and the editors of *Life. Energy*. New York: Time, Inc., 1963. Although this book was recommended for Chapter 1 and the general approach to energy, chap. 4, "The Search for the Ends of the Rainbow," is particularly germane to the present chapter on light energy and visual sensitivity. Like the rest of the book, this chapter is well written, well illustrated, and interesting. These 20 pages are well worth reading.

9. G. DeBeer, *Embryos and Ancestors*, 3d ed. Oxford: Clarendon Press, 1958. A nice little book for the student interested in embryology, especially from a theoretical point of view. In 197 pages the author provides evidence for a refutation of the recapitulation theory, providing his own alternative explanation. Although it is not an easy book, the serious student, by reading selectively, can gain much from it.

10. Israel Abramov and James Gordon. "Vision," in Edward C. Carterette and Morton P. Friedman (eds.), *Handbook of Perception, vol. III, Biology of Perceptual System*. New York: Academic Press, 1973. This highly readable account of vision covers light, the photo pigments, anatomy of the retina, and visual pathways, as well as the electrical responses of the retina and the central nervous system. It is a relatively complete exposition in a well-organized and useful form.

11. G. Adrian Horridge. "The Compound Eye of Insects," *Scientific American*, July 1977. This is an excellent, well-written and well-illustrated article on the insect eye. Good reading for the interested student.

6 /structure of the eye

Before we can examine the functioning of the eye we should gain some understanding of its structure. The reader is referred to Figure 6–1 for an overall schematic presentation of the adult mammalian eye.

Cornea

If the eye is the window of the soul, then the cornea must be the pane in this window. Except for an exceedingly small amount of light that finds its way through the nearly opaque walls of the eyeball itself, all the light reflected from external objects must pass through this window to get to the sensitive retinal layer behind. Developing from the same embryonic layer that produced the dense white protective sclerotic coat, the degree of transparency of this structure is indeed remarkable.

DESCRIPTION

The cornea is a tough, nonvascular sheet of tissue approximately 0.6 mm in thickness. It is formed from bundles of connective tissue fibers, lying one upon the other to form a laminated whole. The external surface of the cornea has a thin epithelial layer that is constantly being renewed by cell division. This epithelial layer provides, among other things, the medium for the elimination of carbon dioxide. This is one of the reasons why you are told not to wear your contact lenses continuously. Carbon dioxide buildup between the cornea and the contact lens might become excessive and the concentration in the trapped fluid would not allow adequate evacuation of the poisonous substance. Superficial to the epithelial layer is a thin (several microns) double layer of tears (oily on the outside and watery on the inside) that forms the optically smooth surface.

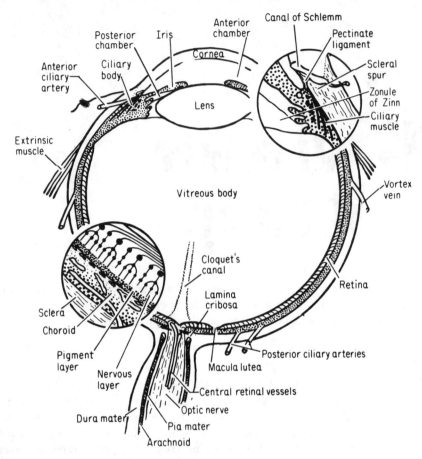

Figure 6–1
Cross section of mammalian eye. Note the sections taken through the retinal and ciliary portions. (From A. M. Ham, *Histology*, 6th ed., 1969, by permission of J. B. Lippincott Company.)

The cornea performs several critical functions. In addition to protecting the delicate internal parts of the eye, it permits light to pass through to the retina, focusing the image on the sensitive surface. Popular belief often holds that the lens of the eye focuses the image on the retina. In animals living on dry land, this is generally not true. The cornea actually does most of the focusing (refraction) of the image on the retina, whereas the lens is responsible for only small adjustments (accommodation) to compensate for changes in distance. As a matter of fact, the cornea acts like a fixed-focus lens, such that about two-thirds of the total refractive power of the eye is supplied by it. In operations for cataract in which the lens of the eye is removed, the cornea (plus some corrective lenses) must supply the entire refractive power for the system.

For fish living in a watery milieu, the converse is true. Differences in refractive index between the fishes' cornea and the water are not sufficient to permit complete image formation. Consequently, for animals living entirely in the water, the lens is responsible for the greater part of the image-formation function. Indeed, gross visual examination reveals a thicker, more nearly spherical lens in fish, as contrasted with most land-dwelling animals. Many fish also appear to have an accommodative mechanism dependent on movements of the lens forward and backward, much like a camera, rather than the shape-adjusting technique employed by most higher-order land-welling animals.

POTENTIAL DISORDERS

The cornea is susceptible to a great many possible defects and physical injuries. As exposed and unprotected as it is, damage from foreign material must be relatively common. Although healing of minor damage is relatively rapid and generally complete, infections, if not treated properly, can result in scar tissue that can greatly reduce or even eliminate corneal transparency. Damage due to scarring, often associated with malnutrition and other metabolic deficiencies, is particularly prevalent in the less well-developed nations of Africa and the Far East, and blindness due to corneal opacity is much more common in these parts of the world.

Although many instances of corneal opacity in well-developed countries may be attributed to infections of a viral, bacterial, or fungal nature, most must be attributed to degenerative or metabolic causes. Although much of the etiology remains unknown, loss of transparency due to metabolic malfunctions with subsequent swelling and opacification of the cornea is of greater significance in this country. It would appear too that genetic causes cannot be eliminated entirely.

When the corneal opacity has reached a point where an insufficient amount of light can pass through it, surgery is generally indicated. Using operating microscopes and delicate "micro" instruments, the skilled surgeon can replace the damaged cornea with a section removed from a recently deceased healthy eye, usually obtained from a so-called eye bank. Although there often remain problems of tissue rejection and the possibility of transplanting a potentially unhealthy cornea, corneal transplant operations are a tremendous step forward in providing "eyes for the blind." Perhaps the comparatively low incidence of rejection in the case of corneal transplants may be due to the lack of blood vessels in the cornea, as contrasted with the high vascularity of other organs which so often resist transplantation. The reduced tendency of rejection probably must be attributed to the relatively low metabolic rate of the adult cornea.

There has also been some progress in replacing diseased corneas with plastic prosthetic devices. The results from these experiments are often less than satisfactory, however, and much remains to be learned to avoid biological rejection and ensure adequate functioning of the prosthetic cornea.

An otherwise healthy cornea can be somewhat misshapen. If the central area of the cornea does not present a perfect section of a sphere to the incoming light, distortion will result and the image will appear blurred. Known as *astigmatism,* this common condition is usually due to an imperfect curvature of the corneal surface. Such a defect, unless very severe, can be corrected by the cylindrical curvature of an eyeglass lens. We will discuss this application in more detail when we examine the use of glasses for correcting visual defects.

Aqueous Chamber

Directly behind the cornea is the anterior or *aqueous chamber* of the eye, containing, not unreasonably, the aqueous humor, a thin watery fluid that contains most of the diffusible substance of blood plasma, and in about the same concentration as plasma. Continuously replenished and absorbed, this fluid presumably provides the nutrient and waste removal function in support of the nonvascular cornea in front and the lens behind. It is believed that the fluid for the anterior chamber is formed in the posterior (vitreous) chamber and enters the anterior chamber between the lens and the iris (see Figure 6–1). Pressure in the anterior chamber holds the iris against the lens, preventing return of the aqueous fluids to the posterior chamber. Fluids from the aqueous chamber eventually leave the eye by way of the canal of Schlemm, ending up in the venous system of the body.

Iris and Pupil

If you have lovely baby-blue eyes, it is due to the pigments in your *iris,* a relatively flat disk with a variable aperture near the center, known as the *pupil.* In humans the pupil has a relatively round configuration, but this is by no means the universal situation. A variety of shapes are found in different species, with the slit-shaped pupil being typical for nocturnal animals. Note, for example, the shape of the cat's pupil.

Along with the *lens,* the iris separates the anterior chamber of the eye from the posterior chamber. But it does much more than this. A highly complex and vascular tissue, the iris contains two sets of antagonistic muscles. One set, composed of smooth muscle fibers, is arranged in a circular or sphincter configuration near the outer edge of doughnut-shaped iris. Innervation of these muscles results in a partial closing of the pupil. Another set of muscles, arranged radially near the back of the iris, serves to dilate the pupil. Both of these sets of muscles are activated reflexively as a result of the level of illumination falling on the retina, and through impulses arriving from the sympathetic and parasympathetic divisions of the autonomic nervous system, as well as light-sensitive cells in the retina itself.

Although changes in the size of the pupil do indeed tend to control the amount of light entering the eye, this is not the primary function of the

iris-pupil structure. A popular misconception tells us that the pupil constricts under conditions of high illumination in order to protect the delicate
interior of the eye. Do not believe this! The total range of light intensity to
which the eye can respond without endangering itself is much greater than
that which can be accounted for by the limited pupillary response. In the
next chapter we will consider the comparative intensity values for pupil
transmission and retinal sensitivity.

An alternative explanation involves the maximizing of visual acuity in
the case of the constricted pupil and the maximizing of "light-catching"
potential for the dilated pupil. Under conditions of high illumination the
pupil is constricted, thus ensuring that most of the light will pass through
the center of the optical system and therby minimizing aberrations due to
improper curvature at the extremes of the cornea and lens. Under conditions of low illumination the pupil widens, allowing a maximum of light to
enter the eye, even though some of it must of necessity pass by way of
the distortion-producing edges of the optical system.

The pupil also tends to constrict for near vision reflexively. This is
fortunate, because a smaller aperture produces a greater depth of field, thus
no doubt reducing some of the wear and tear on the accommodative mechanism that might otherwise be constantly adjusting and readjusting for
small changes in distance.

Can you now see why your eye doctor often dilates your pupils before
performing a refraction? It is not simply to see inside the eyeball better;
there are other reasons. With the pupil at maximum size vision is most
influenced by optical flaws, and a minimum depth of field is found.
Glasses prescribed under such unfavorable conditions can be more precisely selected and are more likely to be accurate than glasses prescribed
under highly favorable circumstances.

The color of the iris is due to a pigment called *melanin* and has little
significance for vision except in its absence. Eyes that are totally lacking
in melanin (*albinism*) are, of course, unduly sensitive to light, because the
basis for iris opacity is lacking, and light may enter the eye through the
peripheral part of the iris as well as the pupil itself. If the melanin is
limited to its posterior surface, the iris will appear blue. On the other hand,
with additional pigments in other layers of the iris, the apparent color may
range from gray to brown. In most Caucasians the development of pigment
often occurs subsequent to birth, so that the blue-eyed baby may later develop eyes of a decidedly brown color. In the case of many non-Caucasians,
the pigment deposition often occurs before birth.

Lens and Ciliary Body

The lens of the eye serves not to form an image on the retina, but to
add, in accordance with changes in viewing distance, increments of curvature to that provided by the corneal surface. Changes in the shape of the

lens are produced reflexively and appear as the result of failure of the projected image to focus precisely on the sensitive surface of the retina. In the normally relaxed state, the slight curvature of the lens contributes just enough positive correction to bring objects at a distance into focus. When nearer objects are to be viewed, the lens must assume a more nearly spherical shape to produce a correspondingly sharp image.

DESCRIPTION

The crystalline lens is a remarkable structure, being composed of both living and ostensibly nonliving tissue. In its young, healthy state it can change its shape to accommodate distances as small as 1 ft to ones as great as infinity, a remarkable range of focus for even our best modern cameras.

As was indicated in Chapter 5, the development of the lens proceeds largely from the inside to the outside. Indeed, after the nuclei-free cells in the core have in effect died from lack of nutrition and isolation from the vascular system, those on the outside continue to grow (at a slower rate of speed). As a result, the mature, overly filled sac with a hard core becomes less pliable and resists assuming a shape either highly spherical, as needed for near vision, or flat, as required for distant vision. The middle-aged owner must then resort to corrective lenses for both reading and far vision, either separate spectacles or, if the person is willing to disclose his or her age, bifocals.

Just how does the lens perform its amazing feat of accommodating for both near and far vision? Although we are reasonably certain that the *ciliary body* and *zonule of Zinn* (see Figure 6–1) are involved in the accommodative process, the complete answer to the question is still somewhat vague. I once heard an ophthalmologist present an excellent description and theory concerning the process. He proposed that the ciliary body did not perform as a muscle, as it is normally described, but rather as a gland. According to his logical hypothesis the lens at rest is in a relatively flat state, adjusted for far vision. When the ciliary muscle (or gland?) contracts, fluid is forced through tiny tubules in the zonule (also called the *suspensory ligament*), thus filling the lens sac and causing the entire body to expand into a spherical or near-spherical shape, much like the process of inflating a balloon. Thus the ciliary body is relaxed for far vision and at work for near vision, consistent with physiological events as we know them. It was a brilliant theory, adequate in every detail except one: No one has ever found any tubules in the space between the ciliary body and the lens!

More generally accepted explanations of the accommodative function assume that the normal resting position of the lens is somewhat on the spherical side and that the attachment of the lens to the ciliary body is such that contraction of the latter relaxes tension in the lens, thereby permitting it to assume its normal near-spherical shape. A relaxed ciliary body, on the other hand, produces tension on the lens, forcing it into its flatter, distant vision configuration. One might ask, "Why not examine a lens after removal from an eye?" To be sure, this has been done, but removal from the eye results in almost immediate changes in the delicate tissue of the interior portion of the lens such that the true shape of the lens in the living organism escapes detection.

One might wonder how such a simple structure as the mammalian lens can produce images so free from serious optical aberration. The old box camera with its simple lens was quite inadequate for eliminating *spherical aberrations* unless only the very center of the optical path was used, thus cutting down appreciably on the light admitting and sensitivity of the system. Even then, chromatic aberration, the differential bending of different wavelengths in the manner of Newton's prism, was inescapable. Optics makers get around the problem by making complex lens systems composed of five or more separate lenses made of materials differing widely in their refractive indices, such as flint and crown glass. The human eye, however, has only a single lens, like the old box camera, and it operates with a relatively large aperture, yet neither spherical nor chromatic aberrations are particularly bothersome.

As pointed out in an earlier chapter, there is an excellent computer behind the human lens, filtering and processing the image; but even without this filtering process the lens, cornea, and retinal combination have several features that tend to mitigate the serious effects of aberration. In spherical aberration, at least three mechanisms may be noted: (1) The cornea and lens are formed from tissues of somewhat different refractive indices, analogous, on a smaller scale, to the camera lens's crown and flint glass. (2) The curvature of the two surfaces tend to compliment each other, with the cornea tapering off gradually at its edges, whereas the lens features an increasing rate of curvature near its edges. (3) Finally, spherical aberration is reduced when it might be most damaging (close work, such as reading) by a reflexive constriction of the pupil, thus limiting the light path to the relatively aberration-free axis of the optical system.

Several mechanisms are also available for the reduction of *chromatic aberration*. Such aberration is most noticeable at the extremes of the spectrum, especially at the blue end, where the light is bent the most. Although the retina itself is sensitive to light over a relatively broad spectral band, filtering provided by the yellowish lens prevents much of the unwanted blue light from reaching the sensitive surface, thus eliminating some of the potential chromatic aberration. Many people who have had their lenses removed in the course of cataract operations must wear yellow glasses to replace the blue absorption function of their missing natural lenses. There is also a concentration of yellow pigment in an area of the retina directly behind the lens. Known as the *macula lutea*, this area is most effective in close, critical vision, and the yellow pigment must, by absorption, prevent some of the undesirable blue light from reaching the sensitive retinal elements. And finally, the sensitive elements of the eye directly behind the pupil (cones) have a greater sensitivity to the red and a lower sensitivity to the blue end of the spectrum as compared to the more peripherally located sensory cells.

POTENTIAL DISORDERS OF THE LENS

Being such a highly specialized structure and consisting as it does of part living and part nonliving tissue, and all on the borderline of nutritional deficiency, the crystalline lens is indeed a delicate organ, poised on the brink of catastrophic disorder. Such disorders frequently take the form of *cataracts*, a term used for any opacity or clouding of the lens. A cataract is not a growth and it does not involve the cornea; it is an opacity in the lens itself.

Cataract-produced opacity takes on many forms: It may be evident at birth, it may develop from an injury or disease, or it may develop apparently as an inexorable result of the aging process (probably the most common form). It may appear in any part of the lens, it may remain stationary, or it may continue to develop until the entire lens is opaque. (Have you ever noticed the disproportionately large number of household pets, especially dogs, with whitish opacity visible in their eyes?)

Although the detailed etiology of most cataract formation still remains somewhat obscure, there does seem to be an underlying relation with systemic disease processes. Apparently the latent protein molecules making up the lens body are subject to significant structural changes under conditions produced by factors associated with diabetes, German measles, radiation, nutritional and hormonal deficiencies, and the general aging process. Recently we have become aware of the cataract-producing potential of microwave radiation. (Note the attention given to microwave ovens and even the ubiquitous television screen.) An occupational hazard of persons working in laboratories where high levels of microwave radiation are encountered is the possible development of cataracts.

Treatment for cataract formation varies according to the situation. When the cause is known, as in diabetes, early recognition and treatment of the systemic disorder may prevent or at least delay the formation of the cataracts. When the cataracts are well developed, surgical removal of the cloudy lens is the only recourse. Even then, surgical removal of the offending lens does not always produce the desired result. Eyes with congenital cataracts are often predisposed to other serious defects, such as *glaucoma* and *retinal detachment*. In children blind from birth the operation may appear to be successful, yet the patient may never learn to fixate properly. In successful cases—and they are many—several devices may be employed to correct the refractive error left from the lens removal. These include spectacles with a relatively large amount of correction (trifocals are sometimes worn to provide correction for distant vision, near vision, and intermediate distances); contact lenses; and plastic lenses inserted directly into the eye. Unfortunately, the latter technique has not been proved to be entirely satisfactory.

For a very interesting discussion of the lens the reader is referred to Bloemendal (1977). Although the stated purpose of this article is to describe the lens as a useful system for the study of fundamental biological processes, it does go beyond this purpose and does provide an excellent presentation of the structure of the vertebrate eye.

Vitreous Body

The main body of the eye that gives it its globular shape is known as the *vitreous body* and is located in the posterior chamber between the lens in front and the retinal surface in the rear. It is a mass of transparent, gelled, amorphous substance whose origin is not known with certainty but is believed to be largely of epithelial origin.

In addition to the gelled substance, liquid similar to that found in the aqueous chamber may also be found in the vitreous chamber. As indicated earlier, the aqueous fluid probably originates in the vitreous body. When parts of the vitreous body have been removed, as in surgery, it may be replaced by the liquid medium.

Along with transmitting light, the vitreous body serves to provide general support for the eye, including holding the lens firmly in place in front and keeping the layers of the retina in the rear in close apposition. Presumably the vitreous body also has a function in the metabolism of the retina.

The vitreous body normally performs its passive light transmission function efficiently and with very little fanfare. As indicated earlier, only a relatively small proportion of the light that impinges on the cornea ever reaches the retina. The remainder is lost through optical scattering and absorption by the various tissues through which it must pass. Furthermore, as an individual gets older the vitreous body tends to lose some of its transparency for reasons not entirely clear. If you look into the eye of an older person with an ophthalmoscope, you may have difficulty in seeing all the way to the retina. Your view will be blocked by an unbelievable number of opaque cells and general "junk" appearing to be either suspended or floating about in the semiliquid medium. Some of these particles are probably dead epithelial cells scaled from the lining of the eye, others are perhaps the result of systemic chemical changes in the normally transparent vitreous tissue. Remarkably enough, however, the presence of a great amount of opaque cells in the vitreous does not seem to bother vision appreciably. With a potential range of 100,000 to 1 in light sensitivity, the loss of even 90 percent or more of the transmissibility of the vitreous medium would scarcely be noticed.

DISORDERS OF THE VITREOUS

Under advanced conditions of diabetes (see the section on retinal disorders) the vitreous may be severely clouded by hemorrhaging and the proliferation of excessive blood vessels. Robert Machener of the University of Miami has developed an instrument that cuts away blood vessels in the vitreous, removes the clouded fluid, and replaces it with a saline solution. The method is still under investigation. Although *vitrectomy*, as the technique is called, can never substitute for the prevention of diabetes, it may prove to be useful when diabetes-produced blindness has progressed too far to be treated by other, less drastic techniques.

Retina

We can, within the scope of this chapter, scarcely touch upon the complex structure and functioning of the retina, the most critical part of the eye. Truly a part of the brain, as indicated earlier, the *retina* is a paper-thin (0.2 to 0.4 mm) sheet of tissue containing the light-sensitive elements (*rods* and *cones*) and an amazing network of nerve fibers and higher-order neural cells. Slightly over one-half of the vitreous cavity is lined by this remarkable organ. Figure 6–2 shows a photomicrograph of a retina in cross section, and Figure 6–3 presents a schematic diagram of its structure. Note that the light transmission appears to be in the wrong direction—that is, the light must pass through the entire nervous structure before reaching the sensitive rods and cones that are juxtaposed against the outermost pigmented layer. In some invertebrates the arrangement is reversed, so that the sensitive elements face the direction of the incoming light.

SENSORY LAYER

Although histologists have identified some ten layers of the retina (see Figure 6–3), we will confine our descriptions to only those layers of significance for our limited purpose. The outermost layer of the retina is the pigment layer, consisting of pigmented epithelial cells that presumably absorb stray light, preventing it from bouncing about in the cavity and activating sensory elements not in the line of vision. The pigment layer does such a good job of absorbing light in the eye that the inside of the eye is virtually dark at all times—so dark that it is impossible to look into the eye without a well-directed source of illumination such as that provided by the ophthalmoscope.

The histologists' second, third, and fourth layers are of interest to us in that they contain the sensitive elements, the rods and cones, their nuclei, and their axonal processes. The size and densely packed nature of the rods and cones are something to marvel at. Some elements are as small as 1 micron in diameter, or about twice the wavelength of red light, some 2,000 being concentrated in an area of about one-third degree of arc. This certainly suggests a tremendous potential for fine resolution and perception of detail. Of the total elements, some 6 million are cones, sensitive to color and able to make color discriminations, whereas perhaps 120 million can be identified as rods, presumably at an earlier stage of evolutionary de-

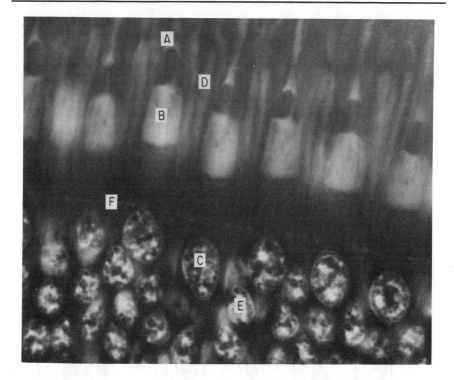

Figure 6-2
Photomicrogram of monkey retina. Portions of both the outer and inner segments of rods and cones can be seen in this photograph. The part labeled A is the beginning or conical portion of the outer segment of a cone. The inner segment of the cone extends to the line at F, representing the outer limiting membrane. The portion of the inner segment labeled B is the ellipsoid of the cone, and C is a cone nucleus. One can see in this view mostly inner segments of rods, such as illustrated by D, with rod nuclei being somewhat smaller and located deeper in the retina (E). The thin line identified as F is the outer limiting membrane, a thick perforated tissue, separating the inner segments of the rods and cones, on one side, from their nuclei on the other. (Photograph courtesy of Mitchell Glickstein, Brown University, Walter S. Hunter Laboratory of Psychology.)

velopment, and sensitive simply to any light within the normally ascribed visible spectrum.

The rods and cones are not distributed randomly throughout the retina. In accordance with evolutionary theory, the color-sensitive (*photopic*) cones tend to be concentrated near the primary optical path, directly behind the lens, whereas the rods occupy the remainder of the retinal surface. At the extreme periphery there are no cones at all, and in a small spot (fovea centralis) directly behind the lens, a slightly depressed area less than 1 mm in diameter contains nothing but cones. To visualize the size of this area, if you hold a dime in front of you at arm's length, the image of it would

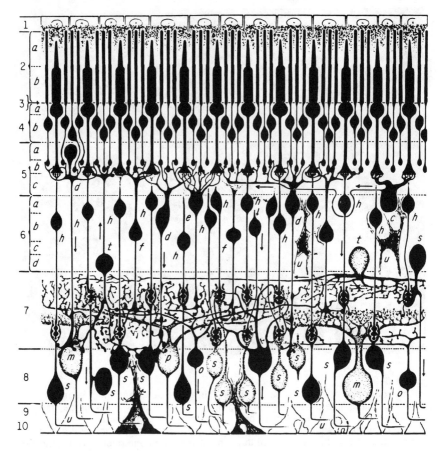

Figure 6–3
Layers of the retina. Note the arrangements of the interconnections and the numbered layers referred to in the text. (From S. Polyak, *The Retina*, University of Chicago Press, 1941, by permission of Mrs. Stephen Polyak.)

just about cover the fovea centralis. This area has a poorer sensitivity to weak light than the rod-filled periphery, but because of the relatively direct one-to-one connections with the higher-order neurons in the retina, the foveal area provides maximum resolution and is the part of the retina one uses for close work. You never read a book out of the corner of your eye, you look directly at it in order to utilize the cones in your fovea to maximize acuity and fineness of resolution detail.

Surrounding and including the fovea centralis is an area of some 5° by 10° known as the *macula* or *macula lutea*, so-called because of its yellow color, which is due to the pigments we considered earlier when we were examining the manner in which the eye mitigates the deleterious effects of chromatic aberration. The macula, although dominated by cones and providing fairly good acuity throughout, contains both rods and cones. As one moves peripherally, the proportion of cones diminishes until, in the outer periphery, only rods are found, and vision is said to be simply light-sensitive (*scotopic*). Perhaps "simply light-sensitive" may be the wrong way to express it, because some rods appear to be as much as 1,000 times more sensitive to light than their more highly specialized cone neighbors. You are probably aware that when you search for a very dim star you can often detect it out of "the corner of your eye" before you can see it directly.

The chemical-electrical functioning of the rods and cones presents an extremely fascinating challenge to the researchers in the area. Although much has been learned of the action of such retinal substances as rhodopsin, iodopsin, and so on, it is best to delay any detailed description of such processes until later in the book. When we discuss color vision, including the development of color theories, we will be better able to grasp the significance of such complex and highly promising work.

NONSENSORY LAYERS

Most sensory neurons, such as those found in the skin, extend uninterruptedly to ganglia of the spinal cord or brain before transmitting their impulses to a higher-order neuron. The sensory neurons of the retina, however, are already a part of the brain, so they find several levels available in the paper-thin retina itself.

We described the histologists' second, third, and fourth layers as containing the sensitive elements and their axonal processes. In the fifth, sixth, and seventh layers we find the *bipolar cells*, with their dendritic and axonal processes. The bipolar cells serve as links between the sensory rods and cones and the deeper-lying ganglion cells. It is at this level that, to a great extent, the functional resolution of the image is determined. Near the fovea centralis a single bipolar cell may connect a single cone to a single ganglion cell; near the periphery, hundreds of rods may feed into one bipolar cell. Thus maximum resolution and precision of the image are available near the fovea, whereas much poorer resolution must obtain for the periphery. On the other hand, the large number of rods supplying a single bipolar cell may mean sensitivity to a much lower level of illumination (because of integration of the separate impulses) for the nonfoveal parts of the retina.

The last three layers of the retina include the *ganglion cells* and are furnished with minute blood vessels as well as nonnervous supporting tissue. Ganglion cells are activated by outputs from the bipolar cells and are in effect, the third level of visual processing. The term *ganglion* as used here is actually a misnomer, the cells being so called only because they resemble the large cell bodies frequently found in ganglia. No true ganglia are found in the retina.

The unmyelinated axons of the ganglion cells are quite long and exit from the last layer, forming a fine network over the inner surface of the eye, before gathering together to leave the eye by way of the optic nerve. The point at which these fibers leave the eye is known as the *blind spot*, as no rods or cones are to be found there. It is a small area on the nasal side of the retina and can be observed by anyone with a little practice. (It is said that one of the former kings of England would use the blind spot to show his subjects how they would look with their heads cut off.)

Several other types of cells are also found in the inner layers of the retina. In addition to the nonnervous supporting cells, both *horizontal cells* and *amacrine cells* are to be found. The purpose of these cells, presumably, is to provide lateral "switching" circuits in the complex computerlike level of the retina. Some of these neurons undoubtedly inhibit the firing of other neurons in some unknown way, thus enhancing contrast effects and light-dark contours, as we will discuss in more detail in a subsequent chapter.

Incidentally, the existence of lateral connections is not limited to the vertebrate eye. Several investigators have demonstrated the existence of lateral inhibition and adaptation mechanisms at the level of the visual receptors in arthropods, and with respect to limulus, contrast enhancement is presumably mediated by pathways between ommatidia. Strausfeld and Campos-Ortega (1977) demonstrated the existence of synaptic connections between amacrine cells and interneurons for insects that appear to mediate neural adaptation and lateral inhibition.

DISORDERS OF THE RETINA

The usually perfect embryological development occasionally falls somewhat short of the ideal. Sometimes the inguinal ring does not close properly after the descent of the testicle, resulting in an inguinal hernia; less often, the bones of the skull and the mouth do not close properly during development, again requiring surgical correction. If you look carefully at Figure 5–6 again you may discover another point where embryological development may fall somewhat short of perfection. When the optic cup is formed from the invagination of the primitive brain wall, two layers, originally with a space between them, fuse to form a single complex layer. These two layers, as we learned in the previous chapter, fuse together, with one becoming the retina and the other becoming the pigment layer. But the fusion is not always perfect. Under normal conditions the existing adhesion and the pressure from the vitreous body hold the retina firmly against the pigment layer. With damage to the eye, such as from a severe blow, the loosely attached retina may separate from its pigmented backing tissue; the disorder known as a *detached retina* is the result. In the violent sport of boxing, detached retinas are not at all uncommon.

Treatment, if the detachment is not too severe and has not been permitted to go untreated too long, consists of refastening the retina to the tissue behind it. This can be done surgically or (more recently) by means of a laser beam. In the latter technique, after the retina is properly positioned, a small, intense beam from a ruby laser is used to "spot weld" the retina back in place. The small burn area and its little scab serve to hold the retina in place until normal healing and tissue regeneration can complete the reattachment.

Another very serious disorder, frequently culminating in blindness, is *glaucoma*. Glaucoma actually includes a number of ocular disorders with hereditary, traumatic, or systemic bases whose common symptom involves an increase in intraocular pressure. Some 13.5 percent of the legally blind persons in the United States have glaucoma as the cause of their affliction.

Presumably, an excessive rate of aqueous secretion and/or an insufficient outflow capability is responsible for the heightened pressure. Detection of the excessive pressure can be made by means of a *tonometer*, an instrument that measures the amount of indentation of the cornea for a given area and known force of the instrument's plunger, thus indicating the eye's resistance of the deformation and hence its internal pressure. An interesting modification of the conventional tonometer has been developed recently by the American Optical Corporation. Called a noncontact tonometer, this instrument measures, by means of reflected light, the deformation of the cornea produced by a calibrated burst of air. It is all done instantaneously and painlessly, with nothing touching the eye.

Blindness from glaucoma is a result of atrophy of the optic nerve at the rear of the eye, which generally progresses from the blind spot outward toward the periphery, but not necessarily in an orderly fashion. The disorder can often be prevented or delayed by appropriate treatment aimed at reducing the intraocular pressure before irreversible damage has been done. As a first step, drugs that either inhibit aqueous production or increase the drainage rate are often employed. Recently, cryosurgical (freezing) techniques have been employed in order to destroy portions of the ciliary body, thus lowering its aqueous-producing capability. Advanced forms of glaucoma may require removal of part of the iris to permit escape of the fluids from the vitreous to aqueous chambers. In some cases the surgical construction of new paths to facilitate drainage of the excess fluid may be indicated.

Diabetes can result in blindness. Diabetic retinopathy, as it is called, is the disorder that, if untreated, may result in the vitreous destruction mentioned earlier. But even if it does not reach that stage, diabetic retinopathy is a very serious condition. It is a widespread problem, being the leading cause of new cases of blindness in the United States among persons between the ages of 20 and 65. According to Maugh (1976), it is observed in half of those individuals who have had diabetes for 10 years, three-fourths of those who have had it for 15 years, and more than 95 percent of those diabetics of 25 years.

The disorder results from the deterioration of tiny blood vessels in the eye. In more severe cases new blood vessels grow on the surface of the retina and even protrude into the vitreous. Eventually, these vessels may rupture and hemorrhage into the vitreous. Finally, scar tissue may form in association with the new blood vessels.

Although it should be apparent that adequate control of diabetes is the best way of preventing diabetic retinopathy, there are relatively recent approaches under study for treating the retinopathic symptoms themselves. Most of the techniques involve photocoagulation, or the destruction of the undesired capillary formations by means of xenon lamps or argon lasers.

Optic Nerve

The fibers from the retinal ganglion cells leave the eye by way of the *optic nerve* and proceed to the brain. In the case of many lower animals (especially those whose visual fields do not overlap), the optic nerve from the left eye goes to the right side of the brain and the optic nerve from the right eye goes to the left side of the brain. In many, the situation is more complex. It might be best described simply by saying that fibers serving the *left visual field* (in both eyes) proceed to the right half of the brain, and the fibers for the *right visual field* terminate in the left side of the brain. There are crossover fibers along the way, but a general contralateral projection of the visual field does obtain.

Figure 6–4 shows in schematic form how this occurs. The temporal half of the left eye's retina goes by a relatively direct path to the left side of the brain, as does the nasal half of the right eye's retina. The latter must cross the corresponding fibers emanating from the nasal portion of the left eye that terminate in the right side of the brain. In effect, the fibers that proceed to the left side of the brain represent the left retinal areas of the two eyes, or since the lenses reverse the images, the right half of the overall visual field. Note that if the left path beyond the *optic chiasma* (crossover point) were destroyed at a point such as A by a tumor or a wound, one would not lose vision in a specific eye, rather, vision would be lost in the right visual field of both eyes, because the left half of both retinas would be isolated from the brain. If damage occurred at point B, the nasal portion of both retinas would be functionally lost and the result would be a loss of peripheral vision in both eyes. The not-too-rare condition of "tunnel vision" is frequently caused by damage to the optic nerves at the point of crossover.

Beyond the optic chiasma the fibers proceed to lower visual centers such as the *lateral geniculates* and the *superior colliculi* and, after various interconnections, terminate in the projection area of the cerebral cortex in the area known as the *occipital lobes*. The tracing of structure and function beyond the optic nerve is another long tale in itself and would go well beyond the scope of this book. However, for the student who is truly interested in just what goes on beyond the retina the work of Hubel and Wiesel (1959, 1968) should prove rewarding. These workers placed micro-

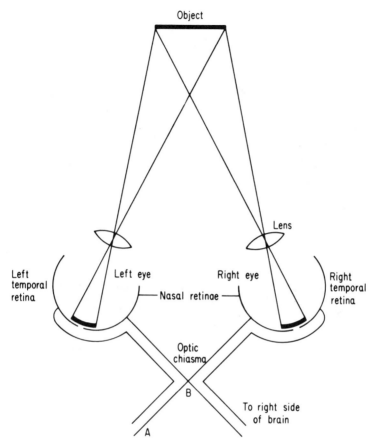

Figure 6–4
Schematic diagram of retinal projection. See text for discussion.

electrodes in various locations within the visual system, such as the optic nerve, the lateral geniculate, and the cerebral cortex, mapping receptive fields in each. Their work is quite exciting but exceeds the scope of this book.

Extrinsic Eye Muscles

The last structure of the eye of significance to the study of sensory processes is actually external to the eye itself. It is the assembly of muscles that position the eyes in their sockets. Three directions of movement appear necessary: (1) up-and-down movements such as raising or lowering the eyes; (2) back-and-forth movements, as used in following a line of print; and (3) rotational movements about the optical axes, as when we tilt

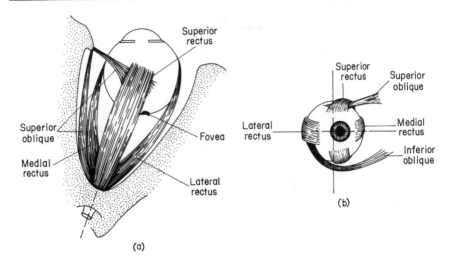

Figure 6–5
Arrangement of extrinsic eye muscles. Note the orientation of the three sets of muscles in three different planes. (Slightly modified from Francis Heed Adler, *Physiology of the Eye*, 4th ed. St. Louis, 1965, by permission of The C. V. Mosby Co.)

the head to one side yet maintain the eyes in roughly the normal orientation to the horizontal.

With three directions of movement three pairs of muscles apparently would be needed, one pair for each plane of movement. This is indeed the situation that prevails (see Figure 6–5). One pair, the *superior* and *inferior rectus* muscles, moves the eyes in an upward and downward direction, a pair of lateral *recti* moves the eyes in the horizontal direction, and another pair of *oblique* mucles is wrapped partially around the ball of the eye at one end, thus producing rotational movements when called for. Failure in the proper functioning of these muscles is often noted and may manifest itself in such forms as squinting or cross-eye, properly termed *strabismus*. When such malfunctions interfere with vision or present cosmetic problems, they may often be corrected through surgery, or, if the condition is not too severe, by means of special training and eye exercises.

Additional Structures

There are many other parts of the eye that have not been mentioned in this chapter. We could, for example, have considered the vascular components and the protective sclerotic membrane in considerably more detail. We could have examined the internal appearance of the eye, as viewed through an ophthalmoscope; we might have included a discussion of the conjunctiva, the eyelids, and the tear glands. The structure of the retina could have been delved into to an almost limitless extent. The aim of this chapter, however, was to provide the student with only enough anatomical and physiological background to enable him to profit fully from the material to be presented later in the book. Where additional material of a physiological or anatomical nature is needed it will be presented at the appropriate point in the discussion. The student who has absorbed the main points of this chapter should now be adequately prepared to grasp the sensory and psychophysically oriented material to be presented later. For those interested in learning more about the anatomy and physiology of the eye, many books are available and college courses with the desired emphasis are not uncommon.

Summary

In this chapter we described the basic structure of the human eye that is of importance to a further understanding of sensory functioning. Examining parts of the eye in a direction of front to back, we considered the cornea, the aqueous chamber behind it, the iris and its pupillary opening, the crystalline lens, the vitreous body, the retina, and finally the optic nerves with their chiasma and subsequent projection fibers. We also mentioned, without providing great detail, several potential disorders of the eye, such as corneal damage, lenticular cataracts, glaucoma, detached retina, and the visual results of damage to various parts of the optic nerves. Finally, we briefly considered the three pairs of muscles that position the eyeball in its socket.

Suggested Readings

Selecting several readings on the structure of the eye that would be relatively easy to read, informative, and not too long has proved to be a most difficult task. Consequently, the following readings fail to meet these criteria. Nevertheless, they are all worthwhile reading for the serious student and should not be ignored simply because of their size or depth of coverage. In addition to these references, any current textbook in the area of neuroanatomy should be able to provide valuable information on the sense organs, especially the one we are interested in here, the eye.

1. S. L. Polyak. *The Retina.* Chicago: University of Chicago Press, 1941. This is still the classical book on the structure of the retina. One would not expect the average student to read its 600 pages as an extra reading assignment. The book does serve as a magnificent source of data and provides interesting descriptions of research technique, as well as 100 superb drawings and photographs of retinal structures. It is a worthwhile book for thumbing through and reading bits here and there as one's fancy directs. The professional investigator in the area should be familiar with the entire book, but the student interested in vision merely as one aspect of sensory-perceptual experience could not be expected to read and master the entire volume.

2. From A. W. Ham. *Histology.* Philadelphia: Lippincott, 1950. Pages 678 to 704 present a highly readable description of the eye, not restricted to histological descriptions, including many structures not described in the present text. Although it directs its emphasis toward histological examination it does not omit important macrorelations. The curious reader is advised to look into this reference to gain more detailed knowledge than was presented in this chapter. (Other sections of the book dealing with nonvisual subjects might also be useful to the interested reader.)

3. From R. L. Gregory. *Eye and Brain: The Psychology of Seeing.* New York: World University Library, 1966. Chapter 4 of this reference includes 25 pages and is one of the simplest presentations available. The last 10 pages of this chapter present material we will later consider in greater detail, but the remaining pages elaborate on topics we tended to treat lightly, such as the functioning of the iris and the relation of eye movements to the extrinsic eye muscles. It is an easy reference to read and will provide some, perhaps not a great deal of, additional information. The entire book (236 pages) is easy and interesting reading, and the enthusiastic student might very well wish to read it in its entirety.

4. From F. A. Geldard. *The Human Senses.* New York: Wiley, 1953. Chapter 2 of this book, "The Visual Stimulus and the Eye," includes 14 pages of relatively easy reading. It includes a discussion of the nature of light and its measurement and treats several subjects we will discuss in a subsequent chapter. It represents fairly easy reading as a background for the material in this and the next chapter.

5. H. Davson. (ed.). *The Eye.* New York: Academic Press, 1962. A large book, an excellent source of information on such topics as physiological optics. It is not a book to read in one sitting, but for general reference application it is perhaps unsurpassed.

6. Haldan Keffer Hartline. "Visual Receptors and Retinal Interaction," *Science* 164 (1969):270–278. Although somewhat technical, this reference, written by a recipient of the Nobel Prize, summarizes in excellent fashion the interaction or "thinking" capabilities of the retina. It is an excellent reading, tracing the history of retinal study as well as contemporary thinking.

7. Mitchell Glickstein. "Organization of the Visual Pathways," *Science* 164 (1969):917–926. Both of the last two readings consider somewhat higher-level functioning, that is, at the level of the retina and higher. This article has excellent illustrations, several in color, and should be of value in gaining knowledge of what happens to the visual impulse beyond the eyeball.

8. From Tom N. Cornsweet. *Visual Perception.* New York: Academic Press, 1970. Several chapters from this brilliant book are of interest to the serious student. "The Action of Light on Rod Pigment," chap. 5, and "The Excitation of Rods," chap. 6, are of particular significance. "Cones and Cone Pigment," chap. 7, is also pertinent, but might be better studied in conjunction with the chapter on color vision. Notice my use of the word *study.* This reading is one of the most advanced included here. It is important for the really serious and capable student; it is not casual armchair reading.

9. Hans Bloemendal. "The Vertebrate Eye Lens," *Science* 197 (1977):127–37. Described in the text, this article is an excellent, well-illustrated description of the morphology and physiology of the lens.

7/ light intensity, brightness, and related concepts

In most experiences the relation between the external world and the resultant experience can be examined in the light of three distinct parameters of the physical event: its *quantity* or intensity, its *quality*, and its *purity*. The latter two characteristics of the visual stimulus, quality (or hue) and purity (or saturation), will be dealt with in later chapters. The subject of this chapter is the first of the three: the intensity of the visual stimulus and the resultant experience that we generally call brightness (often incorrectly).

The Visual Stimulus

Before proceeding to the world of experience we should first gain a preliminary understanding of the physical events that produce the psychophysical or psychological experience of brightness. The amount of light can be expressed in three ways: the amount of light produced by a source, the amount of light falling on a surface, and, finally, the amount of light reflected from a surface to a sensor.

INTENSITY

We might look on a source of radiant energy in terms of its total radiant flux over the entire visual spectrum. This is satisfactory for many applications but it might be more useful for us to consider the effectiveness of the energy in producing a visual experience. This latter approach results in a photometric measure, and is most commonly employed because of its meaningfulness to an understanding of the visual psychophysical function. (If we were developing an intensity system for a specific camera film, we might very well construct it in accordance with the unique sensitivity of the film's emulsion, rather than the sensitivity of the human eye.)

The luminous intensity of a point of light is commonly referred to in terms of *candles*, an arbitrary photometric unit internationally recognized and used by most laboratories. A standard candle is maintained by the National Bureau of Standards in Washington, D.C. If a source of light is twice as intense as the Bureau's standard candle, it has an intensity of two candles, if half as bright, an intensity of one-half candle. In general, the candle is not a measure frequently encountered in the behavioral or biological sciences. Visual stimuli are much more likely to be expressed in one of the following measures, which are derived from the standard candle.

ILLUMINATION

The second approach to light specification involves the amount of light falling on a surface. A standard candle one foot away from a surface provides an *illuminance* (area density of luminous flux) of one *foot-candle*. Illuminance on a surface is, of course, proportional to the luminous intensity of the source, so that a source of two candles provides, for the same distance, twice the illuminance of a one-candle source.

Inasmuch as the light emanating from a point source spreads out in all directions equally, distance influences illuminance exponentially. In technical terms, illuminance varies inversely as the square of the distance from the source to the surface. As an example, doubling the distance from the source to the surface reduces the illuminance to one-fourth its original value. Increasing distance by a factor of 10 reduces the light falling on a surface to 1 percent of the original. A one-candle source 10 ft from a surface provides an illuminance of 0.01 foot-candle, not 0.1 as one might logically believe.

When you use your photoelectric exposure meter as an incident light meter—that is, pointing it at the source of the light rather than at your subject—you are measuring illuminance. You are measuring the intensity of the light falling on your meter's sensitive surface. Indeed, your meter, in order to be used in this fashion, is probably calibrated in foot-candles and has such a scale for your use.

An interesting measure of illuminance, perhaps less often used today than it used to be, is the *troland*, named after the American physicist L. T. Troland. The troland is a measure of illuminance on the retina itself and is perhaps the best-defined measure of direct retinal stimulation we have. It is defined as the light falling on the retina, when viewing, through an artificial pupil of 1 mm^2, a surface whose luminance is one candle per square meter.

LUMINANCE OR BRIGHTNESS

The third approach to measuring light intensity is a measure of the light coming back from a reflecting surface. Formerly called brightness, *luminance* is perhaps a better term for units of this measurement, because it tends to limit subjective influences and can be based on a more rigorous standard. Technically, luminance should perhaps be reserved for the psychophysical correlate of the physical world, with brightness reserved for those situations where subjectivity plays an important role. Brightness should refer to a psychological rather than a psychophysical experience. Occasionally, however, we may in a less rigorous presentation relapse into saying *brightness* when we really mean luminance.

A one-candle source 1 ft from a surface (one foot-candle of illuminance) reflects light at a level of one *apparent foot-candle* if all of the light falling on the surface is reflected back. This is a definitive ideal, because no known surface can ever reflect back 100 percent of the energy falling on it. An apparent foot-candle is, then, a unit of luminance. When you use your photoelectric exposure meter in the conventional manner—measuring the light reflected from your subject's face, for example—you are measuring luminance, and in units of apparent foot-candles if your meter is so calibrated. Automatic cameras also measure luminance, but they make the necessary aperture and shutter settings without requiring you to read the meter and make the adjustments manually.

There are several other measures of luminance, some of which may be encountered in this chapter. *Foot lambert* (ft-L) is the more common expression for apparent foot-candle, and probably the most common unit of luminance is the *millilambert* (mL). Actually, the foot lambert and the millilambert are, for all practical purposes, interchangeable, and

$$1.0 \text{ mL} = 1.076 \text{ ft-L}$$

Before continuing our discussion of light intensity, we will consider the use of a numerical scale, perhaps unfamiliar to some readers, but of great importance to the expression of physical or psychophysical values. Because of their great range, many requirements encountered in sensory studies are expressed in logarithmic units, or logs. A logarithm is that power to which 10 must be raised for it to equal the value in question. For example, what is the logarithm of 100? This is the same as asking, to what power must 10 be raised for it to equal 100? Obviously, 10 must be squared or raised to the second power in order to equal 100. Therefore the log of 100 is 2. If you see the value log 2, it simply means 100. Log 8, as an additional example, means 10 raised to the eighth power, or 100 million. Similar relations hold for values of less than 1; 10 raised to the -1 power (10^{-1}) is equal to 0.1, so the log of 0.1 is -1. Similarly, the log of 0.001 is -3. And because 10 raised to the zero power (10^0) is equal to 1, the log of 1 is

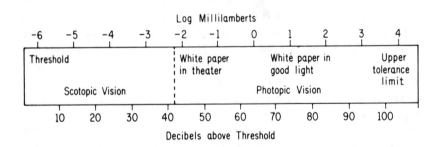

Figure 7–1

Range of light sensitivity of human eye. Notice that the scale is in logarithmic units and that the range as shown is in excess of 10^{10} or 100 decibels.

zero. For intermediate values one must consult a table of logarithms or use a slide rule or electronic calculator.

With this slight digression to explain terminology, let us continue our discussion of light specification and the sensitivity of the eye. The range of light intensity to which the human eye can respond is almost unbelievable. Note in Figure 7–1 that the total sensitivity range of the human eye is in excess of −6 log mL to 4 log mL, or from 0.000001 to over 10,000 mL. This is a range of more than 10 billion to 1! An expensive camera with ten *f*-stops might have a range of 1,000 to 1, but the human eye has the equivalent range of more than 30 *f*-stops. As suggested in the preceding chapter, most of this tremendous range is made possible by the retina, that subsystem of the brain that has been brought out to the periphery to perform just such a miraculous function. Because the scope of this book does not permit us to delve into the mechanisms responsible for this capability, the interested reader is referred to a fine article by Werblin (1973).

As will be seen in the following pages, the various visual capabilities are by no means equivalent throughout this extreme range of light intensity. We can resolve form with high precision only when the illumination is relatively high and we are permitted to use our retinal cones. Under scotopic vision, we can detect low-level sources, but the resultant rod vision does not provide for adequate resolution or acuity. For color we need levels in the photopic end of the scale in order to make confident discriminations. At night, under conditions of scotopic vision, colors are not discriminable and all cats appear to be gray.

Seeing Luminance or "Brightness"

An ability to react differentially to the amount of light falling on a sensitive visual surface appears to be common for all specialized visual organs. Within limits, at least, the manner in which differences in intensity of visual stimulation are registered is determined by frequency of firing of

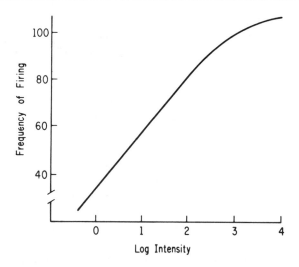

Figure 7-2

Rate of firing of optic nerve of *Limulus*. (Modified from H. K. Hartline and C. H. Graham, *J. Cell. Comp. Physiol.* 1 (1932):277–295.

the sensitive elements. The more intense the stimulus, the more rapid the firing. With more complex systems, since various receptors have different absolute thresholds, the overall magnitude of the visual organ response may also increase with increasing stimulation level.

Figure 7–2 illustrates the relatively simple situation for the *Limulus* eye we referred to earlier. Note that the function is linear over much of the range when rate of firing is plotted against the logarithm of the light intensity. It is a commonly found relationship in the study of sensory-neural action that the sense organ response varies as the logarithm of the stimulus intensity. The common use of logarithmic values for specifying stimulus levels, therefore, serves two purposes: to reduce the tremendous range of sensitivity with its large numbers to workable units and to depict the relationship in an easily visualized and physically accurate manner.

Rate of firing does not suddenly commence with the onset of a stimulus. Contrary to the implicit assumptions behind the early threshold concept, a sense organ is not sitting idly by, waiting to be set into action by a suprathreshold stimulus. To the contrary, it is in a steady state of action, sending out trains of pulses, perhaps maintaining a state of "alertness" or readiness to respond in the higher nervous centers. A stimulus *increases* the rate of firing; and it is the interpretation, at a higher level of functioning, of this increase that is recognized as a sensory event. As indicated earlier, the experimental methods referred to in Chapter 4 that employ detection theory owe much of their acceptance to knowledge concerning the existence of constant ongoing processes.

LUMINOSITY

Although the eye is sensitive to light of wavelengths from perhaps 400 to 750 mμ, it is not equally sensitive throughout this range. When sensitivities are determined for a standard human eye (based perhaps on hundreds or thousands of representative eyes) over the visible spectrum, and plotted on a curve with ordinate values relative to the most sensitive point, the result is a relative *spectral sensitivity curve*, or *luminosity curve*. In obtaining the spectral sensitivity curve of Figure 7–3, a standard light was employed and the observer adjusted numerous wavelength bands until they matched the standard in brightness (hue and saturation ignored). The point on the spectrum to which the eye is most sensitive (555 mμ) was given the arbitrary value of 1.00. Based on the amount of energy required for a match at each of the many wavelengths employed, the *relative* sensitivity for the remaining wavelengths was calculated and plotted, resulting in a relative sensitivity, or luminosity, curve.

The curve shown in Figure 7–3 was obtained with the light-adapted eye and is known as the photopic CIE Spectral Sensitivity Curve, or the photopic luminosity curve of the CIE standard observer. It was developed as a standard by the Commission Internationale de l'Éclairage, more commonly known as the International Commission of Illumination or ICI, and is a result of pooling measurements obtained by scientists in many parts of the world. It is today the basis for the derivation of all photometric units that assess quantities of light. As suggested earlier, light meters have spectral sensitivities closely adjusted to the CIE standard observer.

ROD VERSUS CONE LUMINOSITY

In the preceding section we explored the relative sensitivity of the light-adapted eye, a function based on the response of the cones. Since the time of von Kries and his advocacy of a duplicity theory, we have been aware of the dual nature of vision, the presence of two types of basic receptors, differing in their sensitivities, both quantitatively and qualitatively. As indicated earlier, the rods are much more sensitive to low levels of illumination than are the cones. In addition to a thousandfold advantage in sensitivity, the point in the spectrum where the rods achieve their maximum sensitivity is not the same as that for the cones. Whereas the cones achieve maximum sensitivity at about 555 mμ, the rods are most sensitive to light of about 510 or 512 mμ.

The difference in sensitivity is known as the *Purkinje shift* and is of significance for vision under scotopic conditions. Johannes (Jan) Purkinje's original observation makes an excellent example. In 1825 he observed that of two flowers appearing equal in brightness in daylight, a blue flower appeared brighter than a red flower under night or twilight conditions. That is, when the rods of the eye were being utilized under low-light-level conditions, the point of maximum sensitivity shifted toward the blue end of the spectrum. Figure 7–4 provides a comparison for the two forms of vision,

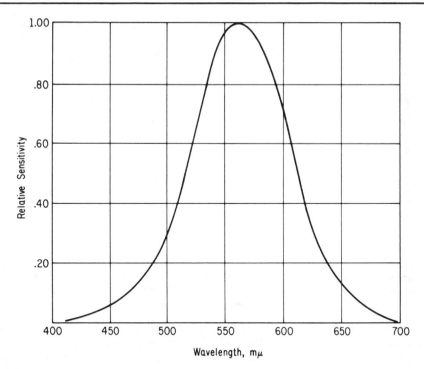

Figure 7–3
Photopic spectral sensitivity (luminosity) curve of standard eye. The ordinate is in units of sensitivity relative to the peak value, which is given the value of 1.00. The abscissa is in units of wavelength (millimicrons).

photopic or cone, and scotopic or rod. It must be emphasized that these are *relative* sensitivity curves. That the rods are 1,000 times more sensitive to light than the cones cannot be determined from this figure. The drawing has been normalized so that the curves for each condition are drawn relative to each point of maximum sensitivity, arbitrarily assigned the value of 1.00 A later curve (Figure 7–5) showing sensitivity at threshold illustrates this difference clearly.

DARK ADAPTATION AND THE ABSOLUTE THRESHOLD

But what about the eye's absolute sensitivity to electromagnetic energy? Perhaps more basic than relative brightness, studies of absolute threshold can become quite complex and require detailed controls and immense precision in the specification of the stimuli and the condition of the observer. Much of what we know concerning the sensitivity of the eye we owe to the monumental work of Selig Hecht and his students, who over many years at Columbia University have produced much of the definitive literature on the subject. Much of our available data is actually based on the right eye of this exceptional research pioneer.

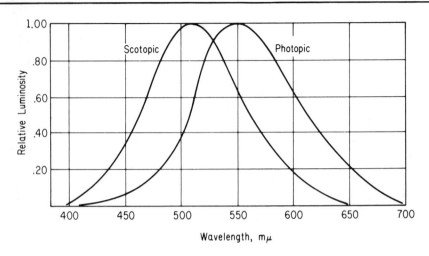

Figure 7–4
Liminosity curves comparing photopic and scotopic vision. Both curves have been normalized so that their points of maximum sensitivity have the value of 1.00.

Sensitivity to light is not an immutable quality of the rods and cones that remains constant regardless of all other circumstances. To the contrary, it is very changeable and is influenced by, among other things, prior activity on the part of the visual system. Sensory elements subjected to strong light stimuli temporarily lose their ability to respond to weak stimuli. Known as *light adaptation*, this loss of sensitivity of the eye has been experienced by anyone who has walked from a lighted street into a dark theater. It takes several minutes before the light in the theater is sufficient to provide anything but the most elemental vision.

For maximum sensitivity to be regained, *dark adaptation* must take place. Both rods and cones have a capability for adapting to light level. There is also a dilation of the pupil in dim light and constriction in bright light, but the magnitude of this adjustment is quite small and rapid in comparison to the neurochemical adaptation of the sensory elements themselves.

Absolute sensitivity of the eye to light increases by as much as five log log units (100,000 times) with a suitable adaptation time. Figure 7–5 is the classical dark-adaptation curve, based on the original work of Selig Hecht. It shows on the abscissa minutes in the dark—that is, adaptation time in total darkness after a two-minute exposure to a light adapting level of 400,000 trolands.* On the ordinate, the absolute threshold in log trolands is shown.

* Adaptation of the dark-adapted eye to light is quite rapid. When you go from the dark theater to the bright street you may be "blinded" for a moment, but the adjustment of your eyes is relatively complete in minutes, or even seconds. Hence the two-minute exposure to a bright light of 400,000 trolands was adequate to form a common standard level from which to proceed with the slower dark adaptation.

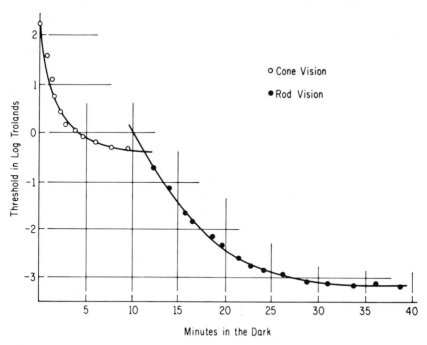

Figure 7–5

Dark-adaptation curve. The data are from research by Selig Hecht and are based on his right eye. They represent changes in sensitivity after exposure to a light of 400,000 trolands for 2 minutes. The circles are for cone vision, where the color (violet) of the test flash was apparent; the solid circles are for the scotopic condition, where the stimuli appeared colorless. (Adapted from S. Hecht, C. Haig, and A. M. Chase, *J. Gen. Physiol.* 20 (1937):731–850.)

Some interesting facts can be gleaned from this figure. Note, for example, that the function cannot be adequately described with a single curve. It is necessary to plot one curve for the threshold of the cones and a second curve for the rod threshold. Even if we did not know about rods and cones before, the location of the points in the distribution would strongly suggest that two "somethings-or-other" must be involved. Whereas the earlier discussion (see Figure 7–4) on relative luminosities did not show the differences in sensitivity between the rods and the cones, Figure 7–5 shows these clearly. It can be seen from this figure that the best threshold obtainable for the cones is about 1 troland (log 0), whereas the rods achieve a maximum sensitivity 1,000 times as great, or 0.001 troland. The range of adaptation is also greater for the rods—something like 1,000 to 1 for increased adaptation for the rods and 200 or 300 to 1 for the cones. Combining both rods and cones the range of sensitivity is over 100,000. That is, the rods, at their maximum dark-adaptation level, can respond to 1/100,000 the light required to obtain a response in the light-adapted cones.

There are marked temporal differences in adaptation for the rods and the cones. The cones require about seven minutes of nonstimulation to increase their sensitivity by a factor of 100 and after roughly ten minutes in the dark, they have achieved their maximum sensitivity. The sensitivity of the rods, on the other hand, does not exceed that of the cones until the latter have reached their limit. After roughly 12 minutes of adaptation the rods are more sensitive than the cones, and this advantage continues to increase, rapidly at first, and later tapering off, for an hour or more. Some investigators hold that dark adaptation for the rods continues to increase for 24 hours or more. For all practical purposes, however, the rods have reached their adaptation limit within three-quarters of an hour.

Our knowledge of dark adaptation has many practical applications. For such tasks as flying aircraft at night in relatively darkened cockpits, pilots may dark-adapt their eyes before beginning the flight. This is often done by wearing dark red goggles, which provide enough light to get around in daylight but block out the shorter wavelengths, thus permitting the establishment of dark adaptation prior to entering the cockpit. Cockpit illumination is often low-level and red so that the occupants can maintain their dark-adaptation level and be more sensitive to lower-level external light.

The results of threshold determinations for the human eye may take on many forms, depending on the methods and stimuli employed. The previous description involved ideal methods and stimuli of maximum efficacy (violet light). Under less favorable conditions the range of adaptation might be closer to 10,000 to 1 or even less, rather than the maximum range of 100,000. We could, for example, determine sensitivity to different hues. Figure 7–6 shows the results of dark adaptation when the stimuli varied in hue. (Thresholds are for detection of light, not recognition of hue; recognition of hue requires considerably more light and is limited to levels adequate for cone vision.) Note that the curve for the red stimulus appears to have no rod component. Rods are essentially insensitive to red; hence there is no red component part of the curve. When the subject is wearing red goggles as described in the preceding paragraph, light adaptation in the rods does not occur, and they consequently retain their high sensitivity to the remainder of the spectrum. Note also that the greatest range in sensitivity is to be found for the violet light, the hue presumably employed by Hecht. Had we included additional hues, they would have been located between the curves for the white and the red. Orange-red, for example, would show only a slight discontinuity caused by rod functioning.

Curves of absolute threshold as a function of light-dark adaptation can take on many other forms as a result of additional variables. If thresholds are determined without the use of an artificial pupil, limiting and keeping constant the effective aperture of the eye, reflexive changes in pupil size will surely confound the results.

The portion of the retina involved is an important consideration. Threshold determinations made with small spots of light limited to the fovea will not show the rod function, because no rods are to be found in that part of

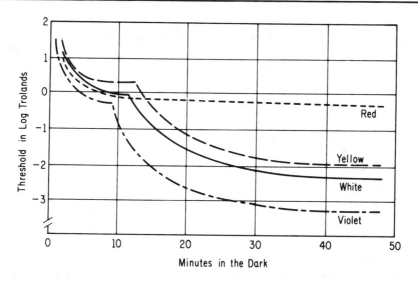

Figure 7–6

Dark-adaptation curves for different hues. Curves show the weakest light that can be seen after entering the dark. Note that we eventually become most sensitive to violet, with our sensitivity to red increasing very little after about 5 minutes. (Adapted from A. Chapanis, *J. Gen. Physiol.*, 1947, by permission.)

the retina. Conversely, a point source in the periphery, where there are no cones, will not show the cone portion of the conventional curves of Figures 7–5 and 7–6.

RICCO'S AND PIPER'S LAWS

Inasmuch as retinal elements, especially rods, integrate over area (approximately 120 million rods and 6 million cones synapse with as few as 2 million ganglion cells), thresholds are dependent on both the location and area of the target, or, more accurately, the location and area on the retina. In the case of foveal stimuli, where interconnections are presumably rather direct and often one-to-one, area and intensity tend to integrate in a simple fashion such that for threshold conditions the product of area and intensity is a constant. This generalization is known as *Ricco's law* and is usually written $AI = C$. It has been found to apply only when the angular size of the test object is no greater than ten minutes. For the periphery, where retinal interconnections are more complex, *Piper's law* ($I\sqrt{A} = C$) applies for visual angles within the relatively wide range of 2° to 7°.

Figure 7–7 shows the preceding relationships in graphical form. The units of measurement are arbitrary, but the relation of area to intensity is clear. Note the linearity when the appropriate area measurements (A or $\sqrt{A}$) are used.

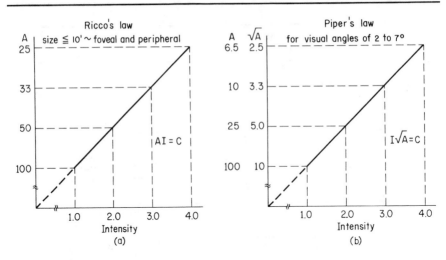

Figure 7-7
Both Ricco's and Piper's laws are illustrated in this highly schematized drawing. Areas and intensities are in arbitrary units to illustrate the principle involved.

The preceding laws and principles are not always as simple as they have been presented here. There are many additional factors at work, and the interested student is encouraged to learn more about the exceptions and limitations from the suggested readings. In addition to integrative effects within the retina, there are also inhibitory effects; there are effects of contours and the intraocular media. Much has been learned concerning the functioning of the eye at or near threshold, but much remains to be learned.

ADDITIONAL ROD-CONE DIFFERENCES

There are other differences between the functioning of the rods and cones that may result in interesting effects. One of the more curious of these is known as the *Pulfrich phenomenon*. Take a piece of string several feet long and suspend a bob on the end of it. If you swing the bob back and forth in front of you in a right-to-left and left-to-right direction while holding a dark (not opaque) glass in front of one eye, the bob will appear to move in an elliptical or even circular direction. Why? The best explanation is based on rod-cone differences in reaction time. The image in the eye without the filter is mediated predominantly by the cones, whereas the lower light level in the opposite eye activates the rods. Because rod functioning is somewhat slower than cone functioning, the image from the partially occluded eye is delayed somewhat with respect to the image from the other eye. The brain "sees" the image from the filtered eye slightly in the past, and the result is different images from the two eyes. If the relationship is right, a pseudo-three-dimensional effect results, not physically unlike the usual stereoscopic vision, in which the images to the eyes do indeed differ.

An interesting example of the effect of the Pulfrich phenomenon has been reported by Enright (1970). He describes distortions of apparent velocity when an observer with one eye partially occluded (neutral density filter over one eye) views a landscape from the side window of a moving automobile. Apparent velocity of the vehicle seems to be reduced when the uncovered eye is in the forward position. Velocity seems to be increased when the partially covered eye is in the leading position.

There may be other practical applications for this difference in response time of the retinal elements. Driving a car at night probably involves considerably more rod vision than daylight driving. Although it is slight, the additional time required for the response from the rods may contribute to the dangers of night driving.

Another difference between the rods and the cones is their directional sensitivity, known as the *Stiles-Crawford* effect. It has been shown that light passing through the center of the pupil stimulates the retina to a greater extent than light entering the eye near the edges of the pupil. Some of the effect may be due to differences in the ocular media, but most of it must be attributed to the cone portion of the retina, because the effect occurs only in the light-adapted eye when cone vision is dominant or when red light, to which the rods are insensitive, is used. The best explanation for the effect suggests that the cones behave somewhat more like waveguides than do the rods. Thus only light from the pigmented layer that enters the cones in a direction parallel to their long axes can have maximum effect. The cones do not achieve the waveguide sophistication purported for the *Copelia* eye, but they do exhibit this characteristic to a greater extent than do the rods.

AREAL AND BINOCULAR EFFECTS

Some interesting effects presumably caused by the "computer" nature of the retina and lower brain centers are to be found. If a single point of light illuminates the retina, the pupil of the eye will adjust accordingly, presumably as a result of the illumination level. However, if a second point of light, dimmer than the first, is inserted into the visual field, the pupil will not constrict as a result of the increased total light. Actually the pupil will dilate somewhat (location and distance between the two points are important), as if it were trying to adjust to the average level. This remarkable phenomenon is generally attributed to inhibitory effects produced by means of horizontal connections in the lower retinal levels (bipolar and ganglion cells).

Indeed, it is probably due to such inhibitory effects that our excellent resolution and acuity is achieved. When one element in the retina fires, there seems to result an inhibitory effect in adjacent elements. Thus contours are greatly enhanced and differences between light and dark areas of stimulation tend to increase.

Although they are not distributed in separate layers, as in the scallop's eye, the mammalian eye does indeed contain both "on" and "off" units,

Figure 7-8
Mach bands. Notice the white and black lines on opposite sides of the separation
between the dark and light gray areas. (From Tom Cornsweet, *Visual Perception*,
Academic Press, 1970, by permission.)

neurons that fire at the onset of a light and those that fire at its cessation.
In all likelihood the interaction of these two types of neurons is also of importance for the inhibitory effects we have mentioned. The importance of
borders and contours to perception has long been recognized, and the significance of inhibitory effects within the retina cannot be tossed off lightly.
Small, almost imperceptible eye movements result in a complex patterning
of "on," "off" responses that apparently maximize the existence of contours and light-dark differences.

An interesting result of inhibitory effects, known as *Mach bands*, can
be observed in Figure 7–8. Near the central division you may notice a thin
darker band in the dark area and a thin lighter band in the light area. The
generally accepted explanation of these Mach bands involves retinal inhibition. It is said that the dark line is due to increased inhibition in the dark
area because of the adjacent light area, and the light band is due to the
reduced inhibition produced by the neighboring dark area.

Another interesting effect, in this instance binocularly produced, and
known as Fechner's paradox, should be described. If you look at a scene
with two eyes and close one, the apparent brightness does not appear to
change. The scene appears to be of equal brightness whether you use one
eye or two. If, however, you use both eyes, but place a filter over one eye,
the scene appears darker than with either both unobstructed eyes or a single
unobstructed eye. The effect, not entirely to be accounted for by pupillary change, must be mediated by some sort of interocular inhibition, either
retinal by way of the optic chiasma, or produced at a higher brain level.

Probably both direct interocular inhibition and higher-level inhibitory effects occur. The amount of "thinking" this subsystem of the brain can accomplish is indeed remarkable.

Chemistry of Visual Function

What takes place in the rods and cones of the eye that can result in such a range of adaptation level and resultant threshold variability as we have reported? Most if not all of the other senses exhibit adaptation and inhibitory effects, but few have the complexity and long-term effects of vision. Perhaps some of the phenomena associated with vision may be due to the additional complexity of the radiant energy–chemical energy–neural energy cycle. For some components of the tactual senses and the auditory sense, mechanical stimulation acts directly to produce a nervous response; hence very little opportunity for adaptation mediated by chemical reaction occurs. With respect to the chemical senses (taste and smell) a chemical reaction with the stimulating material presumably results directly in a neural response.

THE RODS AND VISUAL PURPLE

In the visual sense the situation is more complex. Electromagnetic energy produces a chemical response that is relatively slow, and this chemical response (or an opposing reaction) then results in the firing of the sensory neuron. Such a complicated process takes time and allows for a considerable amount of adaptation or change in the sensitivity of the sense organ. Adaptation is also a quality of the simple chemical senses, and some adaptation is certainly mediated at higher nervous levels, but the exceedingly wide adaptation range of vision indicates the existence of a "dual" chemical process: a chemical reaction in the rods or cones due to the light, and a second chemical reaction to produce the neural discharge.

Although our knowledge of just how external energy can result in the discharge of a sensory neural is not entirely adequate, we do understand rod functioning in the eye to a better extent than is true for most of the senses. Experimental evidence suggests that first of all a quantum of light must be absorbed by a molecule of photosensitive substance in the outer portion of the rod cell. When the pigmented substance of the eye is removed and subjected to light of various wavelengths, it is found that the absorption spectrum of the substance agrees almost perfectly with the scotopic relative luminosity curve shown in Figure 7–4. In other words, the wavelength absorbed best is at about 510 mμ, the point of peak luminosity; and relative absorptions for other hues fall almost perfectly on the rod-function curve. Corrections must be made to allow for discrepancies of the ocular media and the fact that, when determining the relative luminosity curves, light must be measured at the cornea, rather than at the rods themselves. When these corrections are made, the agreement is striking.

What is the nature of the rods that occasions such absorption? In 1876 Franz Boll of the University of Rome discovered in the rod cell of the frog's retina a red pigment that bleached in light and synthesized in the absence of light, thus meeting theoretical requirements for a visual pigment. The substance, which he called visual red, is now known as *visual purple*. It has since been determined that about 30 percent of the entire rod cell consists of visual purple, or *rhodopsin*.

A contemporary of Boll, Willy Kühne of Heidelberg, proceeded with some fascinating experiments in the study of the remarkable light-sensitive pigment. He was able to obtain an image from the retina, known as an *optogram*, demonstrating conclusively that the eye does indeed behave much like a photographic plate. Kühne, after dark-adapting the eye of an albino rabbit, exposed the eye to a barred window for several minutes. After he decapitated the animal, removed the eye, and fixed the retina in an alum solution, he was able to see the image of the barred window in the dried tissue.

By isolating rhodopsin it has been further demonstrated that it has an absorption spectrum identical to the actual rods themselves, and of course, the psychophysically derived luminosity curve. Indeed, recent researchers have removed the sensitive rhodopsin, prepared it in emulsion form, and coated photographic plates with it that actually worked in taking simple pictures. It is clear, then, that it is this substance that produces the relative sensitivity function of rod vision.

Since the discovery of rhodopsin nearly 100 years ago we have learned a great deal about its properties. For one thing, it bleaches under the influence of light: from purple to yellow, and then to transparency. We know too that the unbleached rhodopsin is made up of two molecules, one called the *chromophore*, derived from vitamin A and giving the substance its characteristic color, the other a protein molecule known as *opsin*. Presumably the result of light stimulation is to alter the form of the vitamin A portion and in some manner not yet understood produce an excitation in the neuron. Perhaps the modified vitamin A produces a change in permeability within the cell wall which allows for the passage of ions, much like the neural impulse in a conventional neuron.

After the cessation of the light stimulus it is necessary for the transparent chromophore portion of the substance to revert back to its normal unbleached form. This then, is ostensibly the adaptation we have been discussing. It is probably not the entire story. It has been found, for example, that the entire bleaching-recovery cycle of rhodopsin is not adequate to explain the full range of adaptation. The matter is not settled. Perhaps an interaction of rods such that mutual facilitation and/or inhibition occurs, thereby providing for the unpredicted increase in adaptation range; or perhaps much of the range must be accounted for at higher neural levels. Note again, the earlier reference to Werblin (1973). In spite of much research, the question remains largely unanswered.

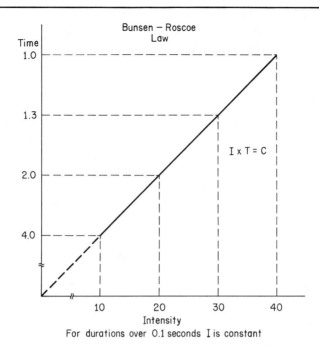

Figure 7-9
The Bunsen-Roscoe law, also known as Bloch's law.

Did you notice the significance of vitamin A in the chemical reaction? Should you eat carrots to see better? To the extent that carrots are rich in vitamin A and to the extent that you have a shortage of vitamin A in your system, they might help you see better in cases where dark adaptation is critical. Under conditions of vitamin A shortage, it has indeed been found that dark adaptation is impaired and that vision under low-level illumination suffers.

The chemistry of cone vision is presumably more complex, since color discriminability must in some way be accounted for. When we come to discuss color vision in a later chapter we will examine what is presently known concerning the chemistry of the cones.

THE BUNSEN-ROSCOE LAW

It was indicated earlier that area and intensity may integrate to provide a threshold stimulation. The manner in which this occurs was described by Ricco's law and Piper's law. If at threshold, the product of area and intensity is a constant (within limits), then an increase in either could be accompanied by a decrease in the other, and the threshold situation would still exist. Inasmuch as the original reaction in the retinal elements is chemical in nature, and since we know that the rate of chemical reaction frequently depends on the concentration of the constituents, we might wonder whether intensity and time might not also integrate and therefore be somewhat interchangeable. In other words, given enough time, could a weak visual stimulus elicit a response that might not occur for a similar stimulus of shorter duration? This is indeed the case, and the law that describes the relationship is known as Bloch's law or the Bunsen-Roscoe law. This law (shown schematically in Figure 7–9) states that a constant photolytic effect is determined by a constant amount of *energy*, rather than intensity or intensity level, energy being a combination of intensity and duration. The law can be written $I \times t = C$, where I is the intensity, t is time or duration, and C is a constant. In photographic emulsions, for example, the law works almost perfectly over a very wide range. As you may know, you can change either the aperture or the shutter speed with equally predictable results (so far as exposure is concerned, at least). In the eye, the law does not apply over all time and intensity combinations. For long duration the critical member of the function is intensity, and time has little if any influence, but for durations up to roughly 0.1 second, intensity and duration are, indeed, interchangeable.

Summary

In the first part of the chapter we considered the specification of the visual stimulus that produces the experience of brightness. We described briefly three approaches to light measurement: intensity, illumination, and luminance, and a few of their more common units of measurement. A large part of the chapter was devoted to the experience of luminance or "brightness" and the specification of the absolute threshold. In so doing we examined differences between rods and cones, including sensitivity, dark adaptation, response time, and the Purkinje shift. In the course of the chapter we described, with a minimum of detail, the known chemistry of rod functioning. Two well-known laws of vision, Ricco's and Piper's laws, were described as well as the Stiles-Crawford effect, the Bunsen-Roscoe law, and the Pulfrich phenomenon.

Suggested Readings

1. M. H. Pirenne. *Vision and the Eye*. London: Chapman and Hall, 1967. This is an excellent little book (205 pages) well worth reading in its entirety. About half of the book is germane to the subject matter of the preceding chapter and the first eight chapters (109 pages) are particularly recommended at this time. Chapters 9 and 10 concern themselves with the limulus and insect eyes and are also worthwhile reading. It is well illustrated and well written, and must be highly recommended.
2. S. S. Stevens (ed.). *Handbook of Experimental Psychology*. New York: Wiley, 1951. Chapters 22 and 24 are applicable to visual sensory processes. These 120 pages are quite detailed and must reading for the serious student. For

others, a more selective approach may be advisable. Chapter 22, written by Dean Judd, emphasizes the physical correlates of the visual stimulus and is therefore recommended for the student with such an interest. The latter half of the chapter might best be read after we have considered color in more detail. A valuable part of this chapter is the glossary of terms at the end as well as several tables that aid in the understanding of the different approaches to light measurement. Chapter 24, "The Psychophysiology of Vision" (60 pages) by S. Howard Bartley is the best detailed elaboration of the material covered in our Chapter 7 that I know of. This chapter also includes considerable material pertinent to later chapters, such as flicker, movement, etc. For the serious or advanced student, these two chapters are highly recommended.

3. S. Howard Bartley. *Principles of Perception*, 2d ed. New York: Harper & Row, 1969. Chapter 4, "Adaptation and Brightness Discrimination," covers most of the material we have presented in a highly readable manner, and these 30 pages are well worth reading. This chapter is especially useful to the reader who wishes original sources, since Dr. Bartley includes references to original research work in most cases.

4. F. A. Geldard. *The Human Senses* (New York: Wiley, 1953). Chapter 3, "Basic Visual Phenomena," includes much of the material included in this chapter. It is easy reading and well illustrated; pp. 28–40 in particular should furnish an excellent supplement to the material just completed.

5. R. M. Boynton. "The Psychophysics of Vision," in R. N. Haber (ed.), *Contemporary Theory and Research in Visual Perception*. New York: Holt, Rinehart & Winston, 1968. Consisting of 17 well-written pages, this article from the 1964 Proceedings of the International Congress on Technology and Blindness is excellent. It includes discussions of physical measurement as well as descriptions of psychophysical methods. It discusses thresholds, dark adaptation, and, in general, most of the topics covered in the preceding chapter. It is highly recommended for additional reading.

6. C. G. Mueller. *Sensory Psychology*. Englewood Cliffs, N.J.: Prentice-Hall, 1965. Chapter 2 of this reference is short, about 11 pages, but it is well worth reading. The presentation of the rhodopsin cycle and photochemistry is particularly lucid and topical. Coverage of the electrical activity of the retinal elements and the nerve impulse is also very illuminating. Highly recommended reading.

7. Frank S. Werblin. "The Control of Sensitivity in the Retina," *Scientific American*, January 1973. Cited several times in this chapter, this fine article should be read by everyone with a serious interest in understanding the manner in which the retina functions. It is well written, well illustrated and certainly worth the expenditure of an hour or so of one's time.

8 / acuity, visual correction

In their quest for new, distant stars, astronomers first recognized the problem of discriminating between small spatial differences in the visual field, and the importance of the resolving power of the eye for this ability. As a result, most early definitions involving visual acuity were originated by astronomers. The early work of the astronomers suggested that the minimum separable difference between two stars that could just be detected was 1 minute of visual angle. This was defined as "normal," with the reciprocal of the visual angle in minutes being the conventional expression for visual acuity. Thus an eye with a minimum separable angle capability of 1 minute was said to have an acuity of 1.0; an eye that required an angle of 2 minutes of arc between two points of light would have an acuity of 0.5 (1 divided by 2).

An acuity of 1.0 was the accepted standard, and even today is the basis for the familiar Snellen chart used by the school nurse and most optometrists and ophthalmologists (see Figure 8–1). We now know that this standard is somewhat too lenient and that a good, healthy eye can resolve a distance of less than 1 minute of arc. Many students may have vision better than 20/20, such as 20/15, which indicates that they can resolve a separable angle of less than 1 minute of arc.* For practical application, however, the use of 1 minute of arc remains the convention.

The more-or-less arbitrary value of 1 minute of arc applies only to man. In spite of his amazing visual ability, in some respects man's capability is inferior to that of some lower animals. The acuity of falcons and hawks, for example, far exceeds that of man (Fox, 1976). When you see a large bird of prey soaring over a meadow, it may indeed be looking for moving creatures

* The meaning of such expressions as 20/20, 20/40, and so on, is considered later in the chapter.

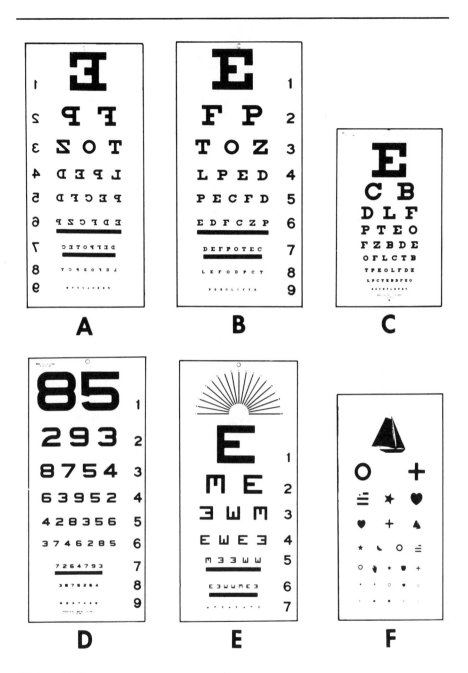

Figure 8–1

Representative acuity charts: (a) is designed for viewing in a mirror, hence the reversed characters; (b) and (c) are the conventional letters; (d) is made up of numerals employing the same spacing; (e) is used for illiterates and also includes an astigmatism detection figure; (f) is for the use of kindergarten-age children and is printed in color. (Courtesy of American Optical Corporation.)

as small as field mice. Considering that its acuity is perhaps 2.6 times as great as that exhibited by humans, the bird probably will locate a mouse.

But enough of birds and mice, let us get back to the subject at hand, the significance of visual acuity for the human. We begin with the subject of resolution—the ability of the eye and its retinal mosaic to discriminate between small spatial distances.

Limitations in Resolutions

Three factors tend to place an upper limit on visual acuity; one of them can, in some cases, be mitigated by means of eyeglasses and one can be improved by means of visual training.

OPTICAL FACTORS

A most important limitation in visual acuity concerns the optical characteristics of the semitransparent media. In the most simple case of improper optical functioning, the cornea-lens combination simply does not bring the image in focus on the sensitive plane of the retina. As in an out-of-focus camera, the image is in focus either in front of or behind the retina. As we show later in the chapter, unless the defect is extremely severe, problems of simple *refractive error* can be corrected by means of corrective lenses.

Another possible difficulty may result from departures from the "true" shape of the cornea and/or lens. As indicated earlier, both the cornea and the lens should have surfaces that represent sections from perfect spheres (at least in the functionally central portion). When these surfaces are distorted or misshapen in any way, projection of an image on the retina is disturbed; this visual experience is known as *astigmatism*. If such distortion involves the portion of the optical path relied on for fine vision, a limitation in acuity must result. As with refractive error, if the disorder is not too severe, corrective lenses can mitigate most of the limitation due to astigmatism.

There are fundamental characteristics in the design of the eye that limit its potential resolving power. As with man-made optical devices, the theoretical limitation based on the wavelength of light can never be attained. Diffraction of light at the pupil margin results in light not perfectly perpendicular to the plane of the retina, and this in turn causes some loss of resolution. Such light may actually bounce around in the eye, resulting in a general "film of light," thus reducing contrast between the image and its background. It is well known that a high degree of contrast between an object and its background is necessary for maximum visibility, and *entoptic stray light* cannot but reduce figure-background contrast. Indeed, some light must enter the eye by way of the sclerotic coat and the eyeball itself. Light may enter by way of the partially opaque iris and contribute to an overall lowering of potential acuity. In the albino eye, with its lack of pigment, this problem is particularly acute.

There are also aberrations due to the nature of the cornea-lens combination. Any lens is in effect made up of an infinite number of prisms. Hence different wavelengths will be refracted differentially, and unless light of a single wavelength is used, chromatic aberration must produce some limitation in resolution. As we indicated earlier, the eye does indeed eliminate some chromatic aberration, but enough surely remains to keep practical resolution well below any theoretically expected level. The nature of the vitreous body probably serves to limit resolution too. It is not as transparent as air, for example, and with the large amount of solid material suspended in it, more diffraction and general clouding of the visual image must result.

RETINAL FACTORS

The size of the individual elements in the retinal mosaic might be expected to limit visual acuity. Many of you are aware of the limitations of resolution in a photographic film due to grain size and clumping of the individual silver molecules. According to figures provided by Polyak, the average cone in the fovea centralis subtends a visual angle of 24 seconds of arc, or slightly less than 0.5 minute. It might therefore be expected that a minimal distance to be discriminated could not be less than 24 seconds of visual angle.

Although "grain size" of the retinal mosaic may provide a theoretical limit, in practice the cross-sectional size of the retinal elements does not appear to limit resolution severely. Under highly controlled laboratory conditions, one can find measures of resolution where the dimensions on the retina are much less than the width of a cone. In vernier acuity (to be described later), differences of 5 seconds of arc, or one-fifth the diameter of a cone, have been reported. We once showed, in a laboratory psychophysical experiment utilizing a constant method, that at a distance of 20 ft, size differences of less than $\frac{1}{64}$ in. could be detected with statistical significance.

How can the eye discriminate distances on the retina that are smaller than the actual size of the retinal elements? Very small, unconscious movements of the eye may result in a moving image, and the "on-off" functioning of the sensitive cones allows for greater resolution than would be predicted on the basis of rod-and-cone cross-sectional size. There are, for example, very rapid eye movement (30 to 70 per second) of quite short excursion that may provide the "scanning" effect that permits resolution much greater than might be expected on the basis of cone diameter alone.

Interconnections in secondary layers of the retina *do* limit acuity. In the nonfoveal regions, where the simple one-to-one connections we described earlier do not exist, acuity is in fact restricted as a function of the retinal mosaic and its bipolar and ganglion cell connections.

NEURAL PROCESSING

The third factor in determining limits of visual acuity concerns the ability of the nervous system to utilize differences in excitation. As mentioned in the preceding paragraph, the lack of one-to-one correspondence from the retinal elements to the optic nerve fibers places a limit on potential acuity. Similar branching at higher levels may also result in loss of visual acuity.

It has been demonstrated that acuity for vertically and horizontally oriented lines or gratings is better than acuity for oblique lines (Howard, 1966). This anisotrophy is not due to the optics of the eye. It has been further established that electrical responses taken from the occipital scalp (evoked potentials) show lower levels for moving oblique lines than for moving horizontal or vertical gratings. But the amplitude of the electroretinogram shows no difference between horizontal-vertical and obliquely oriented lines (Maffei, 1970). It would appear that the effect occurs at a level at least as high as the optic nerve. In support of this supposition, the difference seems to be experientially influenced. Lower animals and humans raised in environments free of oblique lines apparently do not develop a normal sensitivity to nonhorizontal or nonvertical lines (Annis, 1973).

If visual acuity is indeed related to experience, can we not perhaps "learn" to see better? Can we not have improved acuity? Within limits we can. A professor the author once knew emphasized visual training to reduce many visual problems and increase visual skills. He was occasionally accused of teaching people to interpret "blurs." It was said that his training did not improve acuity at all; his patients were merely able to interpret their blurred images better. Is this bad? Indeed, in light of the relatively poor optical quality of the eye, much of our excellent vision is perhaps due to higher mental processes that interpret the relatively inadequate and certainly incomplete retinal image. You have probably seen many examples of how the eye, using the word in a broad sense, fills in details not even present in the viewed image. Perhaps Dr. Renshaw's subjects who learned to "interpret blurs" were just doing what we all do, only doing it better, and in spite of more serious defects in their image-forming structures.

Factors Influencing Acuity

Before considering in some detail the measurement of acuity or resolving power of the eye, let us examine briefly some of the factors influencing it. Acuity, to be described adequately, must allow for the entire accommodative range of the eye. Inasmuch as the lens achieves maximum accommodation for distance at about 20 ft, this distance is normally used for so-called far-point, or distance, vision. For near-point vision, acuity must be measured at the normal reading distance. When your optometrist fits you with reading glasses, for example, he may have you hold a printed page at a distance that is comfortable for reading.

As suggested in the previous chapter when we considered rods and cones, acuity is highly influenced by the portion of the retina involved. Knowing the extent of one-to-one or near one-to-one connections between

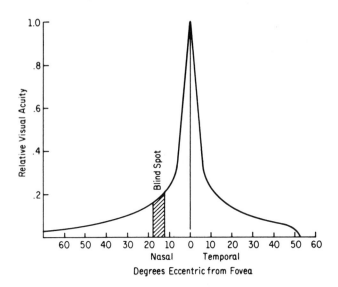

Figure 8–2
Visual acuity on the retina. Note the small blind spot on the nasal side.

the foveal cones and the higher neural centers, we might expect acuity to be better when the central portion of the retina (fovea) is involved. This is indeed the case. Figure 8–2 shows the influence on acuity of angular distance from the fovea. Note the extremely rapid loss of acuity as we progress even 1° or 2° away from the direct line of sight. The curve, of course, is for cone vision, involving relatively high levels of illumination.

Because the rods are more sensitive to light than the cones and because we can best detect a very dim light at a distance of about 20° from the fovea, we might expect that under low-light conditions acuity too would be somewhat better if a retinal area eccentric to the fovea were involved. It has indeed been found that best nighttime acuity is obtained when the direction of regard is on the order of 4° eccentric to the direct line of sight.

As in visual detection, acuity too is influenced by time. Dimmer objects, as well as smaller objects, require more time to be resolved satisfactorily. For a given exposure time, more light is required to see a smaller target than a larger one.

Acuity is influenced by other factors. The brightness of the surround, even the extreme peripheral area, may influence acuity in the central area. Some of this effect may be due to entoptic stray light, which may mask somewhat the area of the retina occupied by the image. There are also, presumably, retinal events that inhibit or sensitize the more central rods and cones. The interaction is exceedingly complex and, like the interpretation of vertical and horizontal anisotropies, cannot be covered adequately in a book of this scope.

Measurement of Acuity

To this point we have been discussing acuity as if it were a single attribute of the visual sense, simple to define and measure, and subject to no controversy. This is not the entire story. Resolution ability and resultant visual acuity can be measured in many different ways, with decidedly disparate results. As in the study of learning, where different experimental materials and methods result in different "types" of learning, different visual stimuli and methods result in different "types" of visual acuity. Let us examine several of the available approaches to the assessment of visual acuity.

VISIBILITY

Basic to any consideration of acuity as a threshold for discriminating differences in areal location of visual stimuli is the concept of *visibility*, or, less rigorously, visibility acuity.* An object must subtend some finite distance on the retina in order to be visible, and the nature of this distance determines visibility acuity. But the matter is not quite that simple. An important factor is contrast—that is, the relative brightness of the object and the background. Except at very high levels of background where light scattering may actually reduce contrast on the retina, maximum acuity is found with maximum contrast. In general, this rule also applies for the more conventional measurements of visual acuity.

Contrast is a relative attribute, since black is rarely the complete absence of light, and white must have some finite limit. Contrast is usually measured in some sort of ratio between the background and the figure or stimulus. In one approach the brighter of the two values is used in the denominator of the contrast ratio fraction as:

$$\% \text{ contrast} = \frac{B_1 - B_2}{B_1} \times 100$$

where B_1 is the brighter of the two and B_2 is the less bright measure.

Another approach results in two different formulas:

$$C = \frac{B_s - B_g}{B_g}$$

and

$$C = \frac{B_g - B_s}{B_g}$$

* Properly defined, acuity refers to the resolving power of the eye, the ability to see two lines or two points as two, whereas visibility is simply the ability to detect a visual stimulus as a function of its size.

where C is contrast, B_g is the brightness of the background, and B_s is the brightness of the stimulus. The first expression is useful for situations where the stimulus is brighter than the background and provides contrasts from 0 to ∞. The second form of the fraction is used when the background is brighter than the stimulus and results in contrasts from 0 to 1.00.

With ideal conditions of contrast the normal human eye can detect a fine wire on a light background when the thickness of the wire is such as to subtend a visual angle of as little as 0.5 second of arc. In terms of the normal visual acuity (as defined by the Snellen chart) such a capability represents a visual "acuity" 120 times greater than the standard 1 minute of arc.

It is also of interest, and germane to our earlier suggestion of higher-level influences, that the length of the line is of some importance. Longer lines can be detected at lower contrast levels than shorter lines, indicating, rather obviously, some sort of summation effect at a level of functioning at least higher than that of the basic rods and cones.

GRATINGS

Another approach, particularly useful for basic research, involves the presentation of gratings made up of dark lines on a light background. (Light lines on a dark background can also be employed, but with somewhat different results.) As most often used, the threshold for acuity is that point at which the subject can identify the area as being a grating, rather than a uniform gray. A modification of the grating technique features alternate squares filled in the manner of a checkerboard and is to be found in a few clinical tests of acuity (see Figure 8–3). Gratings, however, are most often used in research, as, for example, in the studies of hawk and falcon acuity referred to earlier.

The use of gratings combines the more elementary visibility function with the more conventional acuity based on discriminable spatial distances. As a result of this combination, the use of gratings results in acuities poorer than those obtained for simple visibility, but much better than those obtained by the methods normally employed by your optometrist or ophthalmologist for clinical evaluation.

VERNIER ACUITY

Another type of acuity measurement is that of vernier acuity, which indicates the aligning power of the eye, the ability to align two thin lines. Acuity under this condition is about 12 times as good as the Snellen standard, or on the order of 5 seconds of arc. To express it in another way, a misalignment equivalent to one-fifth the width of a cone can be detected. Precision measuring instruments such as micrometers and machinists' calipers capitalize on the remarkable ability of the eye to align opposing lines etched on their metal scales (see Figure 8–4).

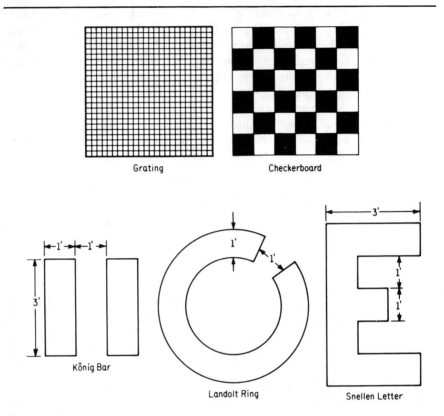

Grating Checkerboard

König Bar

Landolt Ring Snellen Letter

Figure 8-3
Representative acuity-test material. Note the 1-minute dimensions in both the stroke
width and the openings for the bottom figures. Note too that both the König bars and
the Snellen letters have overall widths of 3 minutes of visual angle.

RESOLUTION ACUITY

Probably the most commonly used measure of acuity is that of resolution acuity, defined as the reciprocal of the minimum separable threshold, specified in minutes of visual angle. As discussed briefly at the beginning of this chapter, resolution acuity can be measured by determining the minimum distance (in minutes of arc) between 2 points of light which can just be resolved. In practice, however, it is more usual to use simple geometric figures, with known separations between their components. Three forms of geometric figrues are commonly used and are shown in Figure 8-3.

König Bars. This is probably the simplest test of resolution acuity, and the one which most closely satisfies the definition. The König bar was originated by Arthur König, a brilliant researcher, whose untimely death in 1901 at the age of 45 deprived the world of one of its truly great po-

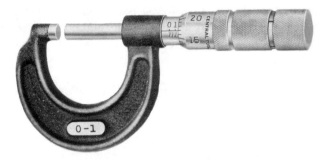

Figure 8–4
Machinist's micrometer. The remarkable precision obtainable with such an instrument is due, partially, to the use of vernier acuity. Aligning one line with another provides the highest measure of acuity possible. (Photograph courtesy of Fisher Scientific Company.)

tential researchers. A König bar for "normal" vision will subtend an overall visual angle of 3 minutes of arc in each direction, consisting of two bars, each 1 minute by 3 minutes and separated by a 1-minute space. The criterion for resolution is not quite as objective as is true for tests such as the Snellen letters, in that the viewer must decide when he can see the two solid bars as separte and distinct. If we mount the display on a track, and bring it from a distance where it looks like a blob up to a point where it is clearly seen as being made up of two distinct bars, interesting subjective reports may result. There will be a stage where the blob looks somewhat "dumbbell-shaped," and then a stage where the ends of the dumbbell will separate temporarily, frequently rejoining and separating, until the target is finally close enough to be resolved with 100 percent precision. Because of the apparent transitional development of resolution and the potentiality for subjective reports, König bars are quite useful for research in resolution.

When used as just described, König bars also produce the most direct measure of acuity in the familiar 20/20, 20/40 terms. When the target has been brought to a distance of 20 feet with a separable angle of 1 minute, and can be resolved by the subject, we can say that he has normal 20/20 vision; that is, he can see at 20 feet what he should be able to see at 20 feet. However, if the observer requires twice the bar sparation of a normal person—that is, he can resolve bars at 20 feet which he should be able to resolve at 40 feet, then he is said to have 20/40 vision.

It is relatively simple to manipulate distance and bar separation to obtain quite precise distance/resolution relations. König bars have been used to study the influence of background area and brightness contrast on resolution. They can also be used to study the influence of figures (noise) in the peripheral visual field at varying distances from the target itself.

Subjective reports concerning the development of the clear separation condition are particularly valuable. König bars are also useful for training, their application being limited only by the imagination of the researcher. On the other hand, the subjective nature of the judgments required make them somewhat less useful for clinical applications than the two following techniques.

Landolt Rings. Landolt rings are intermediate between König bars and Snellen letters in their diagnostic-research potential and in their usefulness for clinical application. A Landolt ring is a doughnut-shaped figure with, for normal vision, a thickness of 1 minute of visual angle and an opening of 1 minute. In practice, the opening can be located at various positions on the circle, and the subject (or patient) indicates the position of the opening in such terms as "north," "southwest," and so on, or perhaps more simply as "top," "left," "bottom," and "right." In some cases the subject may simply indicate the direction of the opening by pointing, thus eliminating the requirement for a verbal response. The underlying assumption is that the subject, in order to locate the opening, must first be able to resolve it.

Landolt rings can be presented individually, as in the König bars, or they may be presented on a card in varying sizes, not unlike the familiar Snellen chart (see Figure 8–1). In practice, some clinicians present Landolt rings of varying sizes in a natural fashion as part of a photographed scene, allowing the patient to view the three-dimensional display by means of some sort of stereo viewer. When using a stereoscopic device distance can be simulated optically, eliminating the necessity for long viewing distances in order to evaluate distant (far-point) vision. Such techniques, utilizing acuity test material in realistic surrounds, may indeed result in more valid measures than the purely artificial office setting with a chart mounted on the wall.

It is probably safe to say that Landolt rings are gradually replacing the familiar Snellen chart as a simple test of acuity. Their greater flexibility and diagnostic potential are being increasingly recognized by modern clinicians.

Snellen Chart. The Snellen chart is still the most commonly used instrument for determining acuity, especially for screening purposes. Like other measures, charts can be used both for distant vision (20 ft) and near-point (reading distance) evaluation. Several possible charts are shown in Figure 8–1. Charts (a), (b), and (c) all utilize the familiar Snellen letters, based on a 5 × 3 minutes of visual angle standard (see Figure 8–3). All characters for a given distance have stroke widths of 1-minute visual angle and spaces between elements of 1 minute. The line on the chart labeled 20/20 would, of course, have the basic dimensions for the 20-ft viewing distance. The 20/40 line would have elements subtending visual angles of 2 minutes at a distance of 20 ft.

In Figure 8–1 charts (b) and (c) are the conventional wall charts with which you are probably familiar. Chart (a) appears to be backward. This is so because it is designed to be viewed in a mirror, and is meant for applications where the viewing room is not long enough to accommodate the nominal 20-ft viewing distance. Chart (d) is similar to the conventional Snellen chart, but utilizes numerals rather than letters. Chart (e) employs figures all in the form of elongated (e)'s and is for testing illiterates. The patient simply indicates the direction of the "arms" by pointing with his fingers. The last chart is for testing kindergarten children and features familiar objects—in color, incidentally—which can be identified by children of this age.

Although the Snellen chart is relatively foolproof, it is not entirely so. When used in the conventional wall card form, dirt, fading, smudges, and so on, can greatly reduce the contrast of the printed material, resulting in acuities with appreciable error. When used for simple screening in schools, in industry, or in the military, uneven lighting and glare may make the results suspect. In the simple wall chart form, the Snellen chart should probably be limited to crude screening and not be relied on for precision measurement unless extreme care is used.

The Snellen chart, as a tool for acuity measurement, is also available in various other forms, similar to those available for the Landolt rings. Outdoor scenes can be photographed with Snellen charts at various distances and viewed (or projected) in stereoscopic form, simulating true binocular vision. Still another possibility involves the use of a zoom type projection system, so that the size of the projected image can be varied continuously over a relatively wide range.

Figure 8–5 shows a device used to screen persons for various visual defects, including acuity. It can provide somewhat more analytic results than a simple wall chart, particularly in the hands of trained nurses and assistants. The Vision Tester, manufactured by Titmus Optical Company, has built-in slides for testing various eye defects. An adjustment for either near or far vision is available, and testing conditions are fairly well controlled. There are several other commercial devices available that make the testing of visual defects much less subject to error in the hands of a nonprofessional than a simple wall chart and test lenses.*

Correcting Visual Defects

We have already discussed some problems in degraded visual ability and the steps necessary for their correction. If the problem is one of unsatisfactory transmission due to ocular media opacities, for example, surgical removal of the cornea or lens may be necessary. Most deficiencies of vision are, fortunately, of a simpler nature and do not require such drastic action. Many of you wear glasses to correct simple visual defects. Did you

* These include the Sight-Screener by American Optical Company; the Telebinocular by Keystone View Company; and the Ortho-Rater by Bausch & Lomb Optical Company.

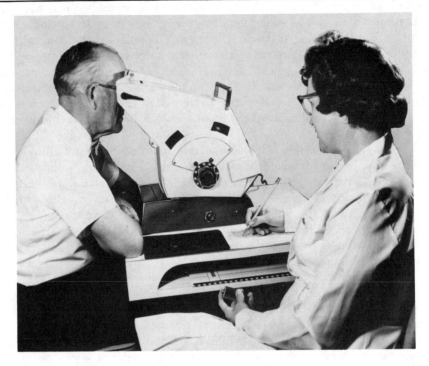

Figure 8–5
A visual testing device. This and similar equipment by other manufacturers provide built-in stimuli and controlled conditions for testing basic visual skills such as acuity, phoria, stereopsis, etc. (Photograph courtesy of Titmus Optical Inc.)

know that spectacles were first used over 650 years ago, and that their invention is generally credited jointly to a Dominican friar named Alessandro della Spina and a native of Florence, Salvino d'Amato? Of greater importance, do you know just what your glasses do for you?

Exclusive of such features as tinted glass, tempered glass, and special frames, your optometrist can provide as many as 12 instructions to the lens grinder—six for your distant-vision glasses and six for your reading glasses, or if you wear bifocals, all 12 for a single pair of glasses. Half of the instructions on your prescription will apply to the left eye, half to the right. But you probably won't see "left" or "right" on your prescription. The "S" you may see at the top of the prescription is the doctor's way of saying "left," and is short for *sinister*, the Latin word for left. For the other lens, the letter "D" is used and is short for *dexter*, meaning "right." "S" and "D" are simply in the tradition of using Latin in all doctors' prescriptions, even medicine for the common cold. Figure 8–6 shows a sample prescription blank.

Each lens (or each half of a bifocal lens) can provide as many as three

_____ 19 ___

M _____

Age _____   FORM A   936A

		SPH.	CYL.	AXIS	PRISM	BASE	V.
DISTANCE	O.D.						
	O.D.						
	FRAME					EYE	
						PRICE	
READING	O.S.						
	O.S.						
	FRAME					EYE	
	DR.					PRICE	

Figure 8–6
Sample prescription blank. (Courtesy of American Optical Corporation.)

basic corrections: a spherical correction, a cylindrical correction, and a prismatic correction. All lenses will not have all these possible curvatures ground into them. Let us examine the significance of these three types of correction.

SPHERICAL CORRECTION

Look at Figure 8–7. In part (a) the point source focuses directly on the sensitive surface of the retina for both far and near vision. As a matter of record (and as indicated earlier), although not shown in this diagram, the cornea of the human eye provides about two-thirds of the refraction necessary to focus an image on the retina. The lens, on the other hand, provides the variability in refraction (*accommodation*) to enable proper focusing with changes in distance. This is possible because the lens is able to assume a thick, relatively spherical shape for near vision and a thin, less "powerful" shape for distant vision. The two extremes shown in the diagram are indicative of a healthy, flexible lens, the sort of lens you were meant to have and once did have. With a lens like this you do not need glasses, at least not to correct a refractive error such as those illustrated in (b) and (c) of this figure.

The refractive error illustrated in (b) is typical of *myopia* or the myopic eye, also called *near-sightedness*. Note that the lens is relatively thick and focuses the point of light on the retinal surface quite adequately at near

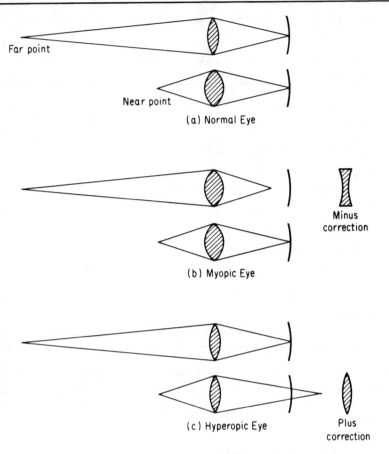

Figure 8-7

Spherical correction. (a) The normal eye is able to adjust its lens shape for both far and near vision. (b) The myopic eye has a lens that does not get thin enough for far vision and a minus or concave lens must be worn. (c) The hyperopic eye has a lens that does not thicken sufficiently for near vision; hence plus or convex lenses must be worn.

point (e.g., reading distance). But when the visual stimulus is at a distance, the lens does not adequately assume its thin, less-powerful configuration. There is too much refraction for distant vision and the point comes to focus in front of the retina. A positive refractive error such as this was once thought to be due to an eyeball that was too long. Today we are inclined to think that the problem is in the lens-cornea combination, rather than the eyeball shape.

In (c) of Figure 8–7 the condition known as *hyperopia* or *far-sightedness* is illustrated. In this condition the lens willingly assumes its thin form for distant vision but is unable to take on the thicker, more powerful shape for near vision. Most young people do not suffer from hyperopia, but in the older generation inability to focus properly at normal reading distances is quite common. Did you ever notice an older person whose "arms were getting too short" to permit him to hold his book far enough away to read?

How does your eye doctor diagnose refractive errors and what can he do about them? One approach to examining accommodation of the lens involves a phenomenon known as Purkinje's images. Noting changes in the relative size and location of images reflected from various interocular surfaces, the skilled optometrist or ophthalmologist can determine with remarkable accuracy the extent to which the lens is accommodating for changes in distance.

More likely, however, and certainly as a final step, trial-and-error procedures will be used. These procedures may involve the physical insertion of trial lenses into temporary frames the patient is wearing, or, in more elaborate setups, manipulation of internal lenses in a device known as a *phoropter.*

It is clear from Figure 8–7, that if you are suffering from myopia—that is, if your lens is too thick—you must make it functionally thinner or less powerful. The answer is obvious: negative or concave lenses to reduce the total amount of refraction in the spectacle-cornea-lens combination. Look through your spectacles at this page. If they make it seem smaller, then you have a concave lens, a negative or *minus* correction for myopia. If your glasses magnify the image, they are correcting for hyperopia, adding curvature or refraction to the total system. They are then *plus* lenses. Your eye doctor determined the type and amount of correction you needed by inserting various lenses in front of you until you said "now it's clear."

When a person gets older, he may suffer from *presbyopia*—that is, he is both near-sighted and far-sighted. His lens works adequately only at some intermediate distance, and he needs negative or minus correction for distant vision and positive or plus correction for reading. Bifocals, invented by that remarkable gentleman Benjamin Franklin, may be called for with minus correction in the top portion and plus correction in the bottom.

All the preceding corrections are called *spherical* because the lenses are, indeed, much like sections sliced from large spheres. If they are to provide plus correction they are not unlike the conventional magnifying or reading glass; for minus correction they are like the inside surface of a large sphere.

The first line of your spectacle prescription will probably specify the amount of spherical correction to be ground into your lens. It will say something like: $+1\Delta$, -0.5Δ, or $+2.0\Delta$. The $+$ and $-$ signs are relatively simple: plus or minus spherical correction. The Δ is the Greek letter delta, and is the symbol for *diopter,* a unit of focal length. The reciprocal of the focal length in meters of a simple lens is expressed in diopters. Thus a lens of 1 m focal length is a one-diopter lens ($+1.0\Delta$ or -1.0Δ). A two-diopter lens has a focal length of 0.5 m, a four-diopter lens a focal length of 0.25 m, and so on. A lens of 0.1 diopter would have a focal length of 10 m and would not be much more than plain glass. For any refractive error less than one-quarter diopter you probably do not need spherical correction.

CYLINDRICAL CORRECTION

The second column on your prescription may specify the amount of cylindrical correction you require. We noted in Chapter 6 that "untrue" shapes or noticeable departures from a true spherical configuration of the cornea can result in astigmatism. If a visual target such as (a) in Figure 8–8 is viewed with an eye that does not present a true spherical surface to the external world, the result may be an image on the retina like (b) of this figure, an indication of astigmatism. Part (a) of this figure is similar to the test target your optometrist uses when he checks you for astigmatism.

Note that there is a directionality to the lack of resolution; the corneal surface is "warped" or "misshapen" in a somewhat systematic way. The obvious correction would be one that would compensate for the corneal distortion, thus restoring an overall spherical aspect to the incoming light.

Part (c) of Figure 8–8 shows schematically the sort of cylinder correction required to counteract the structural distortion. The eye doctor tries various types of cylinders, rotating them until you report that the spokes of the figure are clear and free from blur. Your prescription would then include both the amount of correction, again in diopters, and the angle, or axis, for the flat dimension of the cylinder section. The third column on the prescription blank of Figure 8–6 provides space for indicating the direction of the cylinder.

PRISMATIC CORRECTION

The third entry on your spectacle prescription is that for prismatic correction. As you must know by now, the relation between the eyes and the central nervous system processor is exceedingly complex. The existence of two eyes that see almost but not quite the same thing requires a combining at the level of the brain that is indeed impressive. Presumably, there are "corresponding points" in the two retinas, such that when one looks at a point of light with both eyes, the stimulus activates neurologically analogous loci in the brain. When the images to the two eyes differ slightly, and in the proper manner, the experience of depth, or stereopsis, results. If the images to the two eyes are quite different, the brain may have trouble in combining the two pictures. You may experience *retinal rivalry*, in which the two images are seen alternately, or one image may be repressed and the other accepted as "reality."

Under some pathological conditions the eyes themselves have difficulty in achieving this "corresponding-point" alignment, even though the images to the two eyes are essentially the same. There are imblances, both muscular and functional, that result in the images to the two eyes being slightly misaligned. In the case of severe muscular problems resulting in *strabismus*, or cross-eye, surgery may correct the cosmetic problem as we mentioned

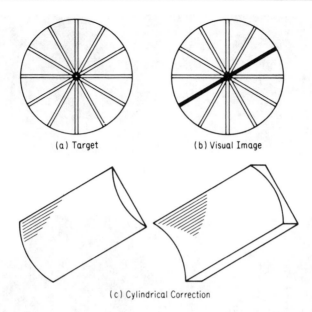

(a) Target   (b) Visual Image

(c) Cylindrical Correction

Figure 8–8
Cylindrical correction for astigmatism. To a person with astigmatism the target shown in (a) appears as shown in (b). Corrective lenses with cylindrical curvature, as shown in (c), are used to correct this problem.

earlier, but the functional problem of combining the images from the two eyes may still remain.

Look at (a) of Figure 8–9, a sample stereogram for testing vertical phoria. When viewed through a suitable binocular device, the horizontal broken line will pass through the note marked "4" if the eyes function properly. If such is not the case, then the eyes are functionally misaligned. In this case it is referred to as *vertical phoria*. If the orientation of the test material is changed, as in (b) of this figure, we can measure *lateral phoria*. Although *heterophoria* is not fully understood, one point can be made. It is not simply strabismus or muscular imbalance. It is a functional, image misalignment, and is not due merely to the direction in which the eye points.

The presence of a vertical phoria is particularly disturbing. Remember, we have lateral eye movements of convergence and divergence that can compensate somewhat (with effort) for lateral phoria. But the muscles that move the eyes in the vertical direction do not work well except in unison. We cannot easily elevate one eye and lower the other. The result, then, of vertical phoria is a blurred image, eye strain, or perhaps even a learned practice of suppressing the image from one eye and relying on monocular vision.

After your eye doctor has determined that you have a phoria problem,

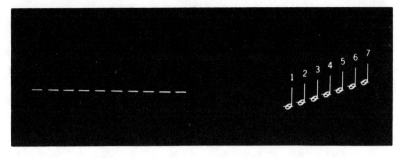

(a) Vertical Phoria

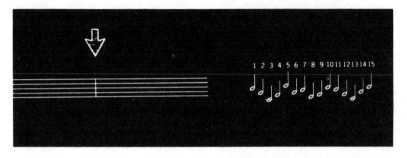

(b) Lateral Phoria

Figure 8–9

Test material for detecting phoria. Illustration (a) is used for determining the presence of vertical phoria, illustration (b) for lateral phoria. (Courtesy of Titmus Optical Inc.)

he proceeds to measure it. As you can see from Figure 8–10, the effect of a prism is to bend all the rays of light entering a flat side. The effect of a prism in front of your eyes would be to shift the image slightly up or down or to the left or right, depending on its orientation. By manipulating prisms in the form of trial lenses, for example, the optometrist determines what prismatic correction is required in order for you to align the images of the stereograms. This is then written into your spectacle prescription as degrees prism and the direction of the required correction, such as "base down 1.0°" or "base left 0.5°" for vertical or lateral phoria, respectively. Prism correction may also be expressed in diopters; in this case a one-diopter prism is one that will deviate an image 1 cm at a distance of 1 m. The eye doctor may place half of the correction in each lens, as, for example, "base up" in one lens and "base down" in the other, to correct for vertical phoria.

These are the three basic corrections for your eyeglasses—spherical, cylindrical, and prismatic. If you wear contact lenses, your prescription

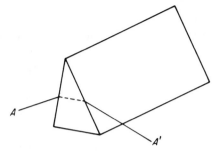

Figure 8-10
Bending of light by a prism. Light enters prism by way of *A* and leaves by way of *A'*.

may be somewhat different. Contact lenses replace the cornea with perfect, precisely shaped surfaces, thereby automatically correcting for corneal-induced astigmatism without the need for separate cylindrical correction. Indeed, for one eye disorder, known as *keratoconus*, the severe bulging of the cornea can be adequately corrected *only* by means of contact lenses. But what about the relatively new soft contact lenses? These marvelous devices fit closely against the cornea; they do not supply a new perfectly shaped surface, so they do not correct for astigmatism. If you have mild astigmatism you may not benefit from soft contacts.

Because their unanchored position on the eye, contact lenses are free to move about (at least rotate) so that the direction of cylindrical correction would be meaningless, even if such correction were included. For the same reason, prismatic correction in contact lenses is difficult if not impossible to achieve unless some means of assuring nonrotation of the lens is employed. Lenses with weighted bottoms have been employed with limited success. Another approach to the problem of rotation is to use larger contact lenses, which cover more than merely the cornea. Such lenses can indeed have tops and bottoms, but they are often uncomfortable and not worth the additional cost. For severe cases of prismatic imbalance conventional eyeglasses are usually superior.

BIFOCALS

The bottom line on many prescription blanks is identified as ADD. This is not a Latin obfuscation; it means additional correction. If this line was filled in on your prescription you probably have bifocals. The prescription blank shown in Figure 8–6, however, has a completely separate section for either reading glasses or the lower half of bifocals. Note, however, because prismatic and cylindrical corrections will most likely be the same for both near vision and distant vision, the bifocal portion of your glasses will need to differ only in spherical correction. Of course, if you do require different prismatic correction for near-point vision, the examiner can so indicate in the appropriate column.

ADDITIONAL CORRECTIONS

Although the preceding three corrections take care of most visual problems of an optical nature, there are a few isolated exceptions. As suggested earlier in the matter of lenticular removal, the patient may wear trifocals. In this case he needs the basic refraction no longer supplied by the lens as well as a fixed accommodative adjustment for both far and near vision.

For patients who have had their lenses removed, ultraviolet absorbing glass may also be prescribed, as was mentioned earlier in our dission of optical aberration. Patients with high sensitivity due to lack of pigment (albinism) may be required to wear dark lenses to limit the amount of light entering the eye.

In some instances, the image produced by the two eyes may differ substantially in size. In these relatively rare cases the patient may wear eyeglasses, one lens of which serves to magnify or reduce the size of the retinal image without changing the focal length of the total combination. Thus the patient has images of comparable size and, presumably, corresponding retinal points for the two eyes. For some even rarer cases the patient may wear magnifying lenses over both eyes, simply to enlarge the image and thereby counteract severe opacities in the optic media, for example.

For children with slight strabismus, doctors may occasionally prescribe prismatic correction, with the hope that forced turning of the eye may eventually result in elimination of the strabismatic condition. For severe cases surgery, followed by visual training, is indicated.

Artificial Vision

Is there any hope for the totally blind? There are about 110,000 people in the United States and Canada who are totally without sight and perhaps 300,000 who are classified as "legally blind" (Dobelle, 1974).

It has been established that direct electrical stimulation of the visual cortex results in photic sensations, or *phosphenes*. At least one patient reported by Dobelle and Mladejovsky was able to recognize simple patterns, including letters, as a result of direct electrical stimulation. Practical application of such exotic techniques is probably in the distant future, but, then, not too long ago such relatively simple operations as corneal transplants were unheard of.

Summary

In this chapter we discussed briefly the meaning of acuity and described three classes of factors that can influence it. We considered optical factors, retinal factors, and the contribution of higher-order neural processing. We then discussed various approaches to the measurement of acuity, beginning with the basic visibility acuity and progressing through the use of gratings and vernier devices, and finally the conventional resolution acuity. With respect to the latter we considered three measurement approaches: König bars, Landolt rings, and the Snellen chart. Finally, we described three basic forms of correction for optical defects: spherical correction for refractive errors, cylindrical correction for astigmatism, and prismatic correction for problems involving phorias and ocular imbalance.

Suggested Readings

1. L. Lewison. *You and Your Eyes.* New York: Trinity, 1960. This is an excellent reference for the material on visual correction. The 235 pages are easy to read, well illustrated, and, to some extent, have a message to deliver. The author emphasizes the importance of the eyes and of taking care of them. His presentation on the use of contact lenses is excellent, as well as his emphasis on the possible value of visual training as a way of eliminating spectacles in many cases. The book is interesting and highly recommended.
2. From S. H. Bartley. *Principles of Perception.* New York: Harper & Row, 1969. This is the same source recommended for the previous chapter. Its chap. 3, however, is quite closely related to the material just covered and includes several topics not included in our Chapter 8. The 30 pages of this reference are relatively easy to read and certainly worthwhile.
3. From Gerald M. Murch. *Visual and Auditory Perception.* Indianapolis: Bobbs-Merrill, 1973. This book is excellent for the entire area of its coverage. Pages 77 to 86 are especially germane to the subject of visual acuity. It is relatively easy to read and interesting.
4. R. M. Boynton. "Some Temporal Factors in Vision," in R. N. Habor (ed.), *Contemporary Theory and Research in Visual Perception.* New York: Holt, Rinehart and Winston, 1968. This is a good reading with a rather restricted content. Although it includes little more than time-intensity relations, it is an excellent example of contemporary research. For the individual with a particular interest in such relations, this article is recommended. Its 11 pages are of moderate difficulty.
5. S. H. Bartley. "The Psychophysiology of Vision," in S. S. Stevens (ed.), *Handbook of Experimental Psychology.* New York: Wiley, 1951. Chapter 24, consisting of 61 pages, probably includes more technical material than any other single reference I can think of. It is recommended as a reference source and for general reading by the interested student.
6. D. Kennedy. "Inhibition in Visual Systems," *Scientific American,* July 1963. This short (7-page) article describes the inhibitory action of sensory impulses, and shows how "off-receptors" improve light-dark discrimination and the perception of contours. It is a short article, easy to read, and worthwhile for the interested student.
7. Floyd Ratliff. "Contour and Contrast," *Scientific American,* June 1972. This article discusses the interaction of contours and resultant contrast. The problem of neural mechanisms underlying the effects are discussed. A very good article for the serious student.

9 / visual flicker and movement

So far we have been describing relatively static relations between the visual experience and the outside world. More often than not the outside world is in a state of change: Lights are alternately on and off, or changing in level, and most visual stimuli move. When objects in the field do not move, the eyes and head move. Movement in some form is central to vision. Some animals are to all intents and purposes "form blind." They can see only moving objects and presumably respond only to movement. As high as it is in the phylogenetic scale, one might expect the frog to have good pattern or form vision. Evidence, however, indicates that the frog responds primarily to movement in its visual field.

We know too that a visual stimulus remaining absolutely stationary with respect to the retina will actually disappear, as the retinal elements reach a state of complete adaptation. Such an experiment requires a highly sophisticated optical system in order that the test object will remain stationary and not be "scanned" by very minute, rapid eye movements such as we mentioned before.

Intermittent Light, Flicker

Research on the effects of intermittent or interrupted visual stimulation has provided considerable insight into the functioning of the visual mechanism. As we learned earlier, the visual response is not an instantaneous event, independent of the temporal and amplitude characteristics of the stimulus. Rather there is a relationship as described by the Bunsen-Roscoe law in which time and intensity of the stimulus tend to summate in producing an experience. The response of the retinal elements themselves occurs over time, and can vary as a function of both the stimulus and the

158

state of the organism (e.g., dark adaptation). It is therefore not unexpected that the experience of an intermittent stimulation need not follow precisely the temporal course of the external event.

In lights or other visual targets that flash on and off at relatively slow rates (under 20 per second) the experience of flicker is obvious, and the activity of the retinal elements must indeed follow closely the alternation of the stimuli. But unlike the ear, which can sense intermittencies of as great as 20,000 per second, the eye functions in such a manner that intermittency rates over 50 or 60 per second are rarely observable. As we increase the rate of alternation from 20 per second to 60, the experience becomes one of a "steady" visual stimulus. For a specified set of conditions, a point known as the *critical flicker frequency* or critical fusion frequency (cff) is reached, often quite abruptly, and the flickering light becomes steady. Recall our earlier discussion of the chemical nature of the retinal response. It should be apparent that complex chemical reactions cannot be repeated at extremely high rates; finite time is required both for the actual reaction and for the recovery phase of the involved physiological structures.

The cff is surprisingly consistent for a single individual, making it a very useful measure of human performance. It has been studied both for a better understanding of how the eye works and for practical applications, such as those described in the following paragraphs.

WAVE PATTERNS FOR STUDYING CFF

Figure 9–1 shows seven forms of intermittent light presentation that might be used in studying flicker. An infinite variety of patterns might be explored, but these seven should serve as general examples.

The first three examples each include three complete cycles. If the total length of the figure represents one second, we should have flicker frequencies of three cycles per second. For rather obvious reasons, these examples are known as *rectangular waves*. Note that they have an instantaneous (comparative, to be sure) rise time and decay time, with an output steady over time. Part (a) illustrates a 50 percent duty cycle, that is, it is "on" 50 percent of the time and "off" 50 percent of the time, and is known as a *square wave*. The second pattern is similar, except that it has a duty cycle of only 25 percent, because 25 percent of each cycle represents the time the light is "on."

Pattern (c) shows a somewhat different situation. It too has a 50 percent duty cycle, but note the height of the "off" portion of the curve. Although (a) and (b) vary in amplitude from 0.00 (no light) to 1.00 (full light), (c) varies from 0.50 to 1.00. This is expressed as *modulation*. The lights for (a) and (b) have 100 percent modulation, whereas (c) exhibits a 50 percent modulation, because the total intensity range is only one-half the potential range. The light has been modulated only one-half as much as it might have been.

Rectangular modulation is perhaps of more academic than practical

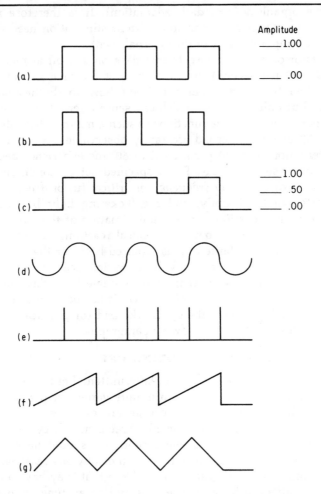

Amplitude
____1.00

(a)____

____.00

(b)____

____1.00
____ .50
(c)____
____.00

(d)

(e)

(f)

(g)

Figure 9-1
Amplitude and temporal patterns for flicker. Here (a), (b), and (c) are rectangular waves: (a) is a square wave; (b) has a 25 percent duty cycle, and (c) has a 0.50 modulation ratio. (d) is a periodic sinusoidal wave and (e) is the result of pulses; (f) and (g) are sawtooth waves, (f) having a slow buildup and rapid decay whereas (g) is symmetrical.

interest in the study of flicker. Few natural or even man-made sources of light exhibit such near-instantaneous rise and decay times, and such steady light output. One example, however, might be an *episcotister disk*, a segmented disk which when rotated at a nodal point of an optical system chops the light in such a fashion as to produce very nearly rectangular modulation (see Figure 9–2). If the opaque sections of the disk are replaced by filters, variable modulation percentages are obtainable, because the "off" cycle will not be the complete absence of light.

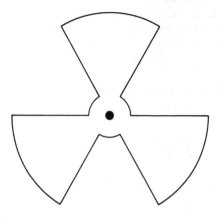

Figure 9–2
Episcotister disk.

If an epicotister disk or other type of moving shutter is placed in an optical system at a nonnodal point, it will result in a noninstantaneous buildup and decay of the light being passed. When properly designed it may produce a light wave of a sinusoidal nature, such as that illustrated by Fig. 9–1d.

Many simple experimental setups in laboratories involve sinusoidal or near-sinusoidal modulation. An incandescent light bulb, because it is basically a thermal device, requires a finite time for the filament to heat up and a finite time for it to cool. Thus when it is powered by an alternating current it follows, in approximately sinusoidal form, the output force (voltage) of the electrical current. Because the filament probably does not cool down completely between cycles, it may result in less than 100 percent modulation, as shown in Figure 9-1c, but with a sinusoidal rather than rectangular form. Only if the alternation rate is quite slow can an incandescent lamp bulb be expected to follow faithfully the alternation in alternating current.

Figure 9–1e illustrates a form of intermittency produced by pulses of light. Using gas-discharge tubes, neon glow lamps, and such devices as stroboscopes and automobile timing lights, trains of pulses that are variable in frequency and amplitude may be produced. Because pulses of exceedingly short duration (microseconds) are generally involved, any further shaping of the light wave must be produced by the chemical-neural action of the visual mechanism. Hence pulsed light is very useful in studying the activity of the chemical-neurological mechanisms of the eye. As both an advantage and a disadvantage, depending on the purpose of the research, such devices usually emit light of a single wavelength, or perhaps several wavelengths, but rarely of continuous spectrum white light.

The last two patterns of Figure 9–1 are examples of sawtooth patterns. Generated by electronic circuits or specially designed episcotister disks, they can be of almost infinite variety. Figure 9–1f, for example, illustrates a wave with a gradual buildup and rapid decay, and the last pattern exemplifies a symmetrical sawtooth pattern.

FACTORS INFLUENCING FLICKER

Many factors influence the cff and determine whether flicker can be seen or not.

Intensity and Wavelength. One of the most important determinants of cff is the intensity of the light stimulation. Figure 9–3 shows the relation between the cff and the intensity of the intermittent light. Notice that the curve appears to level off at around 60 cycles per second; no matter how intense the light is made, the normal human eye cannot detect flicker appreciably beyond 60 cycles per second. Note too that except for lower levels of light, the relationship between the cff and the log intensity of the light is basically linear, and is to all intents and purposes the same for all wavelengths. The curve for lower levels of light (peripheral rod vision was used here) does show differences in cff as a function of wavelength, but when vision is limited to the cones no significant differences due to wavelength are found.

The independence of the photopic cff to wavelength provides the researcher in vision with a very useful tool. Matching two lights of different hue (or wavelength) for luminosity by simple judgments is a very difficult task, producing widely disparate results and a singular lack of consistency. But the cff of a light (all other things being held equal) is solely a function of its intensity, and is not confounded by its wavelength. Hence in a technique known as *flicker photometry* it is possible to match a colored stimulus of unknown brightness with a white stimulus of known brightness. If we know the cff of a colored light we can adjust the level of a white light until its cff is identical. Then, because their fusion frequencies are the same, their luminosities or brightness must be the same, that is, the brightness of the colored light is identical to that of the white light. A principle known as the *Talbot-Plateau law* tells us further that the brightness of a light is due to its total energy, that a light with a 50 percent duty cycle will have the same brightness as a steady light of one-half the intensity. If the standard white light is flickering with a 50 percent duty cycle, then its brightness is one-half its originally known steady-state level. It is this principle that enables us to apply the cff technique to luminosity or brightness measurement of nonwhite light with surprising precision and repeatability.

Size and Location of Stimulus. Both the size and location of the retinal area stimulated influence fusion frequency. Generally speaking, larger areas of retinal activity result in higher cff's than do smaller, point sources. The reason for this, presumably, can be attributed to summation effects

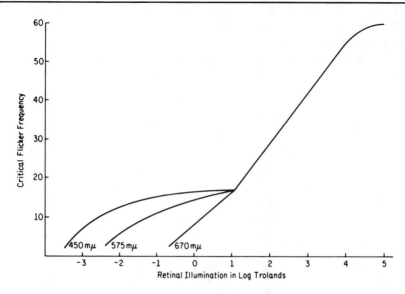

Figure 9–3

Relation between intensity and cff. Note that above about 1 log troland (10 trolands) cff is independent of the wavelength of the light. [Modified from Hecht, Shlaer, and Pirenne, *J. Gen. Physiol.* 19 (1942).]

at retinal levels somewhat higher than the cones or rods themselves. In a similar manner, intermittent stimulation in the periphery requires a higher frequency to achieve fusion, or freedom from flicker, than similar stimulation of the foveal area. This is probably not due to differences in cff between the rods and the cones, because the rods when stimulated by very small point sources may show lower cff's than the cones. But for larger patterns and most practical situations, spatial summation in the periphery may result in a higher critical fusion frequency.

It is significant too that simultaneous stimulation of peripheral areas with steady patterns can have a marked influence on foveal cff. This effect must be attributed to interaction and summation effects, in some cases perhaps at levels much higher than the retina.

Other Factors. There are numerous, almost unlimited, additional factors that can influence fusion frequency. One of these, the modulation pattern of the light, has already been implicitly mentioned, and seemingly owes its effect to its interaction with the chemical-neural functioning of the sensory elements and their interconnections.

As an example of still another factor, if one adapts to a light flashing above the cff (appearing as a steady light) the cff obtained in an immediately subsequent test will be elevated above the normally obtained frequency limit. Thus adaptation is a factor in determining critical flicker frequency.

The size of the pupil has an influence on cff, as do such unlikely conditions as body temperature, fatigue, breathing rate, and even intelligence. Age appears to be a factor, and may be related to normal changes in pupil size that accompany the aging process, as well as systemic or metabolic influences. It is also well known that drugs can have noticeable effects on cff.

APPLICATION OF CFF DATA

But is flicker and fusion frequency only of laboratory interest? Indeed not. Let us look briefly at several instances in our everyday experience where a knowledge of flicker phenomena might be of use. In each case we start out with the tacit assumption that flicker is undesirable, annoying, or even harmful. Let us see how our knowledge of flicker and the cff can lead to better designs in light-emitting devices.

As a first example, commercial motion-picture projectors present 24 frames per second with a dark interval in between; home projectors commonly operate at 16 frames per second. Should we not then see highly undesirable flicker, because we are well below the 50 or 60 cycles per second required for fusion? Indeed we should, if special steps were not taken. Most projectors have a small round shutter, similar to the episcotister disk of Figure 9–2, which rotates in the optical path once per frame, thus providing three exposures or flashes for each frame. The total of 72 (3 × 24) or 48 (3 × 16) flashes per second is high enough that flicker is not likely to be a serious problem. For home movies, lower light output also tends to result in less flicker (lower cff), even though the 48 flashes per second might otherwise be expected to result in an unacceptable amount of flicker.

The 50-cycle current supplied by some power companies, especially in foreign countries, can result in noticeable flicker if conditions such as brightness, size, and direction of view are optimum. Some of you may have noticed flicker in some lights in Canada, where the 50-cycle alternating current is more widely used. The 60-cycle current used in the United States tends to result in much less flicker.

The commonly employed incandescent lamps with their sinusoidal outputs and less than 100 percent modulation tend to reduce flicker appreciably. Flicker is likely to be seen in many gas-discharge tubes, and even in fluorescent lamps. Small neon glow lamps, for example, even with their low light outputs, can be observed to flicker, especially if viewed out of the corner of the eye. Fuorescent lights, with their pulselike outputs, are commonly paired so that when one is on the other is off. The net result then is an overall light made up of 120 pulses per second instead of 60, well beyond the normal cff.

To avoid stimulating your retina with flickering light, your optometrist or ophthalmologist uses ophthalmoscopes and other light-producing devices powered by direct, rather than alternating, current. Note too if you are going to pass light through a rotating episcotister disk to study flicker, you have to start out with unmodulated (continuous) light. Lamps for generating light to be modulated by an episcotister disk have to be powered by direct current for any high degree of waveform specification.

Cff data is also used in the design of cathode-ray tubes for such applications as data readouts, radar scopes, oscilloscopes, and television receivers. The choice of the phosphor to be used on the tube is an important consideration, because the response of various phosphors can vary all the way from pulses such as those illustrated in Figure 9–1e to long, extended sawtooth waves with durations in seconds. If a phosphor has the latter characteristics, flicker may not be noticeable, even at relatively low intermittency or refresh rates. Although slowly changing signals may level out and result in a minimum of flicker, such a phosphor may be quite inadequate where rapid changes in form and position of the displayed signals are required. Rapid changes can result in multiple images, track lines, ghost images, and generally unsatisfactory image formation because of the slow reaction and/or long persistence of the phosphor. To depict rapid movement, phosphors with fast response times and fast decay times such as those in (e) of Figure 9–1 must be employed. In general, for every application some sort of compromise must be made, which often cannot result in completely eliminating the undesirable flicker.

You would probably object if your television picture tube flickered noticeably. Because of the requirements of bandwidth and similar limitations, the maximum refresh rate (frame rate) of your picture is 30 per second. Yet you do not often see flicker. An ingeneous technique known as an *interlace* is utilized to avoid 30-cycle flicker. Every $\frac{1}{30}$ seconds you do indeed get a new frame, but to avoid flicker your set is so designed that you get a half-frame every $\frac{1}{60}$ second. The half-frames are made up alternately of the even and the odd scan lines, which interlace to form the total picture. You get just 30 *different* pictures each second (analogous to the movies' 24 frames), but you get a total of 60 images per second, enough to eliminate most flicker. In color television some parameters are changed, but the principle of interlace is still used to reduce the likelihood of flicker.

ILL EFFECTS OF FLICKER

Although annoyance may be the most common effect and the principal reason for avoiding flicker, it is not the only possible ill effect. There are several electrical waves moving along the surface of the brain (reflecting internal activity) that can be detected and recorded from outside the skull with a sensitive device known as an *electroencephalogram* (EEG). Diagnosis of some forms of brain damage and malfunction can often be made from careful study and analysis of these recordings. One of the well-identified components of the complex EEG is the alpha rhythm. It is known to be associated in some manner with vision and has a frequency of 10 to 12 cycles per second.

When a flashing light is varied in frequency to equal that of the alpha rhythm, a remarkable "locking-in" effect, known as *photic driving*, sometimes takes place; as the frequency of the flickering light is changed, the frequency of the alpha rhythm follows along. One might say "so what— so the alpha rhythm does follow the frequency of the flickering light. Does it have any ill effects on the individual?" In most cases the answer would have to be "no, at least not that we know of." Unfortunately, there does seem to be a glaring exception. For reasons that we do not understand, persons subject to epileptic seizures may be forced into a seizure as a result of such photic driving of the alpha rhythm. Because we do not understand the phenomenon and are not sure that photic driving in the normal individual is completely harmless, it is best to avoid flickering lights within the general range of 8 to 16 cycles per second, regardless of whether the viewer is known to be subject to epileptic seizures.

Real Movement

It might have occurred to you that animals see form and shapes naturally, and when these forms move across their retinas, they "learn" to interpret the moving images as physical movement. If you believed this, you were wrong. Evidence based on phylogenetic analysis indicates that the reverse probably happens: perception of movement is the basic, original visual capability, and form or pattern vision represents a higher level of development. There is a considerable body of modern evidence to support the existence of actual "movement detectors" in the human visual system (MacKay, 1961). Such structures, whatever and wherever they may be, seem to demonstrate reverse aftereffects not unlike conventional adaptation. To go one step further, Regan and Beverley (1973) have demonstrated a similar effect in depth perception. It would certainly appear that the loci for such effects must be at a level higher than the retina.

Note that the earthworm responds to moving shadows and light patterns and that the frog is for all practical purposes blind, except for moving objects. Reflexive responses from the eye are largely based on the perception of movement. A small infant can follow a moving light with his eyes (clumsily at first) long before he gives evidence of anything approaching pattern vision. Even in adults reflexive eye movements result from movement in the visual field. Notice too that the more primitive peripheral portions of the retina are quite lacking in form perception and resolving ability, yet highly sensitive to movement. You can detect the presence of movement out of the corner of your eye, but to see what is moving you must direct your gaze in the appropriate direction.

Eyes that can move in the head appear to have two systems for seeing movement, the more primitive *image-retina* system and a more sophisticated *eye-head* movement system. Although an arthropod, with its compound eye, can detect movement only when a shadow moves across the eye's sensitive surface, activating adjacent and successive ommatidia, the eyes of higher animals can detect movement when the image is steady and the eye is moving. When your eye follows a moving object in the field, you rarely think that the object is stationary and the background is moving. Although you might attribute this discrimination to learning, the ability to recognize movement as a result of the moving or tracking eye is probably somewhat more basic. As evidence, if the background is made homogeneous, movement is still perceived as a result of the eye following a moving target.

The more primitive image-retina system is probably based on the fact that all eyes are originally detectors of movement. Because the retina contains elements that fire at the onset of a light and others that fire at its termination, it is relatively easy to see how contours (leading and trailing edges) or shadows of images can activate retinal receptors as they pass over the surface.

The perception of movement as a result of a moving eye (the eye-head movement system) is not so easy to explain. One explanation, still popular with the modern cybernetic or feedback proponents, holds that impulses arising from sensory endings in the eye muscles and other nonvisual portions of the eye signal the existence of eye movement to the brain, and this complex computer makes the necessary interpretation. Known as the *inflow* theory and espoused by no less an authority than Sir Charles Sherrington, this explanation is now believed inadequate. Based on research involving afterimages and studies of time lags in response, an alternative explanation, originally advanced by Helmholtz and known as an *outflow* theory, appears more consistent with the observed facts. According to this theory, as the signal from reflexive centers is sent to the eye muscles a comparable signal is also sent to the central nervous system computer. Although the brain may indeed receive after-the-fact information from the stretch receptors extrinsic to the eyeball, it is the impulses *directing* the movement that are interpreted at the higher neural centers of the brain.

In effect, one important function of this higher-center interpretation is to cancel the impulses arising from the surround, so that when one views an object moving across a complex background, the background can be effectively ignored and does not appear to rush across the visual field in the opposite direction.

The interested reader is advised to read Derek Fender's article on the visual control system utilized in tracking a moving target (Fender, 1964). The control system was found to be a servomechanism in which the retinal image served as the feedback. Another very fine source of information on movement is Chapter 5 from Rock (1975). This relatively complete presentation discusses both real and apparent movement in a highly analytical manner.

Illusory Movement

The movement we have been discussing to this point has been real, objects actually moving in the visual field, or static objects viewed with a moving eye. But what about movement that appears to exist when no physical change of position occurs, or movement perception that does not truly reflect the antecedent physical movement? Let us examine some instances of movement where the experience does not accurately mirror the external world. We can examine only a few of the many forms of illusory movement that have been documented, and we can examine these only at a relatively superficial level.

AUTOKINETIC MOVEMENT

We will spend most time on this first example of illusory movement for academic reasons and out of scientific curiosity. It is not the most important example of illusory movement, it has no commercial value, the government will not pay you to study it. If you do study it, you do so out of curiosity, "because it's there." It is one of those simple, almost silly phenomena that everyone has seen and no one understands, the most widely accepted explanation still leaving much to be desired. Yet, like Tennyson's flower in the crannied wall, if we understood this simple-appearing phenomena in its entirety, we would be able to explain far more complicated phenomena that do have phychological significance.

Also known as the *autokinetic* phenomenon, or autokinetic streaming (AKS), the apparently random wandering of a point source of light when viewed in a homogeneous field has long been recognized. If you place a glowing cigarette in an ash tray and view it from across a darkened room and if there are no other visible objects in your field of vision, the point of light will appear to move, first to the right, perhaps, then up, down, to the left, all about, and yet not change its position! Sailors and astronomers peering at points of light in black space were intrigued as well as sometimes disturbed by the apparent erratic wandering of a solitary star or a point of light on a distant shore. It is an eerie, disturbing experience, and it demands some sort of explanation.

Despite the fact that dozens of explanations have been offered since the phenomenon was first recognized, AKS still remains something of a mystery. One explanation (many early theories were based on psychologists' introspective reports) suggested that small particles floating about in the intraocular media can be seen, and, as when the stationary moon appears to move as wind-blown clouds scud by, the point of light seems to move rather than the intraocular debris. There are several weaknesses to such a theory: For one thing, you cannot see the minute particles floating about in your eye; they are too small and incorrectly located with respect to any focal plane of your visual system. Furthermore, optical examination of the eye while AKS is in progress does not indicate any directionality to the movements of the particles that can be related to the direction of the AKS experience.

A similar explanation, based on fluids moving on the external surface of the cornea, suffers from the same difficulties.

A more plausible theory, still held by some persons, contend that the eye cannot hold a steady fixation for long periods of time. Consequently, it drifts away from its original line of regard, the experiential misinterpretation being that it is the point of light that drifts away. Such an explanation is untenable. Over 40 years ago Guilford and Dallenbach photographed the eyes while AKS was in progress and found no eye movements to correspond to the subjective reports. What eye movements they did detect were of the small, rapid type we referred to earlier and could in no way account for the relatively large, subjectively reported autokinetic movements with estimated angular distances of 30° or more.

The Gestalt psychologist had an "explanation" for the effect, couched in terms of a pervading spatial framework into which the experience must fit. The quotation marks are intentional because such a theory seems to be little more than a rephrasing of the problem and not an explanation at all.

In a similar vein, some modern psychologists explain away the phenomenon by saying "It's a matter of suggestion." In support of the viewpoint, some investigators have shown that when several individuals of a group report seeing a particular form of movement, others tend to see the same type of movement. Still other persons have had difficulty in demonstrating the efficacy of suggestibility or social pressure. Any such theory tends to beg the issue. Even if suggestion effects were unequivocally demonstrated, the physiological basis for the effect would remain undisclosed. We do not explain behavior by calling it, for example, an "instinct"; we merely give it a name.

The writer once tried a perhaps even more ill-conceived approach to the study of AKS. Having a vague, poorly formulated idea that the direction of movement might have something to do with "directionality" established in the central nervous system, I tried to see whether this "directionality" condition might not be experimentally manipulated before presentation of the AKS stimulation, thus making direction and perhaps rate of AKS movement predictable. Before presenting the point of light, subjects were required to stare at stationary figures (satiation targets) with dynamic qualities, such as aircraft silhouettes or arrows. I anticipated that neural background activity would form a substrate that would determine the direction of movement. The experiment was a failure. Subjects would see afterimages of the satiation figures, and the afterimages apparently served as anchoring points, so that no movement of the observed point of light could occur until the afterimages had disappeared. Had there been a central nervous system directionality effect, it probably would have faded away by then too.

Although it has never been clearly demonstrated, many investigators still feel that there may be something valid in an explanation based on some sort of dynamic directionality in the underlying neural substrate. Such an explanation will be referred to later in the chapter on visual perception when some of the so-called illusions are discussed.

Perhaps a better explanation is one advanced by E. von Holst, R. L. Gregory of Cambridge (Gregory, 1958), and others. It is basically a muscle fatigue theory and involves the eye-head visual system. According to the theory we see movement when the muscles of the eye are fatigued, the erratic movements of the AKS effect being due to the command signals required to maintain fixation despite a tendency for the fatigued muscles to permit the line of regard to wander. There is evidence for this explanation, based on experiments in which the eyes were strained in various directions before the AKS observation. In these experiments the predominant direction of movement of the point of light was predictable as a function of the direction of prior eye strain.

WATERFALL EFFECT

If the striped design of Figure 9–4 is caused to move toward the right for a minute or two, then stopped, the pattern will appear to reverse its direction of movement and move to the left. Similarly, if the spiral design in the same figure is rotated, it will appear to move in the opposite direction when stopped. Even more curious is the fact that, as the spiral design is rotated, it will appear to expand or shrink, depending on the direction of rotation. The experience of reversed rotation that follows the cessation of the physical movement will also be accompanied by the appropriate, and now reversed, expansion or shrinkage. The movement has intriguing paradoxical characteristics. Like the moving point in AKS that constantly moves yet gets nowhere, the constant shrinking or expanding of the spiral results in no change in its size. It constantly gets bigger, yet it is no larger at the end than it was when it started to "grow."

The effect can have a surprisingly long aftereffect. Masland (1969) has shown that, with properly controlled observation, the reverse motion can be obtained as long as 24 hours after the original exposure to the rotating spiral.

This type of illusory movement is as difficult to explain as autokinetic movement. It cannot be adequately described in terms of the eye-head visual system as was done for the AKS movement. If the eye is permitted to follow the movement, the effect is considerably reduced, but when the eye is held stationary and the retina is stimulated differentially, particularly when the stimulus occupies only a part of the retina, the waterfall illusion is at its maximum, thus indicating the importance of the image-retina system in producing this effect.

We referred earlier to the possibility that the sensing of movement may be a primary neurobiological capability, and not simply the result of an inference based on spatial sequentiality. As with insects and frogs, movement per se may be a basic attribute of all visual systems, and, like most attributes, capable of being evoked by a normally "inadequate" stimulus. Just as very cold water may be erroneously perceived as "hot," or a bump on the head may cause you to "see stars," a combination of visual stimuli

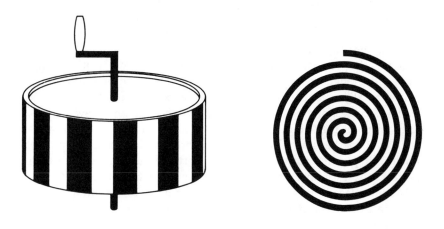

Figure 9–4
The waterfall effect. When the spiral is rotated it seems to shrink or expand, depending on the direction of rotation. When stopped, it continues to shrink or expand in the opposite direction. The left-hand figure appears to turn in the opposite direction when it is stopped.

such as those produced by the targets in Figure 9–4 may result in the erroneous eliciting of the experience of movement: the reverse movement when the real movement is halted and the shrinking and expanding without accompanying change in size.

BETA MOVEMENT AND THE PHI PHENOMENON

The most commonly encountered illusory movement is that based on the *phi phenomenon* and sometimes referred to as *beta movement*. If two similar lights (or any pair of targets, for that matter) with a moderate separation in the visual field are alternated at the proper rate, the experience may be not of two lights alternately flashing, but rather of a single light moving back and forth. If the alternation is too slow, you may simply see the two lights alternately flashing; if the rate of alternation is so rapid that the second light occurs before the image of the first has decayed, then you will see both lights simultaneously, flickering if the repetition rate is below the cff. With optimum alternation rate, however, the apparent movement is quite convincing. Note the effectiveness of motion pictures and television. Both present series of still pictures; you supply the smooth movement by virtue of the phi phenomenon.

The field of Gestalt psychology owed its existence to the monumental work of Max Wertheimer and his 1912 article *Experimentelle Studien über das Sehen von Bewegung*. Appearing in the journal *Zeitschrift für Psychologie*, this article spurred on an entire generation, led by such figures as Kurt Koffka, Wolfgang Köhler, and Kurt Lewin, to investigate molar processes of behavior. Although most investigators today (the writer is not one of them) reject the Wertheimer-Köhler explanation of phi and similar phenomena, you should be familiar with their field-story approach as summarized in the following paragraphs.

Localization of visual functions has been pretty well worked out, and although finer details are still unknown, the principle of spatial localization is generally accepted. It is probably safe to say that every spatioretinal point has a corresponding locus at a higher neuroanatomical level. The locus of a given point may be in the cortex, at a lower brain level, or at a higher retinal level (perhaps at all these levels, with varying complexity). Köhler seemed to imply that it should be in the cortex, but the specific location of the effect is of less importance than the manner in which it behaves.

At some place in this "neural substrate" a locus representing a point on the retina exists, and it will be adjacent to another point representing an adjacent point in the retina. A light activated in visual space will invoke neural activity at some point in the neural substrate. For example, let us say that a visual figure at point A in space produces a response in the neural substrate at point A' and a visual figure at point B in space evokes a response at point B' in the neural substrate (see Figure 9–5). But the neural substrate is, in Köhler's terms, like a *volume electrolyte*. The activation of point A' results in a general spreading of the electrical activity through the electrolytic medium or the "field." If we activate a second light that has its neural projection at B' (see Figure 9–5a), it will appear to the subject that the image from A has simply moved to a new location, B. Note too that if the stimulus had physically moved from point A to point B, the physiological event would have also been an energy movement from A' to B'. Thus apparent movement, according to the Wertheimer theory, is physiologically identical (or very nearly so) to real movement. This is the concept of *isomorphism*, so much a part of the Gestalt approach. According to psychophysical isomorphism there is a relationship, almost one-to-one, between the physical event and the physiological event within the organism. No wonder the movies look so real!

To backtrack a bit, as it was originally conceived by Wertheimer the term *phi* did not simply refer to the movement of the figures from A to B. Rather it included a vague, difficult to express concept of movement. It was, if you can imagine it, movement with nothing moving—movement in the abstract, perhaps movement as a primary experience. In one introspective form, the figures were reported to remain stationary and something (?) moved between them, such as a colorless, amorphous film, obliterating first one, then the other figure. This effect was known as "pure phi" and was at one time the subject of considerable introspective research. Modern usage, however, accepts the term *phi* for the general apparent movement we have been describing, and that has been called *beta movement*, and not just the "pure phi" of Wertheimer.

Time relations for optimum phi movement have been worked out in

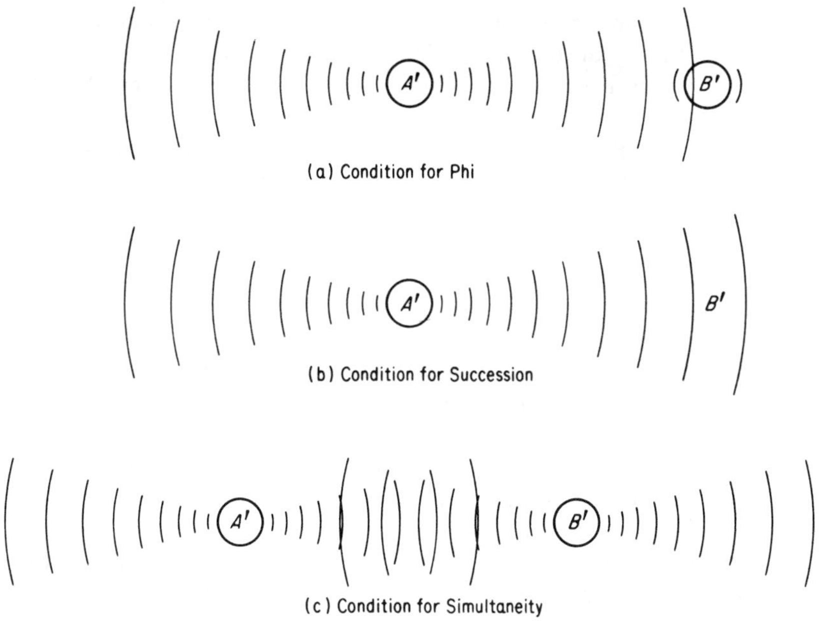

(a) Condition for Phi

(b) Condition for Succession

(c) Condition for Simultaneity

Figure 9–5
Apparent movement. In (a) the temporal condition for optimal movement is shown. In (b) the time interval between the successive stimuli is too great, resulting in successive, nonmoving images, In (c) the time interval is too short, the result being two lights appearing simultaneously and, probably, flickering.

some detail and are not inconsistent with the Wertheimer explanation. For good phi movement to occur, the time relation between the stimulus points (e.g., A' and B') must be consistent with theoretical time requirements for the normal spreading effect in the electrolytic neural substrate. What happens if these time patterns are not met? The second illustration of Figure 9–5 describes the effect when the repetition rate of the two figures is quite low. The spreading from A' reaches the location of B' before the latter is activated. When B' *does* become active, the spreading effect from A' has long gone, faded away perhaps, so that the subject simply sees the two lights, in different positions, and alternating, not one light moving to a new position. In Figure 9–5c, the alternation rate is too fast. Before the wave from A' can reach point B', the latter has been activated. Hence both light stimuli are seen simultaneously, and no movement between them occurs. Rather, the two lights appear to blink or to flicker.

Specific alternation rates required to produce optimal apparent movement cannot be stated absolutely. Rates for phi movement depend on a number of factors. In 1915 Korte presented a series of laws showing that optimal movement depends on (1) the distance between the stimuli, (2) the time interval between them, and (3) their intensity. We might also include adaptation level, and point out that there are large individual differences in the experiencing of the effect. With respect to this last matter, it is curious that when a person has adjusted an alternating pattern to achieve optimum apparent movement, comparatively large changes in the alternation rate can be tolerated before the experience of movement is replaced by one of simultaneity or alternation. There appears to be some sort of "locking-in" effect.

There are several other aspects of the phi phenomenon that make it as interesting to study as the AKS phenomenon. For example, if a vertical arrow is alternated with a horizontal one, the image may appear not only to move back and forth but also to rotate 90°. In some rare cases the movement will appear in the y-axis—that is, the dimension of depth—rather than remaining in the frontal plane.

In another curious example, if a vertical line is replaced by a horizontal line, the visual effect may be one in which the vertical line splits down the middle, the two halves seeming to topple to either side, forming the horizontal line.

Although this effect is not always easy to achieve, targets presented independently, one to each eye, can result in phi if the spatial separations are ideal. Such evidence militates against an explanation of the effect being located in the retina, at least at the rod-cone level. The possibility of interaction at the ganglion-cell level is not completely eliminated, because recent evidence does indicate that there are connections between the two retinas, presumably by way of the optic chiasma.

The study of the phi phenomenon is fascinating. If you set up even a simple experiment, you will probably observe something that no one in the literature has ever mentioned. Introspect a little the next time you see a simple advertising sign employing the phi phenomenon. You may be surprised at the experience; you may even see the "pure phi" the nineteenth-century introspectionists observed.

BOW MOVEMENT

An interesting form of movement, often encountered along with phi movement, is that of *bow movement*, which takes a curved trajectory rather than the presumably straight, shortest distance between two points that might be expected. It comes about presumably as the result of some "interference" in the space between the two stimuli, such that the apparent movement has to "go around."

When I was a graduate student, we once set up an interesting experiment such as shown in Figure 9–6. If we alternate lights at the opposite extremes of a cross as shown in Figure 9–6a, while it is difficult, it is possible to find time patterns that will result in simultaneous left-right and up-down apparent movement. But what happens at the intersection? In every case where we were able to get the antagonistic movements, we found

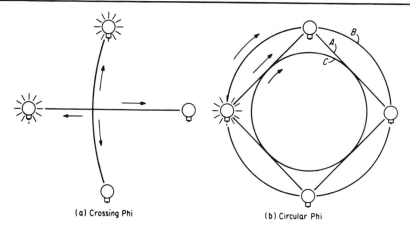

(a) Crossing Phi   (b) Circular Phi

Figure 9–6
Bow movement: (a) shows the result of alternating four lights in such a manner that their apparent movements cross; (b) shows the result of presenting four lights successively to produce a circular movement.

that one of the two movements would assume a third-dimensional aspect, taking a path either in front of or behind, the straight, flat movement of the other pair.

Another form of bow movement is illustrated in Figure 9–6b. If we alternate the four lamps at the proper rate we might expect that the light would appear to move from one corner to the next, forming a clean square (path *A*). But that is not what happens. At the beginning the movement may be similar to *B*, a light moving progressively through the four corners and assuming a circular path. But as we observe the illusory "circle of light," it appears to shrink until it has the path labeled *C*. Notice that the path of the apparently moving light does not even pass through the actual stimuli points!

GAMMA MOVEMENT

Another illusory movement, *gamma movement,* appears somewhat easier to understand. As the intensity level of a figure is increased, its size seems to undergo an increase as well as its brightness. The figure seems to "grow." Conversely, a decrease in intensity may result in shrinking, or decrease in the apparent size of the stimulus. When we are aware of the complexities of the retina network, the lateral connection, and the relatively slow chemical nature of the physiological response, such size-brightness dependency does not seem too unusual.

A somewhat similar, possibly analogous form of movement may occur at the onset and/or termination of a visual signal. A stimulus when suddenly applied seems to "grow" to its full size, and, conversely, when a visible stimulus is turned off suddenly, there is a tendency to see a shrinking or size reduction concomitant with the cessation of the light. A similar process may be at work in both examples.

DELTA MOVEMENT

The last type of movement to be mentioned here is that of delta or reverse movement. It is rather unusual, but occasionally a reversal in direction of the usual beta movement occurs if the second stimulus is appreciably brighter than the first. If in Figure 9–5 we activate *A* slightly before *B*, but the stimulus at *B* is much brighter than at *A*, the movement may appear to go from *B* to *A*, rather than in the expected *A*-to-*B* direction. It would appear that, in spite of the temporal priority of *A*, the neural signal for *B* occurred first because of its greater brightness and the resultant increase in rate of the neurochemical reaction.

The reader may exclaim "Aha, that's why wagon wheels sometimes seem to go backward in Western movies!" Such an effect is *not* an example of illusory movements—the wheels really to go backwards in the projected image. Note that the camera takes 24 pictures per second. If the wheel is turning at 23 revolutions per second (or some multiple thereof) each successive frame of the film will catch the wheel slightly before it has completed a full revolution ($\frac{1}{24}$ of a revolution compared to $\frac{1}{23}$), so that when the film is projected the wheel will appear to be turning in reverse at the rate of one complete revolution each second. The reverse effect has nothing to do with the functioning of the eye: If the wheel were rotating at 24 revolutions per second, it would appear stationary; if it were turning at 25 revolutions per second the projected result would be a wheel rotating in the same direction, but at the rate of one turn per second.

Summary

In this chapter we examined various types of moving stimuli and their phenomenological results. We discussed, first of all, the results of intermittent light stimulation, including factors such as wave patterns of the light, its intensity, and other factors that influence the critical fusion frequency. We mentioned briefly some practical implications concerning knowledge of cff. We dealt briefly with real movement and spent considerable time describing six forms of illusory movement: the autokinetic phenomenon (AKS), the waterfall effect, beta or phi movement, bow movement, gamma movement, and delta movement.

Suggested Readings

1. From E. G. Boring. *Sensation and Perception in the History of Experimental Psychology.* New York: Appleton, 1942. Pages 588 to 602 represent the best presentation of background on perceived movement that I know of. It is historical in nature and should be familiar to the serious student. Its ease of

reading and brevity make it highly recommended for anyone reading this book.

2. From R. L. Gregory. *Eye and Brain: The Psychology of Seeing.* New York: McGraw-Hill, 1969. Chapter 7 consists of 24 pages covering the same general material we included in this chapter. It is easy to read and provides a theoretical approach quite different from that of the present text. Well worth reading.

3. From S. H. Bartley. *Principles of Perception.* New York: Harper & Row, 1969. Pages 241 to 258 discuss the perception of visual movement. Both real and apparent movement are described, with a somewhat different approach than that used in the present book. This reading is well referenced, providing numerous primary sources for the interested student. In addition, pp. 104–111 provide some additional information on intermittent stimulation and the cff.

4. From Gerald M. Murch. *Visual and Auditory Perception.* Indianapolis: Bobbs-Merrill, 1973. "The Perception of Motion, Causality, and Time," chap. 7, is especially appropriate for this chapter. Coverage includes a discussion of theories, such as Gibson's theory of the ambient array, thresholds of movement, the kinetic depth effect (appropriate for the next chapter), and numerous examples of apparent movement. It is a very thorough presentation of the subject.

5. Gunnar Johansson. "Visual Motion Perception," *Scientific American,* June 1975. An excellent article that examines the remarkable manner in which the eye is able to "freeze" motion without the shutter mechanism utilized in cameras. The article points out that the visual mechanism works more like a computer than a simple camera. This is a well written, excellently illustrated reference.

Chapter 2 of Haber's *Contemporary Theory and Research in Visual Perception* includes eight articles on the subject of movement perception that are all worthwhile reading. The following three articles are representative and particularly useful.

6. I. M. Spiegel. "Problems in the Study of Visually Perceived Movement: An Introduction," in R. N. Haber (ed.), *Contemporary Theory and Research in Visual Perception.* New York: Holt, Rinehart and Winston, 1968. A brief survey of visual movement, including real movement, induced movement, and apparent movement. Bases for the experience of movement are discussed with extremely liberal use of references. An excellent article of 16 pages, providing many primary references for the serious student.

7. P. A. Kolers. "Some Differences Between Real and Apparent Visual Movement," same source as (6). Consisting of 13 well-referenced pages, this is an excellent thought-provoking article that purports to show that the underlying mechanisms for real and apparent visual movement are *not* the same.

8. J. H. McFarland. "The Influence of Eye Movement on a New Type of Apparent Visual Movement," same reference as (6). These three pages describe a form of apparent movement resulting from successive presentation of the three sides of an equilateral triangle. The author shows that eye movements may be a factor in this type of apparent movement.

9. Derek H. Fender. "Control Mechanisms of the Eye," *Scientific American*, July 1964. This is a rather specialized article, being a report on the application of systems analysis to the study of visual tracking. Although rather technical, it is well written and well illustrated. It is recommended for the serious student.

10. From Irvin Rock. *An Introduction to Perception.* New York: Macmillan, 1975. "The Perception of Movement and Events," chap. 5, has 66 pages of useful information on visual movement. Also including an excellent and modern bibliography, this is a very important reading for the interested student.

10/binocular vision and depth perception

Up to this point we have been considering the functioning of the eye primarily as a unique sensory device, and what might be said for one of our two eyes should apply equally to the other. But we do have two eyes, not one, and they normally function not independently but as a well-coordinated team. Let us consider in this chapter situations in which two eyes are used, and where meaningful integration of the images from the two eyes occurs and subsequent spatial perception may result. Moreover, the extent to which a single eye can provide satisfactory and adequate depth perception must be examined.

Nature-Nurture Question

As we concluded in the last chapter, it would appear that the perception of movement is based on fundamental physiological and anatomical properties of the organism and is not simply an inference based on learning or experience. What about the experience of depth or three-dimensionality? Is it learned or the result simply of maturation?

The emphasis of the behavioristic theories of psychology, which arose as a reaction against early structuralism, was on the importance of learning, the development of stimulus-response relations as a function of experience. Behaviorists emphasized that the infant "learns" to see depth, largely by manipulating his environment. The Gestalt psychologists, on the other hand, tended to consider depth as a primary attribute, rather than something inferred as the result of learning or experience. To some extent both proponents have been proved right.

The problem has been under investigation by numerous persons for many years, with varying results, but with the general conclusion that at least some recognition of depth is a basic capability of the visual mechanism and is not entirely the result of learning.

In 1913 Shepard and Breed published the results of their research on the pecking ability of newly hatched chicks. They showed, for example, that chicks kept from pecking for five days subsequent to hatching required only one day of "practice" to achieve the same pecking accuracy achieved with two to five days practice by chicks that had been kept from pecking for only three days. Because of the small size of their samples and their inadequate controls, the experiment has been repeated, with modifications, by numerous other persons, including Moseley, Bird, and Cruze. On the basis of Cruze's most definitive study it can be concluded that the pecking response in chicks includes both learned and unlearned behavior and that some perception of spatial relations exists purely as a function of maturation and is not dependent (except for refinements) on learning. As a matter of fact, Bird found that some chicks, when reared in the dark for greatly extended periods of time, never did "learn" to peck.

In 1934 Lashley and Russell showed that young rats previously deprived of normal visual experience could make crude distance judgments. These experimenters placed rats on a small platform and forced them to jump to a second platform at varying distances from the first. A spring arrangement measured the force exerted by the rat when it leaped from the first to the second platform. Although the rats did not jump very accurately, of greater significance was the fact that the farther the distance to the opposite platform, the harder the rats tended to jump.

A few years later Arnold Riesen of Yale University and later of the University of Chicago was to demonstrate the need for visual stimulation, and indeed actual patterned visual experience, for adequate development of form and spatial vision to occur in the primate. Riesen's evidence indicated that when young animals have been reared in the darkness some visual reflexes may develop, but prolonged withholding of visual stimulation can have profound effects on the subsequent development of visual skills.

More recent experiments have also pointed to, or hinted at, the "unlearned" basic nature of depth perception. The phenomenon of brightness or lightness contrast referred to earlier and generally attributed to lateral connections at the retinal or higher level provides a good example. It has been shown that the extent of the effect is influenced not only by the relative lightness of the adjacent areas, but also by their position in the third dimension. Gilchrist (1977) suggests that, "If perceived lightness of surfaces depends on their perceived location in space, depth perception must occur first and be followed by the determination of surface brightness." This sounds as if the perception of depth must be quite basic.

Recent experiments on the nature-nurture issue have utilized a device

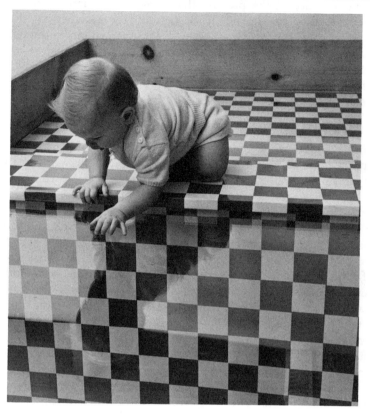

Figure 10–1

The visual cliff. The child is being tested on the visual cliff. A sheet of glass rests directly over the checkered pattern at one end, and at a distance of several feet above the pattern at the other end. (From "The 'Visual Cliff,' " E. J. Gibson and R. D. Walk. Copyright © 1960 by Scientific American, Inc. All rights reserved. Courtesy William Vandivert.)

known as the *Visual Cliff*. Pioneered by Eleanor J. Gibson (Gibson, 1960) and others at Cornell University, this device seems to indicate that various species of animals are able to perceive and avoid a sharp drop-off or cliff, as soon as they are able to move about. Using an apparatus such as that shown in Figure 10–1, Gibson and Walk showed that human infants (6 to 14 months of age), kids, lambs, and baby chicks when first placed on the device refuse to crawl onto the glass and over the imaginary cliff. These same authors found that species that apparently do not rely on visual depth perception for their everyday behavior (rats, turtles) are not disturbed by the visual cliff and will crawl out on the glass with no alarm at the chasm below. A slight physical displacement, however, will prevent the rat with his vibrissae-moderated spatial sense from crossing over.

If one can accept the premise that these young animals have had no prior opportunity to "learn" depth (admittedly a somewhat dangerous assumption), the conclusion is clear: Depth perception is an unlearned, natural attribute of higher-order animals. Whether it should be attributed to factors of motion parallax (as suggested by Gibson and Walk, and to be described later) or other innate capabilities is a matter for further conjecture and research.

PRIMARY AND SECONDARY DETERMINANTS OF DEPTH

With all this smoke there must be some fire. Some aspects of depth perception must be unlearned, a result of the physiology and anatomy of the organism. We refer here to these effects as *primary* as contrasted with *secondary* "cues" for distance. Our categorization may be proved to be in error, but for the purpose of classifying depth determinants let us consider those with a definite, known physiological basis as primary and those that appear to be learned as secondary. For example, we probably have to learn that of two images of people differing greatly in size, the smaller is probably farther away, or that when one object covers (obscures) another, the former is probably the nearer of the two. We may have to "learn" that railroad tracks converge in the distance and that colors viewed from a distance tend to lose much of their brightness and saturation.

On the other hand, it may be that those effects shown to result in demonstrable physiological changes are interpreted as distance without a prolonged learning process. The difference in images to the two eyes, the activation of receptors in the muscles of the eye when we accommodate to a near object or when our eyes converge, are perhaps direct cues that require no lengthy learning process. It is probably such primary cues that enabled Cruze's chicks to develop pecking skill so quickly, or Lashley's rats to jump with a degree of skill not consonant with their past experiences.

Monocular Cues for Depth

Although it is indeed true that two eyes provide a richer, more natural appreciation of the three-dimensional world, persons who have the use of only one eye are by no means devoid of depth perception. There are many ways, using monocular vision, that the three-dimensional world can be recognized and spatial orientation maintained.

PRIMARY CUES

Accommodation or the adjusting of the lens for varying distances is perhaps the only primary cue provided by monocular vision.* When one

---

* Persons who have lost the sight of one eye may still, in effect, converge the two eyes, thus providing a primary cue of convergence. This, of course, is actually a binocular cue, since the relative position of the two eyes and the resultant activation of stretch receptors in the extrinsic eye muscles and ligaments are involved.

adjusts (reflexively) the lens for varying distances, stretch receptors in the ciliary body and the suspensory ligaments presumably send "messages" to the higher centers indicating the degree and direction of the adjustment. This point of view is quite old, having been advanced as early as 1709 by George Berkeley, Bishop of Cloyne, in his *A New Theory of Vision*. Bishop Berkeley, however, did not presume that accommodation resulted in an unlearned, primary cue for depth. Rather he felt that it had to be learned, integrated into the tactual-physical perception of depth.

Even today the efficacy of receptors in the accommodative muscles for indicating distance is in doubt. There is even some evidence that the *apparent* distance of the object rather than the real distance may determine the degree of accommodation.

In any event it is clear that feedback from the accommodative mechanism cannot be effective except for very restricted limits. For all intents and purposes the lens does not change shape for distances beyond 15 or 20 ft, and depth perception beyond such distances must be mediated by other means.

It has been further suggested (originally by the same Bishop Berkeley) that the "blur" arising form inadequate accommodation may not only serve to activate reflexively the accommodative mechanism, but also act as an indirect cue for distance. This again must be a relatively restricted cue, serving, if at all, for distances of less than 20 ft.

SECONDARY CUES

In contradistinction to the primary, or unlearned cues, most visual cues that do not require binocular vision are probably learned, hence, secondary cues. (Note the Gibson and Walk reading for a somewhat divergent point of view.) Let us examine some of the visual effects that might be interpreted as depth.

Size. When one has learned the normal, expected size of a familiar object, one can presumably estimate the distance of the object as a function of its apparent size or its size on the retina. A man has a known size. When two men are in the visual field and one is distinctly smaller than the other, the smaller figure is assumed to be farther away. Indeed, in visual illusion demonstrations, this effect of size can be shown to be more important than most other cues. We are familiar with the relative size of people, and if a man towers over, for example, a locomotive, we rarely see a "large man" and a "small locomotive." We tend to see a man nearby and a locomotive far away. Size differences were among the first cues for distance successfully employed by early artists. Before its use to depict distance, however, size difference was employed to indicate the relative importance of the various characters. The dominantly large figure in early Egyptian drawings, for example, indicated the importance of the character, rather than distance, which was apparently not recognized by these early artists.

Texture. A comparison of near and distant objects may also be observed as gradients in *texture*, as emphasized by James J. Gibson, and illus-

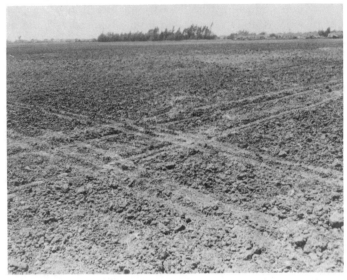

Texture

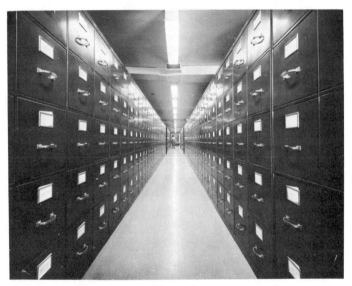

Perspective

Figure 10–2

Texture and perspective as cues for distance. [(*Top*) From *The Perception of the Visual World* by James J. Gibson. Copyright © 1950 by James J. Gibson. Reprinted by permission of Houghton Mifflin Company. (*Bottom*) Photograph courtesy of Herbert Gehr, *Life* Magazine, © Time, Inc.]

trated in Figure 10–2. For example, as a pilot brings an aircraft in for a landing, the closer terrain exhibits considerably more variety or texture, which gradually disappears in the textureless (relatively speaking) distance. As the texture builds up in front of him it must be clear that he is approaching the ground and moving in a forward direction. Note too that for the upright individual texture tends to decrease in an upward direction in the visual image. If the visual image were to be reversed 180° (with lenses, for example), texture gradients might very well provide confusing information as to distance.

Linear Perspective. Also related to size differences, parallel lines tend to decrease their separation as they recede into the distance, thus converging at some point known as the *vanishing point*, which may or may not be visible in the scene. The construction of drawings of satisfactory perspective for use in architecture, for example, is highly dependent on the location and use of various vanishing points, frequently positioned on the draftsman's drawing board, well beyond the limits of his actual drawing. Note in Figure 10–2 how all the parallel lines in the third dimension tend to converge. Linear perspective is one of the most convincing and most resistanct to misinterpretation of the large number of distance cues.

Partial Overlap. When one object appears to overlap a second object, it is generally assumed that the former is closer than the latter. Although this is most certainly a learned cue, it is again subject to error. If what appears to be the distant object is actually closer, but with a portion removed to fit the contour of the nearer but seemingly more distant object, perception of the true relationship is indeed difficult. Note in Figure 10–3 that the image seen (top) could result from either of the two stimulus situations below.

Shadowing. Both attached shadows—that is, where the shadow is part of the object—and cast shadows, in which the object produces the shadow, provide important cues for depth. Figure 10–4 illustrates these two forms of shadowing. The renowned Leonardo da Vinci recognized the efficacy of both attached and cast shadows as cues for distance, and used them profusely and with remarkable success in his paintings. They indeed present a convincing indication of distance.

In the lower part of the illustration of Figure 10–4 the quonset huts turn into towers when the picture is inverted. This must be a learned relationship. We recognize unconsciously that light normally comes from above, and we interpret our visual images in light of this anticipation. A metal tank with rivet heads protruding will normally have attached shadows on the bottom surface of the rivet heads. Were we to invert such a picture, the rivet heads would now look like dents in the surface, the shadow being on the upper surface of the dents where they logically belong.

Aerial Perspective. This cue for distance is in no way similar to the linear perspective discussed earlier. *Aerial* is really the key word in this cue for distance. Light from distance objects must pass through a much greater

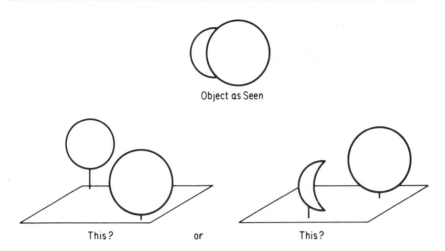

Figure 10–3
Overlap as a cue for distance. The figure as seen at the top could be produced by either of the two bottom arrangements.

amount of the atmospheric medium than light from nearby objects. Consequently, light arriving from a great distance has been subjected to considerable absorption and scattering from molecules of air, water vapor, and the minute solids suspended in the atmosphere. One result of this scattering is a lowering of the saturation or purity of color of distant objects. Pure or nearly pure colors appear to be weakened as if by the addition of white or black, resulting in tints or shades rather than the original pure hues. Such a hue can easily be incorporated in a painting by painting distant objects with less-saturated colors.

In addition, distant objects tend to take on the color of the ambient light, regardless of their own reflexive characteristics. In the daytime, distant objects tend to be bluish like the sky, or in the evening, reddish like the prevailing light at that time.

Movement Perspective. Another cut, also related to size, is that of movement perspective and related monocular parallax. It can be induced both by moving objects in the visual field and by head and eye movements on the part of the observer. Perhaps in the same way that size indicates distance, relative velocity of moving objects can also indicate distance. If you see a locomotive moving slowly along the horizon, you interpret this as great distance, whereas a locomotive moving across your visual field much more rapidly would be interpreted as being nearer. When you try estimating distances of flying objects such as airplanes or balloons, you have a great deal of trouble, largely because the actual speed of the objects is often unknown.

When you drive along in a car, the utility poles that seem to flash rap-

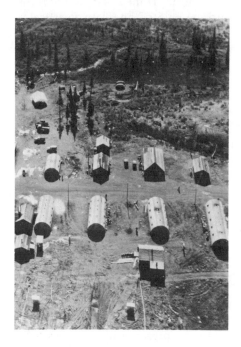

Figure 10–4
Shadows as a cue for distance. Rotate the photograph 180° to see the quonset huts change into towers. (From *The Perception of the Visual World* by James J. Gibson. Copyright © 1950 by James J. Gibson. Reprinted by permission of Houghton Mifflin Company.)

idly by are recognized as being closer than those that move by at a slower rate.

When you see objects moving by (or you move by them) you see more surface than for a stationary object. To the extent that the object is near, you see part of the leading surface as the object approaches, and the trailing surface as it recedes from view. Thus the degree of monocular parallax depends largely on distance. Near objects may even appear to "rotate" as you move past them, viewing them with an ever-changing line of regard. The fact that you can see some of the side of a solid object as you move past it is a strong indication of proximity.

Height in Visual Field. The cue of height in the visual field is often overlooked by investigators in the field. For terrestrial animals, nearby objects are usually located near the bottom of the visual field, and distant objects occupy a higher position. In many cases the gradation goes from bottom to center (horizon) and from directly above to center (horizon). Such cues have long been recognized. Indeed, the vanishing point we referred to earlier is frequently located on such an imaginary horizon. In early examples of prehistoric art the artist did not recognize the significance of a horizon or vanishing points; the relative vertical position of objects on the drawing is frequently the only indication of depth provided. The artist who wished to show objects farther away would simply place them higher in the picture.

Height in the visual field may also be related to the cue of cast shadows referred to earlier. Most vertical objects cast shadows, and in almost all cases the shadows are at the base of the object, or, generally speaking, in the lower part of the visual field.

Such a cue, like most others, is subject to misinterpretation. For example, the illusion in which the moon appears to be larger when near the horizon has been attributed to a misinterpretation of this cue. The explanation goes something like this: Being near the horizon, the moon is presumed to be at maximum distance. But, since it subtends the same visual angle regardless of where it is, the size-distance confusion produces an erroneous perception of large size.*

Binocular Cues for Depth

Although the preceding so-called monocular cues can be and surely are employed with binocular as well as monocular vision, the following cues owe their existence to the presence of two eyes—located spatially apart, which might, under normal circumstances, not be expected to view identical scenes. Our classification of primary and secondary cues is particularly tenuous in binocular vision. Perhaps all binocular cues are primary, perhaps they are all the result of learning; the matter is not settled. Let us, however, take the approach that convergence and retinal disparity serve as primary cues, the result of inborn structure and maturation, whereas binocular parallax as a cue for distance must be learned. The writer tends to lean in this direction, although the evidence is still controversial.

PRIMARY CUES

The two most commonly recognized unlearned cues are those of convergence (the eyes either converging or diverging as a function of distance) and retinal disparity (the fact that the two eyes receive different images from the same stimulus object).

Convergence. The theory that distance is indicated by sensations from receptors located in the extrinsic muscles of the eye employed in convergence was also a product of Bishop Berkeley's fertile mind. As with accommodation, he felt that cues based on convergence are learned, associated with body movements involved in reaching, positioning, and so on. But as in accommodation, the efficacy of feedback from the extrinsic muscles as a cue for distance is still open to question.

* For a modern, more complete analysis of the "moon illusion" the interested reader is referred to Restle (1970).

In line with Gregory's theory concerning the sensing of eye movements referred to in the last chapter, it may be that the cue is not impulses arising from the stretched or constricted muscles, but rather a parallel output from the effector nerves that evoke the convergence.

In any event, it is doubtful that convergence is an important cue for distance. At distances of 15 or 20 ft or so the lines of regard for the two eyes are in effect parallel, so the effect can at best be useful only at comparatively short distances. Perhaps, as in accommodation, the blur due to lack of registration of the two images may be as important as the muscular-evoked impulses, and may be the true basis for convergence as a cue for depth perception.

Retinal Disparity. What happens when the two eyes do not "see" the same thing? Any one of three effects can result from such a situation. As we noted in Chapter 8, ocular imbalance and phorias can be detected and measured by using a pair of stereograms such as shown in Figure 8–9. In this case the different views to the two eyes are *fused* into one picture containing the elements from both the right-eye and the left-eye view. In another demonstration often seen, an outline of a bird is presented to one eye and an empty bird cage to the other. The result, for the individual with normal vision, is a bird in a cage. In general, if the views can be meaningfully combined, fusion of the two images will result and the ultimate experience will be a combination of the two views. The key word for this effect is *fusion;* the organism must fuse the two images into a meaningful third image.

But what if the combination is not as logical as a bird in a cage or an arrow under a row of numerals; then what happens? In effect, the eyes simply refuse to function as a coordinated pair, and revert to independent operation, each on its own. If figures such as shown in the stereogram of Figure 10–7 are employed, the eyes "take turns" seeing. Known as retinal rivalry, and to be discussed later in this chapter, the result is an alternation between the left- and right-eye views. Sometimes there is partial fusion and part of the scene has a checkerboard pattern; sometimes one eye's view may predominate, but generally the result is an alternating of the two views.

In normal binocular vision, however, neither of the preceding situations predominate. The images produced by the two eyes are, indeed, slightly different because of the location of the eyes in the head, but these images, although slightly different, are capable of being fused.

The most significant feature of binocular vision that leads to depth perception is probably retinal disparity. The eyes are separated some 3 or 4 in. As a result, they do not "see" the same thing. The right eye sees a little of one side of an object and the left eye tends to see a portion of the other side. As early as 1838 the physicist Charles Wheatstone pointed out the importance of disparate images to the two eyes for the production of depth. As a result of his development of the stereoscope it was possible to show that a strong depth effect (*stereopsis*) can be produced when disparate images are presented to the two eyes. He further showed that the effect is destroyed if identical views are presented to the two eyes, or if the views are reversed—that is, the right-eye view presented to the left eye, and the left-eye view to the right eye. He was also able to demonstrate that if the disparity is increased (as if the interpupillary distance were greater than 3 or 4 in.), the illusion of depth is correspondingly enhanced.

The manner in which disparate images arrive at the retina can be seen from Figure 10–5. In this figure the observer is looking down on the truncated surface of the pyramid. Note the direction taken by the rays of light proceeding from the object to the eye. The right eye sees more of the right surface of the pyramid, and the left eye sees more of the left surface. The images on the retina would be much like the view drawn as (c). Indeed, if a stereogram were prepared like (c), with the correct images being presented to the left and right eyes, the visual experience would be identical to that obtained by looking directly down at the truncated surface.

This is all there is to the construction of stereograms and the experimental evocation of depth by means of disparate images, but the underlying physiological mechanism of the effect is much more illusive. As indicated in an earlier chapter, fibers from the retina do not appear to terminate in the brain in a manner replicating the retinal surface. Rather, if anything, they tend to replicate visual space. Note from Figure 6–4 that fibers to the left side of the brain arise from these portions of both retinas representing the right half of visual space. Conversely, potentials arising from stimuli in the left visual field are combined in the right side of the brain. This is a highly simplified description, but in general, it is about what happens.

Looking at Figures 6–4 and 10–5, we can see then that points represented by 2, 4, 6, and 8 in Figure 10–5 will fall in the left half of each retina, and hence be projected to the left side of the brain. But if we assume that points 2 and 8 are the same for both eyes, then points 4 and 6 will stimulate slightly disparate loci in the brain projection area. It is this disparity in the brain that presumably results in the most convincing stereoscopic or three-dimensional vision.

Indeed, it appears to be the fusion of corresponding points on the retina that makes retinal disparity work. If we present the top drawings of Figure 10–6 to the eyes by means of a stereoscope we can see depth. The left figure is that of a bar tilted in the third dimension, the right figure is of two circles, lying at slightly different distances from the viewer. If we supply anchoring points such as are shown in the lower figures, fusion occurs with less effort and the effect of depth is easier to obtain.

Although we can create an illusion of depth at will and understand many of the factors related to such hypothetical constructs as "corresponding points" on the retina, the underlying physiological mechanism in the

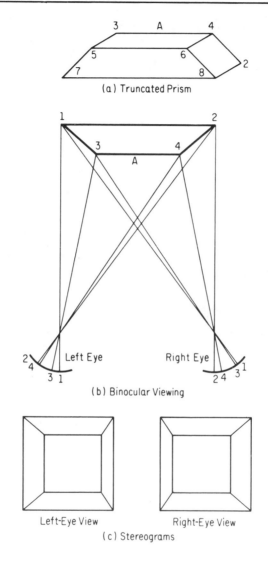

(a) Truncated Prism

(b) Binocular Viewing

Left-Eye View   Right-Eye View
(c) Stereograms

Figure 10-5
Stereoscopic vision: (b) shows the results of observing the truncated prism from a
point directly opposite the surface *A;* (c), when viewed in a suitable stereoscope,
would produce the same visual effect of depth.

brain remains an enigma. In some manner or other it works. One would be
hard put to design a computer that would carry out the operations accomplished so quickly and efficiently by the brain.

Utilization of disparate imagery to test an individual's depth perception or stereopsis is an important laboratory and clinical procedure. Your

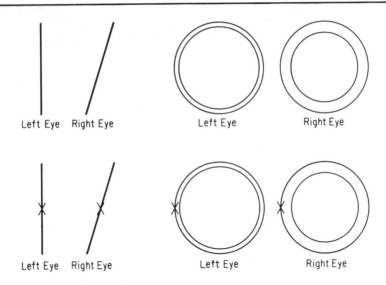

Figure 10–6
Anchoring points in stereopsis. The bottom figures with their anchoring points (shown by X's) are more easily seen in three dimensions than the top figures.

optometrist may, for example, give you tests with stereograms that result in a score in terms of percent stereopsis—a measure of how well you can utilize retinal disparity as a cue for distance. Another mensuration technique, somewhat more precise and more useful in research, determines the amount of disparity in angular distance required to produce stereopsis.

Persons to whom depth perception is of particular importance, such as athletes and airplane pilots, may be studied to determine their degree of depth perception. Most devices used to screen persons for inadequate depth perception are based on the ability to perceive depth as a function of disparate images.

When depth is utilized to enhance the realism of visual presentations, retinal disparity is the technique most often employed. You have all had some experience with the common stereoscope and the stereo camera, which simultaneously takes two pictures from slightly different angles. Means of presenting the results of such stereo photography to the respective eyes vary. One technique employs polarizing filters over the two projectors, and similar polarizing lenses in front of the eyes, so that the image meant for the left eye is delivered to that eye and the right-eye image finds its way to the right eye. In some cases colored filters are used, one image red and the other geren. With appropriate red and green filters over the eyes an illusion of depth can be created.

In many instances the depth effect can be enhanced by increasing (effectively) the interpupillary distance. Most binoculars have a somewhat wider separation than the human eye alone. In photography for stereo effects the cameras (or lenses) are often separated by a distance somewhat greater than the normal interpupillary distance, thus increasing the disparity between the left- and right-eye images.

Incidentally, visual stereopsis has been demonstrated for at least one bird. Fox et al. (1977) demonstrated the existence of stereopsis in the falcon, a bird that, unlike many of its kind, has binocular vision. Such a finding suggests that stereopsis may be a general attribute of vertebrate vision, and not limited to mammalian evolution.

SECONDARY CUES

The only secondary cue that depends on binocular vision for its existence is that of binocular parallax.

Binocular Parallax. We discussed under the heading "Movement Perspective" a form of parallax that presumably contributes to depth perception. With monocular vision we can see some of the sides of objects as a function of time if either the object or the viewer is in motion. With binocular vision we can see a bit of the sides of objects without time or movement, because the separation of the eyes permits us in effect to "see around" the object, at least if the distance is not great. It is quite possible that we learn to infer distance partially as a result of the amount of binocular parallax available—that is, the amount of the sides we can see.

Note too that objects at distances other than the fixation distance will not be optically superposed. Objects closer than the fixation point will result in crossed images, whereas objects at a distance will be separated on the retinal surface. Such an effect was hinted at when we were describing the effects of convergence, but probably should be included with binocular parallax effects.

Retinal Rivalry

We have discussed two of the effects that can result from the presentation of different images to the two eyes: (1) a combination of the two images to form a third, as illustrated by Figure 6–4, and (2) the perception of depth as a result of the neurological combining of the disparate images. The third possibility was also mentioned briefly, the alternation phenomenon known as retinal rivalry.*

If patterns such as those illustrated by Figure 10–7 are presented to the respective eyes, the result will be the alternate perception of the left-eye image and the right-eye image, with quite limited fusion and combination. The alternations may vary from several a minute to 50 or 60 a minute, depending on the pattern and factors inherent in the observer. What causes this alternation and of what significance is it? An answer to the first

---

* Actually the term *retinal* rivalry is probably a misnomer, since it is likely that the basis for the rivalry is to be found at a higher neural center.

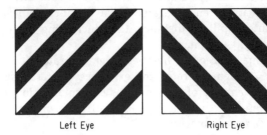

Left Eye   Right Eye

Figure 10-7
Retinal rivalry targets. When the targets are exposed to the respective eyes the result is alternating impressions of the two figures.

question is not possible in light of our present knowledge of the visual system. Presumably there is some physicochemical process, perhaps a metabolic-suppression cycle, that requires refreshing at frequent intervals. Just what it is eludes discovery.

We are fairly sure, however, that rivalry *does* have significance for depth perception. It appears likely that the fusion of disparate images is not a simultaneous perception of the combined images, but rather, at some neurological level, an alternation of the impulses from the two retinas. It is known that persons with rapid rivalry rates tend to have better stereopsis than those with slower rates. The more rapid suppression of the image from one eye and subsequent replacement with the image from the other goes along with superior depth pereception.

Which is cause and which is effect is not entirely clear. Does high rivalry rate produce improved stereopsis, or does good stereopsis result in high rivalry rate? In some severe clinical cases where the two eyes are markedly different optically, thus preventing normal fusion, no rivalry may exist. The patient, although he has two eyes providing two images, uses the image from only one eye, effectively suppressing the image from the other. To be sure, such people tend to have poor depth perception, because they must rely largely on such secondary cues as partial overlap, shadowing, and so on. We might also wonder if the permanent suppression of one eye by such people is physiologically the same as the alternate suppression by normal individuals.

With respect to the cause and effect question, many experts feel that good stereopsis is the result of high rivalry rate. Consequently, they use devices that present conflicting images alternately to the two eyes, slowly at first, and gradually increasing in alternation rate until the "normal" rivalry rate is simulated. As a result of such training, patients, it is said, increase their own true rivalry rates and at the same time their depth pereception is appreciably improved. For people with severe defects, resulting in complete monocular suppression, it would be necessary first to correct the physical defect for fusion of disparate images to be optically possible.

Although they do not really understand the basis for retinal rivalry, most practitioners *do* recognize its significance for adequate vision.

Summary

We have discussed in this chapter the recognition of depth and the use of binocular vision. We suggested that depth perception is both a matter of learning and a fundamental property of the visual mechanism. We described numerous indicators or cues for distance, some of which are presumably primary and some of which appear to be learned. Cues that do not require binocular vision include accommodation and blurring, size, texture, linear perspective, partial overlap, shadowing, aerial perspective, movement perspective, and height in the visual field. Cues based on the coordinated performance of two eyes included convergence, binocular parallax, and retinal disparity. In addition to describing the use of two eyes in producing depth, we also discussed binocular vision that does not result in depth, such as fusion of paired images and retinal rivalry.

Suggested Readings

1. E. J. Gibson and R. D. Walk, "The 'Visual Cliff'," *Scientific American*, April 1960. A short (9-page) article summarizing the recent literature on the nature-nurture issue with respect to visual depth perception employing the "visual cliff." It is an easy-to-read, interesting summary concluding that all animals seem able to avoid the drop as soon as they can move about.
2. From D. J. Weintraub and E. L. Walker. *Perception*. Belmont, Calif.: Brooks/Cole, 1966. Chapter 4 (18 pages) of this paperback is the best short summary and description of visual depth of which I am aware. It discusses depth perception from the philosophical and artist's approach as well as from the physio-psychological approach. It is well illustrated and makes quite interesting reading. It is not highly technical, but rather takes a "you are there" point of view.
3. A. H. Riesen. "Arrested Vision," *Scientific American*, July 1950. This is a short (five pages), concise summary of the early work on the influence of arrested vision on the development of form and spatial vision in the primate. It is certainly worthwhile reading and is highly recommended.
4. From J. J. Gibson. *The Perception of the Visual World*. Boston: Houghton Mifflin, 1950. Chapter 3 of this book, "The Visual Field and the Visual World" (18 pages) is relevant to the present chapter. Chapters 6 and 7 which consider the stimulus variables for visual depth and distance are particularly germane and are highly recommended. These 68 pages include many excellent illustrations of the cues we discussed, as well as a large number of variations. This entire book (230 pages) is highly recommended for the serious student.
5. Frank Restle. "Moon Illusion Explained on the Basis of Relative Size," *Science* 167 (1970): 1092–1096. This short article presents a modern approach to the explanation of the moon illusion, suggesting that the effect is a result of the broad extent of the horizon, rather than its apparent proximity.
6. John D. Pettigrew. "The Neurophysiology of Binocular Vision," *Scientific American*, August 1972. This is an excellently illustrated and well-written

article, worth any student's time. It traces the ability to locate objects visually to the activity of single nerve cells in the visual cortex of the brain.

7. From Gerald M. Murch. *Visual and Auditory Perception.* Indianapolis: Bobbs-Merrill, 1973. Pages 167 to 200 present visual space perception. It is easy to read, relatively thorough, and worth the student's time. Highly recommended.

8. From Irvin Rock. *An Introduction to Perception.* New York: Macmillan, 1975. One chapter of this excellent book was suggested for the preceding chapter. Several other chapters are quite appropriate for the material just covered. Chapters 3, 6, 7, 8, 9, and 10 are particularly relevant to our discussion of binocular vision and depth perception. This is a rather advanced book, but thorough in its presentation of more perceptually oriented topics.

11/color vision

Background

Contrary to a popular misconception, mammals are not the only animals capable of color discrimination. Man does have a very well-developed capability, possibly with a broader spectral sensitivity than most lower animals. Remember, however, the ultraviolet sensitivity of some insects, mentioned in Chapter 1. For all we know, many lower animals may have a sensitivity to wavelengths beyond one or both extremes of the human spectral range. In many invertebrates this is certainly true, at least at the violet (short wavelength) end of the spectrum (Wasserman, 1973).

But can lower animals make discriminations within their range of sensitivity? Common sense tells us that many can. The wide variety of coloration in flowers must have some survival value for insects, and the range of birds' plumage must be of use to them. Blue birds can probably recognize other blue birds, at least partially by their coloration. And a girl ladybug can probably recognize a boy ladybug somewhat more easily because of his color.

Accepting the near universality of color vision, let us now answer the questions, "What is color?" and "How is it sensed by the human?"

Nature of Color

Lights, paints, filters, and so on, are *not* colored. They merely produce, reflect, or transmit visible radiation in a selective manner, generating or passing some wavelengths, reflecting some, and absorbing others. Color, like beauty, is in the eye of the beholder. It is an experience that depends primarily, although not exclusively, on the wavelength of the light that stimulates the eye, light being simply electromagnetic radiation within a highly restricted range, as indicated earlier, from about 400 to 700 mμ (see Figure 1–1). Light can be measured physically in terms of its dominant wavelength, its overall composition, and its intensity. The eye and its associated computer see the combination of these physical parameters as "color." In addition to the attribute that varies as a function of the wavelength and is identified as *hue*, there may also be an attribute of *saturation* as a function of the purity of the light, and one of *brightness* as a result of its intensity. These three psychological attributes—hue, saturation, and brightness (sometimes called *lightness*)—serve to identify *any* color, and in this sense both black and white must be considered to be colors. Hues other than black and white (and, of course, gray) are considered to be *chromatic* colors, whereas those in the white through black range are *achromatic*. Let us examine these three attributes of color with the intent of relating the psychological experience to the physical characteristics of the light.

HUE

The most obvious characteristic of any color is its hue. Is it red, yellow, green, blue, or some intermediate hue? Or is it achromatic—that is, lacking in hue, such as black, white, or some shade of gray? If a color has a recognizable hue it may be located on the visible spectrum of Figure 11–1. Note that a light consisting of a single wavelength of 510 mμ will be seen as green; one of 520 mμ will also be green, but a slightly different green, whereas orange will result from a wavelength of roughly 600 mμ, the precise location depending on the rather arbitrary standard of the individual. As a matter of fact, the number of discriminable hues that can be identified on the scale of Figure 11–1 is in the hundreds for the person with average sight.

Colors as normally observed in nature, however, are rarely produced by a single wavelength such as in these examples. Although sunlight and incandescent light are made up of a continuous spectrum, that is, energy continuous throughout most of the visible spectrum, there are a few sources of monochromatic, or near monochromatic light. Sodium vapor lamps, often employed as street lights, produce visible energy of several specific wavelengths, primarily in the yellow portion of the spectrum, and mercury lamps, often employed for the same purpose, have their line spectra in the blue. Ordinarily fluorescent lamps produce light of several wavelengths, depending on the chemical deposition on the inside surface of the tube, but not continuous throughout the spectrum. Known as a *line spectrum*, the output of this common light source is seen as white, because the visual mechanism performs an integrative function on the various independent wavelengths.

Most colors are combinations of many wavelengths, and the resultant experience of hue arises from complex activity of the visual mechanism. We refer, then, in the case of complex patterns of wavelengths to the *ap-*

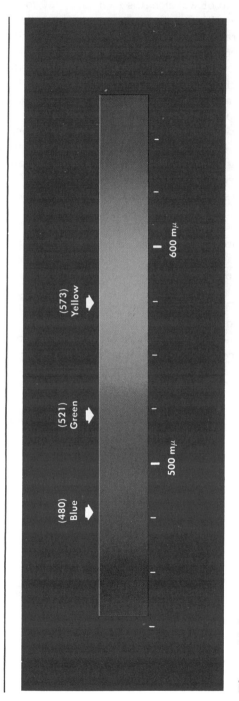

Figure 11-1
Approximate spectral colors.

parent hue or perhaps the *dominant wavelength* of the color. If, for example, a light is made up of wavelengths from, say, 560 to 640 mμ (yellow to red), unless the intensities of the components differ greatly, the color will look like the general center of the wavelength distribution. In this case the result would be much like that produced by a 600-mμ stimulus, and we would refer to the experience as orange. We would say the color has a dominant wavelength of 600 mμ and an orange hue.

Suppose we have only two equally intense wavelengths, one of 560 mμ (yellow) and one of 640 mμ (red). Will we see orange now, even though no 600 mμ orange light is present? Indeed we will. In this case the apparent or dominant hue will be orange, the midpoint of the distribution, even though no wavelengths normally associated with orange are present. We can generalize: for wavelengths relatively close in the visible spectrum, the visual experience will be equivalent (in hue) to some "balance" point within the range of the individual components. If the yellow hue in our example were much more intense than the red, then the apparent hue would shift toward a yellowish orange (equivalent to 590 mμ, perhaps) and, conversely, if the red component were more intense the experience might be one of reddish orange. Note too that a similar orange could be produced by many different pairs of reds and yellows. Pairs of colors that produce the same apparent third color are known as *metameric* pairs. The combinations look alike but the composition differs.

What happens if the component hues are *not* nearby in the spectrum? To understand and predict the results of such combinations we need a so-called color circle, such as is shown in Figure 11–2.

SATURATION

Figure 11–2 shows the influence of the second psychological attribute, saturation, as determined by the purity of a color. When we obtained an orange by combining red and yellow light, we did indeed obtain an orange of the same hue as we could have produced with a pure wavelength. But it was not the same orange. The orange of a 600-mμ apparent wavelength would be less pure, less saturated, than a similar orange produced by an actual wavelength of 600 mμ. We can explain this in terms of the complementary nature of colors.

The circumference of the color circle of Figure 11–2 shows the relative location of pure spectral colors from red at one extreme to violet at the other.* A unique feature of many hues is that, when paired, they produce achromatic colors. As the color circle is drawn, any diameter of the circle will connect complementary colors, colors that when combined produce white or gray. Specifically, as examples, red and blue-green when com-

---

* What about the purple, shown between the red and the violet in Figure 11–2? Purple is a nonspectral color. It does not exist in the spectrum and therefore cannot be extracted from white light by means of prismatic refraction. It can be created by mixing spectral red and violet and is necessary to an understanding of the complete color cycle. Hence its inclusion.

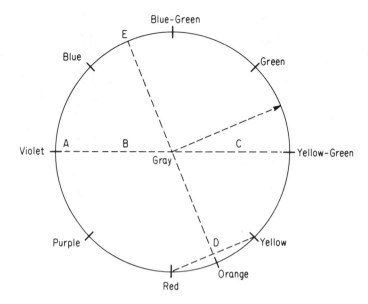

Figure 11-2
The color circle. The circumference represents saturated, pure colors. Broken lines shown as diameters of the circle represent variations in saturation. Note that the orange indicated at *D* could be produced either with a mixture of red and yellow or orange plus gray.

bined in the proper ratio produce an achromatic gray or white, as do violet and yellow-green, or blue and yellow.

But blue and yellow make green, don't they? The answer to this question is both yes and no. When we combine blue and yellow pigments, we do indeed get green, but when we combine blue and yellow light (of the proper wavelength and intensity), we get gray or white. The former is called *subtractive* color mixing, the latter, *additive* color mixing. Note the schematic illustration of additive and subtractive color mixing shown in Figure 11-3. The colors are not true in this example, but the principle of color mixing should be apparent.

In subtractive color mixing, a surface or filter is yellow not because it produces yellow light, but because it absorbs the blue end of the white ambient spectrum. The blue pigment is blue because it absorbs the red portion of the ambient light. If we remove both the red and blue ends of the spectrum, what is left? Only the center, or green, portion of the spectrum remains. Hence blue and yellow pigments result in green, not white, as with additive mixtures. Note too that when we additively combine all colors, we produce white. But when we systematically remove all colors, in subtractive color mixing, what is left? Nothing—or in terms of the visual experience, black.

Let us return to Figure 11-2 and the concept of saturation. As just

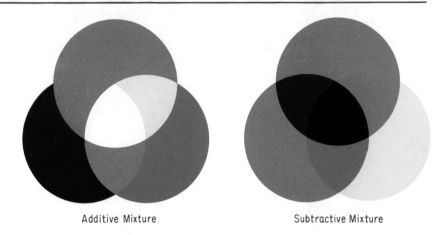

Additive Mixture   Subtractive Mixture

Figure 11–3
Color mixture. The figure on the left illustrates the results of combining lights of three
colors. The figure on the right indicates what may happen when pigments or colored
filters are combined. The figures are merely illustrative, and the actual colors shown
in the figure would probably not be obtained in practice.

mentioned, if we combine a violet light and a yellow-green light in the
proper proportions (depending on the relative spectral sensitivity of the
eye) we get a gray, indicated by the center of the color circle. But with
anything other than perfect proportions, the result will be a location on a
line between the two primaries—not at the center of the circle—resulting
in either a violet of less than perfect saturation (< 1.00) or a yellow-green
of a saturation less than 1.00. If, for example, our mixture is predominantly
violet, resulting in a color at A, the experience will be almost pure violet;
if we have only slightly more violet than yellow-green, the result may be
found to occur at B. This experience would be of a very low saturation of
violet, perhaps just gray with a violet cast to it. If our proportions were
such that the composite fell at C the result would be a yellow-green of intermediate saturation, perhaps 0.50. In a similar manner, any hue can be
"desaturated" by adding to it its complementary. Remember the hue does
not change, only the saturation or purity.

With respect to our example of combining spectral red and yellow, assuming equal effective intensities, the resultant hue will be orange, halfway
between the red and the yellow at a point indicated by D. But this point
has a saturation of less than 1.00. It is no longer on the circumference of
the circle where the spectral hues must be located. It could have been produced by adding a bit of the blue hue between blue and blue-green (E) to the
pure, spectral orange. The experienced colors would have been indistin-
guishable to the normal human eye.

An important fact may be observed. Although any hue can be obtained
by combining two noncomplementary hues, resultant saturations must

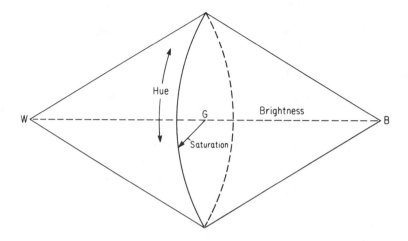

Figure 11–4
The color solid. Hue is located around the circle, saturation is the distance from the central line to the surface, and brightness or lightness is shown as the longitudinal axis.

always be less than 1.00. Note that we could produce violet by combining red and the spectral color indicated by E. But note too that the line for violet would cross the red-greenish blue line at about B, where we have already indicated the experience would be little more than gray with a violet cast to it. The hue would indeed be violet, but the saturation would be so low as to make the color useless.

This limitation poses a problem to those who deal in color-mixing applications. When one is limited to three primaries, such as in color films or color television, only three hues can have maximum saturation, and all other hues must be tints or shades of the resultant composite colors. We will discuss this problem again when we consider methods for specifying colors for commercial application.

BRIGHTNESS

Terms such as *white, gray, black, tint,* and *shade* have been used without adequately defining them. To understand the concept of brightness we must add a third dimension to our circle. The result, shown in Figure 11–4, is a color solid, a double-ended cone with *brightness* (the psychological correlate of intensity) running along the longitudinal axis. In this figure the center axis represents achromatic colors from white at one end to black at the other. All pure colors are located on the surface, with saturation diminishing as the center axis is approached. Thus any color can be located in the three dimensions of the solid by simply stating its apparent hue, saturation, and brightness.

Those colors found to the left of the midpoint—that is, of higher brightness—and approaching the gray center line are called *tints*. Pastel colors are colors of relatively low saturation and high brightness. *Shades* are simply darker colors lying to the right of the midline of Figure 11–4.

Color Specification

The utilization of the color experience can range all the way from the prosaic matching of pastel colors in milady's boudoir to the spectral analysis of radiation from distant stars. Although many primitive tribes may have gotten along quite nicely with only three or four words to describe color, our complex civilization utilizes literally millions of color differences describable by words. The number of actual color words is far less, but there are an enormous number of the possible visual experiences and compound verbal expressions. Deane Judd, for example, has estimated that there are 10 million distinguishable color differences describable by words.

In spite of the possibility of such a large number of terms, a simple classification, based on the names people give to their experience of color, should be useful from a practical standpoint. Such a classification would, to be sure, depend somewhat on the culture of the persons involved. Whorf (1956) and others have shown clearly how linguistics and culture influence color naming and even color recognition. One rather simplistic example of color naming is given in Table 11–1. Although this table gives a rather long list, note the many colors that are not there: nile green, teal blue, canary yellow, shocking pink, navy blue, fuchsia. Artists, of course, have another language classification, sometimes based on the content of their pigments: cobalt blue, Prussian blue, chrome green, and so on. Certainly our recognition of color is greatly influenced by our culture.

It should be obvious that popular color names are not sufficiently precise for scientific and technical application. If two companies made a paint called sea green would they be highly similar in appearance? Surely not.

In addition to the physicists' spectral analysis and specification of dominant wavelength and physical composition of the light, several other approaches to the specification of color are available. Based on the experience of colors, and including therefore the behavior of the normal human eye, these approaches are of great value in commercial applications from color television to the design of textiles.

THE MUNSELL SYSTEM

The Munsell system utilizes sample "chips" of color, varying in hue, chroma, and value. The sample plate included as Fig. 11–5 is one page from the Munsell *Book of Color* and is for a hue defined as 5YR, with a dominant wavelength of 589 mμ.

The Munsell and similar systems plot the *appearance* of the color, not its composition. Munsell reasoned that the appearance of color is apparent in objects, so the result is a series of surface colors varying in appearance, with a well-defined nomenclature. The system identifies color in terms of

TABLE 11-1
Typical Hue Names Associated
with Spectral Energy Bands

Approximate Wavelength (nm)	Associated Hue
380–470	Reddish blue
470–475	Blue
475–480	Greenish blue
480–485	Blue-green
485–495	Bluish green
495–535	Green
535–555	Yellowish green
555–565	Green-yellow
565–575	Greenish yellow
575–580	Yellow
580–585	Reddish yellow
585–595	Yellow-red
595–770	Yellowish red*

* A pure red with no tinge of yellow requires some blue. That is, a "pure" red is extraspectral and cannot be produced with a single wavelength.

From R. W. Burnham, R. M. Hanes, and C. J. Bartleson, *Color: A Guide to Basic Facts and Concepts.* Copyright © 1963. Reprinted by permission of John Wiley & Sons, Inc.

three attributes: hue, value, and chroma, ordered into scales of equal visual steps. These scales are employed for the specification and description of color under various conditions of illumination and viewing. Based on the *Atlas of Color*, published in 1915, a continuous development and refinement of the system has resulted in a highly workable and almost universally accepted method for color specification.

Notations in the Munsell system include hue (H), the position of a color in relation to a visually equal-spaced scale of 100 hues. Thus the 40 hues, each on a single page of the Munsell *Book of Color*, represent less than one-half the total hues of the system. The 100 hues are grouped into ten major hues: Red, Yellow-Red, Yellow, Green-Yellow, Green, Blue-Green, Blue, Purple-Blue, Purple, and Red-Purple. Symbols used to indicate hue may be such as R, YR, Y, GY, and so on, or if greater precision is required, identification numerals from 1 to 100.

A second notation is that of value (V), which indicates the degree of lightness or darkness of a color in relation to a neutral gray scale extending from absolute black to absolute white. With respect to notation, numerals from 0/ to 10/ are employed to represent value, with 0/ being absolute black, 10/ absolute white, and 5/ a middle gray and with all

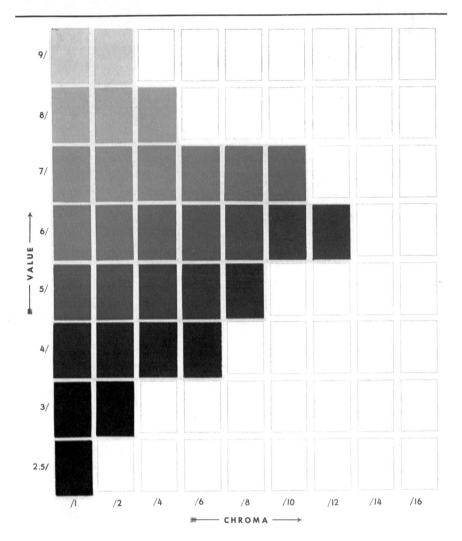

Figure 11–5
Sample page from the Munsell Book of Color. The hue for this sample is 5YR, the 5 representing a Munsell code and the YR yellowish red. (Courtesy of Munsell Color.)

chromatic colors between black and white. In Figure 11–5 value is expressed on the vertical axis.

The third, and final notation is that for chroma (C) and indicates the distance of a color from a neutral gray of the same value. The horizontal dimension in Figure 11–5 represents the chroma. Notations are in the form of /0 for a neutral gray or achromatic color up to as high as /16. For example, a particular red hue of intermediate value might have a chroma of /4 and be called "rose" or a chroma of /14 and be recognized as "vermillion." For specifying any specific color the value of these attributes are combined in the notation, for example, 5R 5/4 for "rose" and 5R 5/14 for "vermillion."

THE OSTWALD SYSTEM

The Ostwald system of color specification is in many respects similar to the Munsell approach. It, however, is based more directly on the double-cone depiction of Figure 11–4 with, for example, equal numbers of steps in the saturation dimension for all hues. It is, presumably, based more on psychophysical than psychological variables. Its variables appear to be more like dominant wavelength, purity, and relative luminosity, rather than hue, saturation, and brightness. As a result, its forced symmetry, in contradistinction to the asymmetry of the Munsell system, leaves it vulnerable to the accusation that it does not truly depict color experience.

ICI SYSTEM

The system of specifying color, or chromaticity, developed by the previously mentioned International Commission on Illumination is probably the most useful approach from the standpoint of technical design and application. It is *not* based on psychological experiential data, as are the Munsell or Ostwald systems. Rather it is based on a series of international agreements defining a luminosity curve for a standard eye (see Chapter 7), color-mixture curves for three imaginary standard lights, energy distributions for three basic ambient light sources, and other necessary appurtenances.

The system is quite precise and exceedingly useful for defining and describing such things as filters, pigments, color combinations, and ambient lighting, and their ultimate visual result for the hypothetical standard observer. The system can predict the appearance of various pigment mixtures under differing ambient conditions. Three sources of light known as illuminants A, B, and C ranging from the red incandescent to the bluish north sky are defined, and can be used in the diagram to predict their visual result. It is an excellent, well-developed technique for indicating the psychophysical results of visible energy.

We cannot, within the limits of this chapter, go into the ICI system in any great detail. The interested reader is encouraged to consult the pertinent sources at the end of the chapter.

Let us examine briefly how the system defines color. The ICI chromaticity diagram, as utilized for several purposes, is shown in Figures 11–6 and 11–7.

If we look back at Figure 11–2, we see that we can define a hue by two primaries; in our earlier example of producing orange, we used red and yellow. But if we wish to locate a color anywhere within the circle, we must utilize a third primary. Again returning to Figure 11–2, to produce lower saturations of orange, with the same red and yellow primaries, we would have to add some of the primary indicated as E. Hence, three primaries are needed to make any desired color.

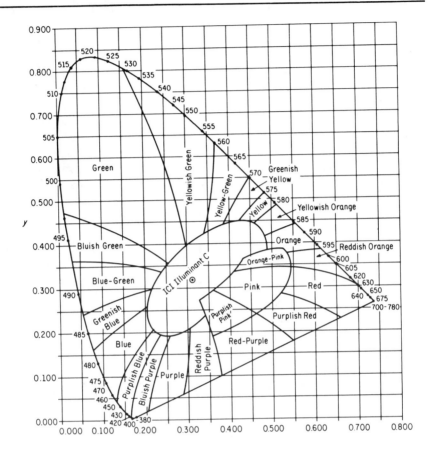

Figure 11-6
ICI chromaticity diagram showing approximate location of colors. The abscissa *x* is the ratio of the tristimulus value *X* to the sum of all three (*X* + *Y* + *Z*); the ordinate *Y* is the ratio of *Y* to this sum. (From NBS Circular 478, National Bureau of Standards.)

The three hues selected by the ICI for universal primaries were previously referred to as *standard lights* and their proportions needed to match a given sample are known as *tristimulus values*. The numerals along the side of the figure and identified as *x* and *y* are the tristimulus values for *x* and *y*, respectively. But what about the value of *z*? The total light can be defined as the sum of the *x*-, *y*-, and *z*-components. In proportinal units, the value of any one is, obviously, one minus the sum of the other two. Hence if we know the values of *x* and *y* (the red and green primaries, respectively) the value of *z* is determined and need not be plotted separately.

The numerals on the curved portion of the perimeter represent spectral hues, and nonspectral purples and magentas fall on the straight-line portion at the base.

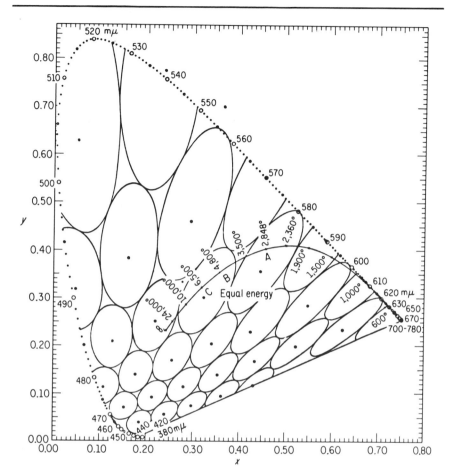

Figure 11–7

ICI chromaticity diagram showing equally perceptible differences. The distance from points on the boundary of each ellipse to the indicated point within it all correspond, approximately, to 100 times the just perceptible chromaticity difference under certain specific viewing conditions. (From NBS Circular 478, National Bureau of Standards.)

Approximate location for various colors and the location of the ICI illuminant C are shown in Figure 11–6. Although this specific diagram is based on work by Kelly, involving the description of colored lights on a dark background, it is acceptable as an aid to understanding the general ICI diagram. Note that the wavelength we referred to as orange (600 mμ) is classed as "reddish orange" in this diagram. Notice too the tints, or pastel colors (such as pink) as one moves in a direction of lower saturation and approaches the "white" center of the ICI diagram.

Figure 11–7 illustrates several different additional properties of the diagram. Note the curved line passing through the three illuminants. This line shows equivalent chromaticities for various color temperatures. If you know the color temperature of your camera flashbulbs or your movie lights, you could locate their chromaticity on this line. Would this be of value to you? If you knew, further, the tristimulus values of your subject, you would know just how the subject would look under your own special illuminant. Manufacturers can predict how a given enamel surface on a refrigerator will look under a known form of illumination in the purchaser's kitchen.

Notice, too, the location of the three standard illuminants and the point of equal energy. At this latter point the tristimulus values are all .33—in other words, equal amounts of the red, green, and blue primaries are indicated for this point. Illuminant A, as indicated earlier, is representative of incandescent light, heavily weighted with red (roughly 45 percent), whereas illuminant C, corresponding in a general way to light from the northern sky, is made up of only a little more than 30 percent of the red primary.

The oval areas represent another useful application of the ICI chromaticity diagram. They show, in pictorial fashion, equally perceptible differences in color or chromaticity. Actually the distance from each point to the circumference of the respective oval represents 100 times the just perceptible chromaticity difference; in our earlier language, 100 jnd's in chromaticity or color.

THE LAND EFFECT

Although it is in no way as complete a color classification system as the preceding three, the system of color production demonstrated by Edwin Land (1959, 1964) should be mentioned. The Land system is intriguing in that it purports to produce most color experiences by means of just two primaries instead of the three required in other systems. One example follows: A colored scene is photographed twice with black and white film; once with a red filter and once with a green filter. The film is processed as black and white transparencies, later projected and superimposed on a screen. The slide taken with the red filter is projected through a red filter but no filter is employed with the other transparency. It is hard to believe, but the full range of colors in the original scene (or nearly so) can be observed. It would appear that under some circumstances fewer than three primaries are needed to produce the normal range of hues.

Color Vision Theory

Any theory of how the organism "sees" color must take into consideration the phenomenological experience of color. Most people have agreed on the existence of fundamental hues. Red, green, blue, and yellow "appear" to be basic hues, and all color theories attempt to account for the basic color experience of these so-called primaries.

There are two basically antagonistic groups of theories to explain color vision. One of these, the *opponent* theory, first advanced by Ewald Hering in 1874, holds that there are antagonistic systems at work; thus, white and black are opposites, red is the opposite of green, and blue is the opposite of yellow. According to these theories, there must be some sort of antagonistic neurochemical behavior as the base of the experience.

The *component* theories, first advanced by Thomas Young in 1801 and elaborated by Helmholtz, Ladd-Franklin, and others, considers that there are individual components—cones, if you will—"tuned" for different wavelengths, and that the chemical-neural response is basically the same for all hue experiences.

Let us examine these two approaches in more detail, noting some of the evidence for both.

THE OPPONENT THEORIES

In the opponent theory, paired colors are said to elicit opposing responses. Thus the sensation of red is, chemically and neurologically, the opposite of the green experience. Presumably, one might be considered to be an anabolic process and the other essentially catabolic. They are not entirely unlike the reversible reactions found in chemistry.

Evidence in support of such theories was once largely phenomenological. For example, negative afterimages and simultaneous-contrast effects can both be explained quite nicely with an opponent-type theory. When one gazes at a red figure for some time and then looks away at a gray surface, he sees a negative afterimage of the red figure. The afterimage is green, the complementary color for red as plotted on the conventional color circle. Similarly, gazing at a yellow figure results in a blue afterimage. According to opponent theory, when the "red" process is active one sees red, when the red stimulus is removed the process reverses itself and the effect is a green afterimage produced by the reverse chemical reaction.

Simultaneous-contrast effects, such as when one gazes at a green figure on a gray background and the latter tends to appear reddish, can also be accounted for by the theory. The only requirement is the presence of lateral connections in the retina, and these have long been known to exist.

Historically, there has been a severe weakness in the opponent theories. Like the ophthalmologist who could find no tubules between the ciliary body and the lens, early researchers were unable to identify, or even conceive of any physiological mechanism by which such color effects might be achieved. With the advent of microelectrode technology in recent years, however, evidence for an opponent theory has somewhat greater support. DeValois (1965), for example, has shown antagonistic wave patterns from a single nerve cell in the lateral geniculate nucleus as a function of the color of a stimulating light. Red and green result in opposite reactions, as do yellow and blue. Moreover, responses of the cells in the lateral geniculate are greatly influenced by prior adaptation of the retina. After a prolonged adaptation to a green light, the "red" neural response can be evoked by a much wider range of spectral stimuli than before.

Subjective Color. An interesting phenomenon best explained by an opponent theory and the temporal factors of DeValois is that of subjective color.* It has long been recognized that the viewing of certain patterns consisting of high-contrast stripes, herringbone designs, and so on, may result in the sensation of color, especially if the patterns are moving. It is indeed difficult to conceive how "tuned" receptors in the retina could be activated differentially to such monochromatic stimuli.

A well-known example of subjective colors is that produced by the Benham disk, illustrated in Figure 11-8. If the disk is rotated at optimum speed (on the order of 8 to 12 rotations per second), the four sets of thick lines will take on four different hues. The outside set may be blue, the inside set red, with the other two sets taking on intermediate hues. If the direction of rotation is reversed, the location of the hues is reversed, the outside set being red and the innermost lines blue. Paradoxically, it makes little difference what sort of light is used to illuminate the rotating disk. Even with red light the lines appear colored from red through blue. Saturation is poor, and some practice may be necessary in order to identify the colors. But with practice in the effect, the appearance of the "subjective" colors is astonishing.

The only explanation which seems reasonable is that when the "on-off" responses of the retinal elements are such as to produce pulse trains in the neural fibers that duplicate those of colored stimuli (note the work of DeValois), the experience is one of color.

An entrepreneur in California with a scientific bent adopted the Benham top principle to black-and-white television. In a commercial for a well-known soft drink, he produced an alternating or flashing signal, presumably duplicating the time relations of the lines on the Benham disk. The result was supposed to be the soft drink trademark in color, and all on black-and-white television. In spite of the fact that the signal flickering at 10 to 12 cycles per second proved to be rather distracting, a few astonished viewers did notice the "color" and wrote or called their respective television stations.

COMPONENT THEORIES

As a class, component theories all hold that there are different kinds of receptors in the retina. Some cones are "tuned" to one color, some to another, the finer nuances in the ultimate color experience being mediated through stimulation of combinations of these "tuned" receptors. Until recently the nature of structural or chemical differences in the receptors was unknown and presented the greatest difficulty for the component theory adherents.

The Young-Helmholtz Theory. Traditionally the most popular theories for color were those based on the original work of Thomas Young and developed by Hermann Helmholtz (a contemporary and rival of Ewald

---

* The interested reader is directed to the Cohen and Gordon reading at the end of the chapter for numerous examples of subjective color, their history, and possible explanations.

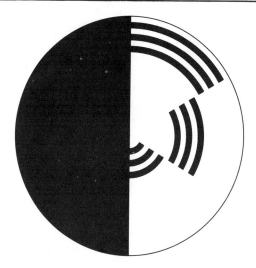

Figure 11–8
The Benham disk. When the disk is rotated at the proper speed, the sets of segmented lines are seen in color, ranging from an unsaturated red to a deep blue.

Hering), Christine Ladd-Franklin, James Clerk Maxwell, and others. Young's original primaries of red, yellow, and blue were replaced by red, green, and blue, but the original theory of Young remained essentially unchanged.

Phenomenological results of color mixing agree closely with the hypothesis of individual receptors in the retina for red, green, and blue. Moreover, the phenomena of color adaptation and afterimages mentioned before do not disprove the theory. Whatever color vision may be, it *is* trichromatic. There are three fundamental hues, and whether their recognition depends on constructs of a component theory or an opponent theory, their existence cannot be denied.

Recent work on the chemistry of vision tends to support a component theory. Just as rhodopsin was demonstrated to be the substance of importance for rod vision, so was *iodopsin* identified as the chemical ingredient of the cones. Wald first isolated this substance from cones of the chicken eye, gave it its name, and showed that it underwent a bleaching action similar to that of rhodopsin. Iodopsin was shown to have an absorption spectrum with its maximum at 565 mμ as contrasted with rhodopsin's 500 mμ maximum. In light of the Purkinje shift, such a difference was just about what might have been expected.

Wald, Rushton, and others proceeded to analyze iodopsin, further breaking it down into two constituents, one known as *chlorolabe* ("catch the green"), the other, *erythrolabe* ("catch the red"). Rushton found that persons unable to perceive red are lacking in erythrolable and persons with green color blindness have an insufficiency of chlorolabe. Persons with normal color vision, on the other hand, have both of these substances in their iodopsin.

There still remained the identification of a "blue catcher" to be named *cyanolabe*. It was not until 1964 that several workers independently were able to demonstrate conclusively the existence of a "catch the blue" substance. The substance finally demonstrated by Marks, Dobelle, and MacNichol at Johns Hopkins and Brown and Wald at Harvard had an absorption maximum at 450 mμ, most definitely in the blue region. These researchers also showed that the three substances were not mixed indiscriminately within a single cone. They found that one and only one of the three substances was present in a single cone. Thus after 160 years the original hypothesis of Thomas Young that three types of "tuned" receptors exist was finally proven.

The Ladd-Franklin Theory. Both phylogenetic and (to some extent) evolutionary evidence tend to support the component theory. The theory of Christine Ladd-Franklin is especially interesting. She reasoned that when vision first developed it was little more than sensitivity to light, and primitive eyes were essentially scotopic devices, probably limited to the elements we now recognize as rods. To creatures with such eyes, light was simply light, and color did not exist.

However, by a mutation (more likely very many mutations) some animals developed the ability to distinguish not only light from darkness, but the extremes of the visible spectrum. That is, they could distinguish between the high and low ends, or what we might refer to loosely as "blue" and "yellow" light. Presumably some organisms developed two kinds of "cones" while still retaining their rods; others (e.g., birds) did not retain their rod vision, their retinas containing only cones.

Still later in evolution the elements sensitive to yellow underwent a further division, making possible a discrimination between "red" at one end and "green" at the other. Thus the animal had three kinds of cones, those sensitive to blue, those sensitive to green, and those sensitive to red. Any intermediate colors (including yellow) could, of course, arise from the simultaneous stimulation of more than one of these three types of receptors.

There is at least a modicum of evidence in support of the evolutionary theory. Evidence in general supports the notion that color discrimination improves as one goes up the phylogenetic scale. Man, in contrast with many lower animals, has excellent color vision. The relationship between position on the phylogenetic scale and color vision sophistication is not perfect: mammals other than man appear to be lacking in color vision, in general possessing no cones; some insects appear to have excellent color vision; and birds, as indicated previously, have retinal elements consisting exclusively of cones. Nevertheless, there is a general trend toward increased color discrimination with higher position in the phylogenetic scale. The possibility of discontinuities in the evolutionary process and the branching out and specializing by lower species can account for the lack of a simple linear progression from the simple one-celled animals to man. No one has ever claimed that evolution must follow an orderly, single path from simple to complex.

If color vision did indeed develop through evolution in this manner would there not be additional evidence? There should be and there is. One might expect that the first mutations from scotopic to photopic vision would take place at the fovea of the eye, with further development proceeding in a radial direction. Later mutations would likewise start in the center, developing outward from the fovea. In support of this supposition, we find that the more highly developed cones are indeed located in the fovea, whereas rods are more peripherally located.

If we map the color-sensitive areas of the eye with a device known as a perimeter (Figure 11–9), we can determine the areas of the retina sensitive to different spectral radiation. In line with the theory we would expect that the "older" color zones would have migrated out from the fovea and that the "newer" areas, those sensitive to red and green, would be smaller. Results of such experiments are also shown in Figure 11–9. Note that the area sensitive to blue is much larger than that for red or green, as if it perhaps has been developing for many more eons than the johnny-come-lately red-green vision. The area sensitive to yellow is approximately the same as the blue-sensitive area.

As with most theories, there are weaknesses in the original Ladd-Franklin approach. The specific wavelengths for the primaries as originally defined have since been proved unsatisfactory, and some data based on knowledge of color blindness fail to support the theory in its details. As a general approach, however, the emphasis on evolutionary development seems to be useful. But some details and discrepancies in the theory must be worked out and/or eliminated before it can receive universal acceptance.

What about color blindness? Can this condition be accounted for with the constructs and language of component theory? The answer to this question is, in general, yes. In fact, its ability to account for color blindness and color weakness is one of the theory's greatest strengths.

MODERN THEORY

Before looking at color blindness, let us give some attention to several recent developments in color vision research, much of which seems to cast doubt on the relatively simplistic theories previously described. Although much of the following does not bear directly on color theory, it does involve colored stimuli and seems to be more appropriate for this section of your text than any other. Vision, especially color vision, is not as simple as Hering and Helmholtz seemed to believe. Indeed, the title of this paragraph is probably misleading: There is no modern, comprehensive theory. There are many findings, many facts, most of which do not dovetail into classical theory in a simple and logical manner. We cannot go into these findings in great detail or in a highly critical manner, but the interested reader should find the references to be excellent jumping-off

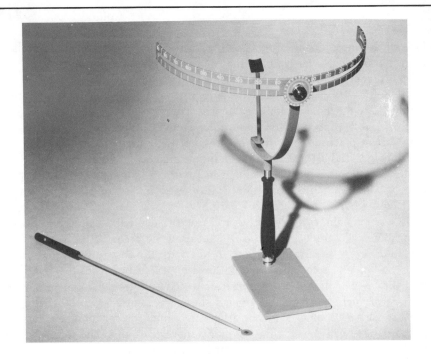

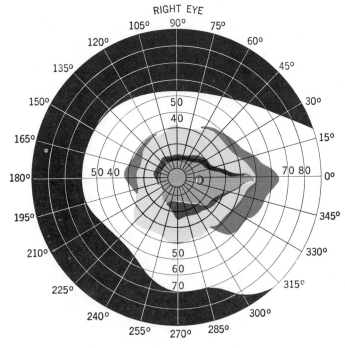

Figure 11-9
Perimetry. (*Top*) An instrument, the perimeter, used to determine color zones of the retina. (*Bottom*) The results of such a determination, with the four color zones and the rod-mediated achromatic zone identified by the appropriate colors. [(*Top*) Photograph courtesy of Lafayette Instrument Company. (*Bottom*) From *Psychology*, 5th edition, by Norman L. Munn. Copyright © 1966 by Norman L. Munn. Reprinted by permission of Houghton Mifflin Company.]

points for more serious inquiry. Let us look into some of these recent findings.

Considerable recent research on color vision focuses on portions of the visual system higher than the retina. Note the earlier reference to the Benham disk and the work of DeValois. As a further step Gouras (1970) has identified all three cone mechanisms of rhesus monkeys in single neurons of the striate cortex.

Kolers and von Grunau (1975) studied a phenomenon we might call "apparent movement" for color. If disparate shapes are flashed under optimal temporal and spatial conditions, an observer will see a gradual transition from one figure to the next. If the two figures are, for example, a square and a triangle, alternation of the two figures at about three or four per second will result in apparent movement from square to triangle and back again. In the case of two differently colored rectangles the transition is not gradual, but is characteristically an abrupt change from one color to the other. Should there not be a gradual transition of color as well as shape? Why, if the two colors are complementary, do we not see an intermediate achromatic color in the transition? Apparently the neurophysiology for color discrimination is different from that for form.

A recent development in vision has been the rather frantic search for, and discovery of, so-called *feature specific detectors*. Numerous aftereffects of visual experience have been observed that can best be understood as arising from fatigue in some specific neural or chemical-neural structure. We alluded earlier to color-sensitive pigments such as chlorolabe, erytholabe, or cyanolabe. What about effects mediated presumably at higher neural levels? Are there, perhaps, detectors in the visual system for shape, movement, orientation, and other phenomena?

The individual most responsible for releasing this Pandora's box or can of worms, depending on how you look at it, was McCullough (1965). She presented a grating of vertical black lines on an orange background, alternated with a similar grating of horizontal lines on a blue background. Two to four minutes of alternation resulted in a fatigue effect that was specific to the orientation of the contours of the pattern. The simplistic assumption is that there are "receptors" selectively tuned to both color and orientation. The effect, first demonstrated by McCullough, has been replicated and extended by numerous other individuals, some of whom have advanced quite contrary explanations for the phenomena (see, for example Harris 1968; Held 1971; May 1976; Green 1976).

Another possibility is the existence of "curvature" as a specific feature of human visual perception. Riggs (1973) and Stromeyer (1974), utilizing similar techniques, seem to come to opposite conclusions in explaining the aftereffects of curvature.

Many other specific neural detectors have also been argued for. Size-detecting mechanisms have been proposed by Blakemore and Sutton (1969). Movement-specific feature detectors were found by Hepler (1968) and by Farveau, Emerson, and Corballis (1973). These latter used rotating,

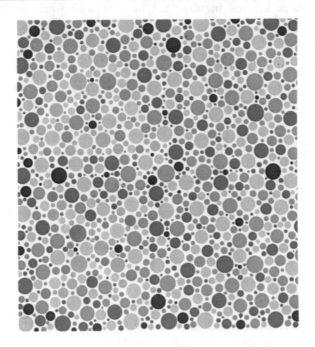

Figure 11–10
Pseudoisochromatic plate used for color-blindness testing. (Courtesy of American Optical Corporation.)

red contracting and green expanding spirals to adapt their subjects. When a subsequent stationary spiral was shown, a red spiral or a green spiral appeared to contract or expand in an opponent-type movement.

These studies seem, on the surface at least, to indicate the presence of differentially sensitive specific feature receptors. But there are other possible explanations, centering on the computerlike nature of central nervous system processing. Much more must be known about the functioning of the brain before we can say with certainty that feature-specific detectors do indeed exist. Perhaps we may still be able to apply the principle of parsimony, accepting feature detectors as useful constructs but not expecting to tease them out of the nervous system with sharp little scalpels.

Defects in Color Vision

Color vision is commonly evaluated by means of a simple screening device employing *pseudoisochromatic* plates such as those illustrated in Figure 11–10. Subjects with serious color vision deficiencies are unable to discriminate between the dots of a given color and the background color. If plates containing different color schemes are employed, the nature of the color deficiency can be determined as a function of what colors are confused.

Another method of detecting and identifying color blindness involves the use of an *anomaloscope*. With this device the patient adjusts the amounts of two colors in a two-color mixture to match a third color. For example, the subject may adjust the amount of red and green light needed to make a match with a known yellow. The extent to which this is impossible, or the extent to which the subject requires more or less of a given primary than the normal subject, is then a measure of his color blindness or color weakness.

Color vision is trichromatic; hence in theory there might be a weakness or even total absence in any one, two, or all three of the color sensitivities. A classification of color blindness is given in Figure 11–11. Although this figure may not be complete, it does show the more common forms of color blindness. Let us look at this table in more detail.

The most benign form of color vision defect is simply a "weakness" in the ability to see one of the three primary colors. Such people have, like the rest of us, *trichromatic* vision—they can see red, green, and blue, and they require three colors in order to match all the colors in the spectrum. However, in the preceding example of color mixing, the anomalous trichromat needs more of the one component (e.g., red) than the normal individual in order to match a given mixture containing red.

Although there is probably a continuum from the normal trichromat through the true color-blind, about 5.6 percent of the male population exhibit enough defect to be classed as *anomalous trichromats*. Most of these cases (4.6 percent) are *deuteranomalous*—that is, they require more green in a red-green mixture to match a specified yellow than the normal person. Deuteranomalous persons are probably deficient in chlorolabe. About 1 percent of the male population is presumed to be deficient in erythrolabe, because they require more red in the red-green mixture. These individuals are classed as *protanomalous*. The third type of trichromatic anomaly, *tritanomalous* vision, should in theory exist as a result of a shortage of cyanolabe. As a matter of fact, such cases are relatively rare and not at all well documented. Gregory (1966) indicates that the entire theory attributing anomalous color vision to shortages of chlorolabe, erythrolabe, and cyanolabe is in error. He has no alternative explanation, but is most definite in saying that the problem is not simply a pigment shortage.

The second major breakdown of color vision deficiency includes the *dichromats*, persons who can match any color of the spectrum with varying amounts of only two primary colors. As in anomalous trichromats, the condition (at least with respect to the red-green deficiency) appears to be largely hereditary, specifically a sex-linked recessive characteristic appearing ten times as frequently in males as in females. Three subgroups can also be identified for the dichromats. Known as *protanopes, deuteranopes*, and *tritanopes*, the complete absence of erythrolabe, chlorolabe, and cyanolabe, respectively, appear as underlying causes. Amout 1.2 percent of

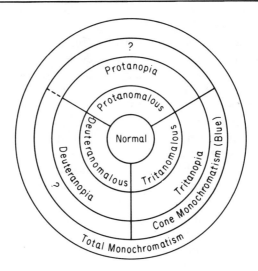

Figure 11-11

Classification of color blindness. The inner area of this figure represents normal color vision. The second area includes persons with three-color vision, but with some weakness or anomaly. The third level is for persons with two-color vision, and the last two levels represent monochromatism, or one-color vision.

the male population can be classed as protanopes and 1.4 percent as deuteranopes. As a result of a picture-magazine survey in Great Britain, in which a pseudisochromatic chart was included, it has been further estimated that about from 1 in 13,000 to 1 in 65,000 persons in Great Britain are tritanopes.

The most serious, and fortunately most rare, color deficiency is that where no color vision at all exists. *Monochromats* have no color vision; to them, all cats are gray, regardless of the time of day. In theory, of course, four possibilities suggest themselves. A retina could be composed exclusively of cones of a single color sensitivity, red, green, or blue; or a retina could contain no cones at all, providing pure rod vision. Pure rod monochromats have been identified, and one form of cone monochromatism has been documented. Presumably, the other two forms of exclusive cone vision are possible.

Did you notice how nicely the Ladd-Franklin theory fits in with colorblindness data? Simple red-green color blindness is the most common form, and red-green discrimination was, in theory, the last to develop. A simple mutation could rather easily destroy this evolutionary johnny-comelately. Older discriminations, such as blue-yellow, would be expected to be more resistant to throwbacks to earlier forms of development.

As a final conclusion in the age-old opponent-component theory controversy, we must acknowledge that both approaches have merit. Both theories are needed to explain all color phenomena adequately. Modern investigators tend to feel that a component theory is needed at the cone chemistry level, but for the transmission of the nervous impulse and its higher-level interpretation, some sort of opponent theory demands recognition.

Summary

Chapter 11 has aimed at obtaining an understanding of the manner in which color is experienced. We started out by describing the nature of color and its three attributes: hue, saturation, and brightness or lightness. We then described several approaches to the specification of color, including the Munsell and Ostwald phenomenological techniques and the psychophysically oriented ICI system. In the final half of the chapter we discussed color vision theory, describing both opponent and component theories and the experimental evidence in support of each. Such evidence included research results on afterimages and color adaptation, subjective color, the chemistry of cone functioning, color blindness, and evidence based on evolutionary findings. The ultimate conclusion was that both an opponent and a component theory are required to describe color vision adequately— a component theory at the retinal-cone level and an opponent theory at higher levels.

Suggested Readings

1. R. M. Evans. *An Introduction to Color.* New York: Wiley, 1948. Although relatively old, this is still the best general book on color. It is well written, beautifully illustrated, and not overly technical. Chapter II of this reference has already been suggested for reading in support of our Chapter 5, and the remainder of the book might well be read at this time. Most of what has been included in this chapter can be found in expanded form in the 324 pages of this reference. In addition, interesting chapters on paints and pigments, colorimetry, color photography, and color in art are included. It is the sort of book that can be read at leisure, almost like a novel.
2. Optical Society of America, Committee on Colorimetry. *The Science of Color.* New York: Crowell, 1953. This reference is the "bible" of color. Much of the book is highly technical and is scarcely to be read like a novel. It presents much of the technical elaboration omitted, for the sake of ease of reading, from the Evans reference. As a reference book it is highly recommended, and every scientist seriously interested in color should have access to this book.
3. D. B. Judd. *Colorimetry*, NBS Circular 478. Washington, D.C.: Government Printing Office, 1950, or I. Nimeroff, *Colorimetry*, NBS Monograph 104 (same source). Either of these references is suggested for the reader interested in the technical aspects of color production and mensuration. Of minimal interest to the student with a purely biological or psychological inteerst, the 50 or so pages of either of these pamphlets provide the most nearly complete, yet not extremely complex, explanation of colorimetry and the use of the ICI Chromaticity Diagram.
4. From M. Alpern. "Vision," in M. Alpern, M. Lawrence, and D. Wolsk, *Sensory Processes.* Belmont, Calif.: Brooks/Cole, 1967. Although the entire part of this book written by Alpern is worthwhile reading, several pages are par-

ticularly useful to an understanding of color vision. Pages 27 to 48 discuss in an excellent fashion the chemistry of rod and cone vision, color blindness, the component and opponent theories of color, and the present status of color vision theory. For gaining an understanding of color vision, I know of no better short reference.

5. J. Cohen and D. A. Gordon. "The Prevost-Fechner-Benham Subjective Colors," *Psychol. Bull.* 46 (1949), 97–136. This is an interesting, even fascinating, history and analysis of subjective color. The reference includes many examples of designs suitable for producing subjective colors. For the student interested in getting at the "root" of the problem, this reference is particularly recommended.

6. E. F. MacNichol, Jr. "Three-Pigment Color Vision," *Scientific American*, December 1964. This is an excellent summary describing the nature and history of the three-pigment theories of cone functioning, written by one of the pioneers in the field.

7. G. S. Brindley. "Afterimages," *Scientific American*, 209 (October 1963). There are eight pages of textual material in this reading, which is highly recommended. With demonstrations and examples printed in color, this short article supplies some of the information on afterimages that had to be omitted from Chapter 11 in the interest of brevity. The relating of the phenomena of afterimages to photochemistry is a particularly valuable contribution of this reading.

8. R. C. Teevan and R. C. Birney (eds.). *Color Vision.* Princeton, N.J.: Van Nostrand, 1961. An excellent little book of 214 pages, consisting of selected readings from original sources. From Thomas Young to Edwin H. Land, the gamut of information on color vision is sampled. I am not recommending specific readings from this book, but rather that you read what interests you.

9. C. H. Graham, "Color Theory," in S. Koch (ed.), *Psychology: A Study of Science*, vol. I. New York: McGraw-Hill, 1959. These 150 or so pages present one of the most nearly complete descriptions of color and color theory that I know of. It describes color mixing in great detail, systems of color notation, and includes detailed analyses of numerous color theories. It is not a simple or elementary article, but is worth looking into by the serious student. Its bibliography of 209 entries is especially complete.

10. From H. R. Schiffman. *Sensation and Perception: An Integrated Approach.* New York: Wiley, 1976. Pages 249 to 253 provide a nice summary of the problem of feature-specific detectors. Numerous references are provided, enabling the interested reader to delve more deeply into the matter.

11. From Tom N. Cornsweet. *Visual Perception.* New York: Academic Press, 1970. Chapter VII to X of this excellent book are of particular significance for our current chapter. Professor Cornsweet's book is not easy to read. It contains a very large amount of information and comes close to being the definitive work in the area. Highly recommended for the serious and able student.

12. Olga Eizner Favreau and Michael C. Corbalis. "Negative Aftereffects in Visual Perception," *Scientific American*, December 1976. This is another of the series of finely illustrated, well-written articles appearing in *Scientific American*. It is must reading for the intermediate student with a serious interest in visual aftereffects.

12/sound waves and hearing

Let us first examine some terminology* and consider the nature of the external stimulus that gives rise to the experience of "sound." Sound is not something that happens "out there." To the contrary, sound is a psychological and behavioral experience. If the proverbial tree were to fall on the deserted island with no one to hear it, there would be no "sound." There would be rapid vibrations in the air that we might call sound waves, but to have sound we would have to have an experiencing organism. Similarly, the airborne vibrations would have no loudness, because loudness is also an experience. The sound waves might have amplitude or intensity or power, but they would not have loudness. Loudness is the psychological, experiential correlate of sound amplitude; hence no listener, no loudness. Just as brightness was in the eye of the beholder, so is loudness in the ear of the beholder. Incidentally, the so-called loudness meter used to measure the applause of an audience in response to an entertainer is not a loudness meter at all; it does not measure loudness, it measures the amplitude or power of the sound waves produced by the applauding audience. More accurately, the meter in question is a sound level meter.

Just as light can be varied in three primary dimensions—intensity, leading to the psychological experience of brightness, wavelength with its resultant experience of hue, and purity, which is experienced as saturation—so can sound waves vary in three dimensions. For intensity of sound waves the experience is known as *loudness*; the quality or frequency of the sound wave we recognize as *pitch*; and purity evokes the psychological experience of *timbre*. As in vision, we can also recognize temporal variations. Alternating or flickering lights can form temporal patterns not en-

* See the reference by Martin Sonn (1969) for psychoacoustical terminology.

tirely unlike the rhythms and tempos of acoustic stimuli. And finally, to some limited extent, the excellent spatial character of vision can be approximated by the normal, healthy auditory mechanism. The spatial capability of hearing does not match that of vision. In some cases we may even have to "infer" direction of an acoustic source, and often we may be seriously in error. There is, however, some spatiality in audition that to a limited extent mirrors the three-dimensional world of vision. Let us examine in more detail the physical events leading to the experience of "sound."

The Nature of Sound Waves

If we imagine that a wheel is rolling along a flat surface, as shown in Figure 12–1, a point of the circumference will, in effect, follow the path shown by the curve at the right of the wheel. Note that the point will gradually rise to its maximum height or amplitude as indicated by *B* in the adjoining curve. Note too that the rate of vertical climb of the point is gradually decreasing, until at point *B* it is, for an infinitesimally short instant, stationary. For an infinitely short time the point is neither rising nor falling. Then the point returns toward *C*, reaching its maximum downward speed as it passes through its original level, again slowing down and pausing at *D*, and accelerating as it passes its origin, *A'*. The curve generated by such a point on a rolling wheel is known as a *sinusoidal function*.

As another example, note the pendulum of Figure 12–1, which will also generate a sine-wave function. When the pendulum is at point *A'*, it is, for an infinitesimal instant, stationary. It has a velocity and hence, amplitude, of zero (point *A* on the curve above). But at point *B'* it reaches its maximum velocity, an amplitude indicated by point *B*. As a result of gravity, the swinging pendulum will slow down gradually, reaching this time at point *C'*, another instant of motionless or velocity of zero as indicated by *C* on the sine-wave curve. When the pendulum has returned to point *A'* it will have completed one complete cycle, or the distance from *A* to *A'* on the curve.

As a third example of sine-wave production, a tuning fork vibrates in such a fashion that it alternately compresses and rarefies the adjoining air in a sinusoidal manner. The progressive movement of such alternate compressions and rarefactions through a compressible medium, such as air or water, is known as a sound wave. It is precisely this sort of activity that results from any sound-producing source, be it the vibrating strings of a Stradivarius violin, the reed of a clarinet, the air columns of an organ pipe, or the exceedingly complex vibrations of a cymbal.

FREQUENCY AND PITCH

The primary determinant of perceived pitch (high, low) is the frequency of the impinging sound wave. Before examining in detail and in a later chapter, the matter of pitch, let us first consider the physical concept

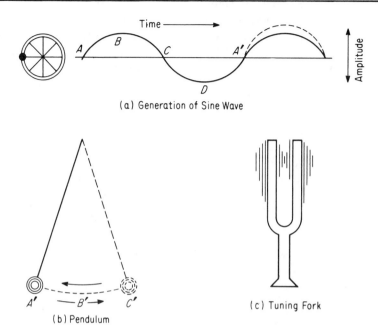

(a) Generation of Sine Wave

(b) Pendulum

(c) Tuning Fork

Figure 12–1
The nature of waves. The sound waves generated by the tuning fork are representative of the wave action illustrated by the rotating wheel and the swinging pendulum.

of frequency. If we thing of the *x*-axis (horizontal axis) of the sinusoidal curve of Figure 12–1 as time, we can see that the time for the wheel to make a complete revolution (360° rotation) is represented by the distance from *A* to *A'*. Similarly, the pendulum or tuning-fork action can be shown to complete a single cycle, also represented by the distance from *A* to *A'*. (Remember, *A* to *A'* is a pictorial representation of time, not distance!)

But we know that the alternate rarefaction and compressions produced by the tuning fork do not simply remain alongside the fork's prongs. Like the waves emanating from a pebble dropped in the water, the alternate rarefactions and compressions in the air move steadily away from the tuning fork. They form a progressive wave in all directions.

Happily they move at a known speed. At 0°C sound waves travel in air at a velocity of 1,087.5 ft per second. At moderate ambient temperatures, and under certain other specified conditions, their speed is on the order of 1,130 ft per second. Although the velocity differs in different media, such as water, air, or steel, it is this standard of 1,130 ft per second that is normally specified as the speed of sound. Expressed in miles per hour, instead of feet per second, the number becomes something like 730 miles per hour, the familiar Mach I of jet airplane interest.

If we know the speed the sound travels and the frequency of the vibrations—that is, the number of complete cycles in a given unit of time (normally taken as 1 second)—we can calculate an additional parameter of the physical wave, its wavelength. If a source is producing a sound with a frequency of 1,130 cycles per second, it is clear that any point on the curve of Figure 12–1 will repeat itself 1,130 times per second. Furthermore, because the resultant wave is progressing through the medium at a velocity of 1,130 ft per second, the successive points of corresponding amplitude will be exactly 1 ft apart. The wavelength of an 1,130-Hz tone in air of normal temperature and certain other specified characteristics, is 1 ft. A 2,260-Hz tone would complete each of its cycles in half the time; hence its wavelength or distance traveled per $\frac{1}{2,260}$ second would be on the order of 6 in.

For general application, the relation between wavelength and frequency can be expressed in the following forms:

$$f = \frac{1,130}{\lambda}$$

$$\lambda = \frac{1,130}{f}$$

and

$$\lambda \times f = 1,130$$

where f is the frequency in cycles per second, λ (the Greek letter, lambda) refers to the wavelength, and 1,130 is the velocity of the transmission. Note too that the time required for each cycle can be expressed as

$$t = \frac{\lambda}{1,130}$$

For media and conditions other than the typically defined air, the velocity figure of 1,130 would have to be replaced by the appropriate value.

The preceding expressions are general and apply to any wave phenomenon. In Figure 1–1 we showed the electromagnetic spectrum with both wavelength and frequency identified. But the preceding formulas when used with electromagnetic radiation involve the tremendous speed of transmission of these waves (about 186,000 miles per second), rather than the relatively slow velocities of sound waves. Note, however, that the *only* similarity between sound waves and electromagnetic waves is the wavelength-velocity-frequency formulations. Sound waves are *not* a part of the electromagnetic spectrum. They simply are alternating compressions and rarefactions in a physical medium. They cannot exist where there is no molecular medium, such as in outer space or in a laboratory-created vacuum.

Although most of us have lost much of our hearing ability above 12,000 Hz, the range of 20 to 20,000 Hz is generally recognized as the frequency limits of hearing for man. These limits might also be specified as wavelengths from roughly 0.75 in. to 56 ft. The significance of these values will be discussed later in the book.

Frequency of acoustic signals is of importance to us in that the pitch of sounds, from the low hum of the honeybee to the shrill squeak of a rusty hinge, depends largely on the frequency of the physical signal. A low musical note such as C below middle C on the piano has a basic frequency of about 128 Hz, while middle C may be tuned to about 256 Hz, and C above middle C has a frequency of 512 Hz. An octave higher is represented by 1,024 Hz, and so on, each octave representing a doubling of frequency, until the limit of hearing is reached. The manner in which we are able to discriminate different frequencies and their psychological attributes of pitch is a fascinating problem and will be explored in a later chapter.

PURITY AND TIMBRE

The sound from the honeybee and the squeaking door may also differ in another important respect. Note that the middle C you strike on the piano does not sound the same as the middle C played on a trombone. Some of the difference may be due to temporal factors such as the rise-and-decay characteristics or the steadiness of the tones, but much of the apparent difference between presumably identical notes produced by two different instruments has a more subtle basis. The sounds produced by the two instruments are not the same, even though they are both producing the same note on the musical scale.

Musical instruments do not produce pure tones like the sinusoidal curve of Figure 12–1. Rather, they generate a principal wave, known as the fundamental frequency (for instance, the middle C in our example), and numerous variations on this fundamental frequency known as overtones or harmonics.

In Figure 12–2a the fundamental vibration of a stretched string may be seen. The string bounces back and forth, much like the tines of our tuning fork, alternately compressing and rarefying the air adjoining it. If the string vibrates at a rate of 100 times per second it will produce a tone of 100 Hz. But a string is not as rigid as a tuning fork; it also vibrates in the manner shown in Figure 12–2b, that is, generating an acoustic wave of twice the frequency of the fundamental (second harmonic). If the string in (a) is vibrating at 100 Hz, then the one in (b) will be emitting waves at 200 Hz. Similarly, the string at (c) will be producing a 300-Hz tone. A single string tuned to 100 cps will simultaneously produce all these frequencies, plus 400, 500, 600 . . . in varying degrees of strength (12–2d). It is the experienced quality of the tone, produced by the relative strengths of the various harmonic frequencies, that we call *timbre*. Because of differences

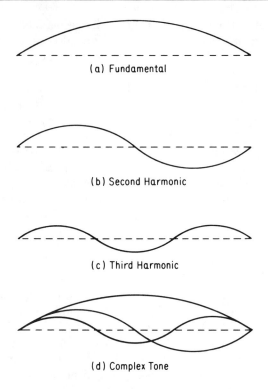

(a) Fundamental

(b) Second Harmonic

(c) Third Harmonic

(d) Complex Tone

Figure 12–2
Vibrating strings. This figure shows the nature of the first, second, and third harmonics and the pattern resulting from their combination.

in absorption, resonance, and other factors, different musical instruments produce different patterns of complex waves, thus a cornet sounds different from a French horn. A Stradivarius has a different, presumably more pleasant tone than a less expensive violin. And some voices appear more pleasing because of the richness of their harmonics produced by the resonances of the various cavities of the mouth, larynx, and nasal passages. Timbre, analogous to saturation in vision, is a result of the complexity of the auditory signal.* It is the psychological experience of purity or, perhaps more accurately, the absence of purity that we refer to as timbre.

Random Noise. As an example of a complex sound carried to an extreme, the "whispering" sound, such as produced by the wind, represents

---

* The advanced student may very well recognize the oversimplification of the preceding section. Tones may be produced by both longitudinal and transverse vibrations, the action of columns of air is often quite complex, and in practice the simple harmonic relations we have described do not always obtain. In the interest of brevity and simple exposition, however, it is hoped the serious student of acoustics will find this simplified presentation adequate.

a special case in which all (or nearly all) of the audible frequencies are present at the same time. Somewhat analogous to zero-saturated light, or white light, such sounds are, not unreasonably, known as *white noise*. Variously referred to as a Gaussian noise, random noise, or white noise (depending on the actual form and distribution of the total components),* such signals are commonly employed in the testing of hearing and in research on the functioning of the ear. When you last had your ears tested, the otologist may very well have "masked" one ear with white noise while he mapped your hearing acuity in the opposite ear with a series of pure tones. Random generators, as used in auditory research, commonly generate frequencies limited to the range of 20 to 20,000 Hz, because these are the general limits of hearing.

AMPLITUDE AND LOUDNESS

There is a third primary quality of sound waves that is derived from the amplitude or intensity of the waves, and is experienced as *loudness*. The concept of loudness is not simple, and, as suggested before, resides in the experiencing organism. It will be examined in much more detail in Chapter 14. In the meantime we should gain an understanding of just what amplitude or sound intensity is, how it is measured, and what broad ramifications it may have for our understanding of the auditory function.

Let us look again at the pendulum of Figure 12–1. It is a law of physics (fortunate for the designers of pendulum-controlled clocks) that a given pendulum always makes a complete cycle in precisely the same time. That is, if the pendulum were to start swinging at a point slightly to the left of A and therefore complete its first half-cycle at a point to the right of C, the time required for the extended excursion would be the same as that for the distance A to C. This time, a function of physical parameters such as the weight of the bob and the length of the string from which it is suspended, determines, in accordance with a formula similar to our last formula on p. 226, the primary or fundamental frequency of the oscillation. Note that you change the frequency of a metronome by changing the position of the weight on the vertical shaft. The fresquency of the individual waves, and therefore their wavelengths, is determined by the time required for each individual excursion.

A similar situation exists with respect to the tuning fork. As a result of its physical construction it can vibrate (in a given medium) at only one frequency, the one to which it is tuned. If we strike it extra hard the tines will make larger back-and-forth excursions, but always at the same frequency.

---

* Strictly speaking, the term *white noise* should be reserved for the situation in which all the frequencies are included in strictly sinusoidal form, such as when one combines a very large number of outputs from differentially tuned audio oscillators. Random noise is truly random, and the outputs of the various components may vary in time from zero to maximum.

What difference results then from starting the pendulum with a harder push, or striking the tuning fork with a little extra energy? Because the pendulum travels a greater distance in the same time, it must be traveling faster. Similarly, the tuning fork must be alternately compressing and rarefying the adjacent air with increasing amplitude. The movement of the wave through space in the longitudinal direction remains fixed, but the velocity of movement of the indivdual molecules increases as the excursion distance of the tuning fork's tines is increased.

Such a variation is known as the *amplitude* or *intensity* of the sound wave. It is represented schematically by the height of the wave in Figure 12–1. The broken line at the right of this figure represents a tone of the same wavelength and frequency, but of a greater amplitude. Psychological loudness, then, is the psychological experience of the amplitude of the sound wave.

Definition of Sound Amplitude. The strength of a sound wave (and many other wave forms as well) is generally specified in terms of power—that is, the amount of work done in a unit of time. In somewhat technical terms we might say that the power of an energy flow through an area 1 centimeter square (1 cm^2) can be expressed as pressure times velocity. It follows then that the power of a sinusoidal wave is proportional to the pressure caused by the sound wave times the velocity of the air molecules produced by the wave. Can we express this in somewhat simpler language?

The unit known as a *dyne* is a unit of force or pressure, being that force that when acting on a body of 1 g mass for one second will impart in the body a velocity of 1 cm per second. The commonly accepted measure for sound is in terms of dynes per square centimeter (dyne/cm^2). When we express this force over time, we have *power*.

When we use a microphone or similar device for the measurement of sound intensity we take advantage of the fact that a body suspended in space (or of adequate flexibility) will be moved by any alternate compressions or rarefactions in the medium impinging on it. The diaphragm of a microphone will follow the frequency of the impinging molecular vibrations as well as their instantaneous velocity or pressure. If we feed the output of our microphone into an oscilloscope we can see the actual form of the impinging wave. Furthermore, the greater the intensity of the impinging force the greater will be the excursions of our microphone's diaphragm, and hence its output in volts or fractions thereof. In a high-quality microphone, and over a limited frequency range, output will be proportional to the force of the acoustic wave rather than its power. Furthermore, the output of the microphone will be in volts, a pressure unit. We are in no trouble, however, since we know that power varies as the square of the voltage. Thus when the output of the microphone increases from 0.01 to 0.02 volt (V) (doubling), we know that the power input to the microphone must have increased by a factor of 4. Increasing a sound-pressure level from 1 dyne/cm^2 to 10 dyne/cm^2 is a tenfold increase in pressure but a hundredfold increase in power. It is important to remember that power varies as the square of the force. This is an important concept, necessary for the complete understanding of the decibel scale to be considered in the following section.

Sound Power. When we were discussing the electromagnetic spectrum we noted its tremendous width, and pointed to the necessity for referring to both frequency and wavelength in terms of powers of 10. Indeed, the value shown in Figure 1–1 are expressed in this form.

Although the wavelength and frequency of sound waves in the audible range do not encompass such a great range, variations in amplitude do. The most intense sound that man can tolerate without excessive pain is some 10 trillion times more powerful than the weakest sound he can hear—a factor of 10 million million to 1!

Obviously, handling such long numbers for the various values between the upper and lower limits of sound intensity would be extremely clumsy. As in the electromagnetic spectrum we must resort to a system involving units expressed as powers of 10. For example, 10^0 would equal 1, 10^1 would equal 10, 10^2 would equal 100, and so on, until the long number referred to earlier describing the most intense sound that can be tolerated would be expressed as 10^{13}.*

Also, the concept of zero power with respect to measurement of air-molecule movement is difficult to grasp (Brownian movement occurs constantly in any case), and furthermore there is no way to express zero in a logarithmic form. There is no power to which 10 can be raised to equal zero. The solution to this enigma is to adopt a scale that has a starting point, identified as 10 to the zero power (equivalent to 1), and base all measurements on this anchoring point.

Various anchoring points or scale bases have been used at various times by different disciplines. Engineers commonly use 1 dyne/cm^2 (also referred to as 1 microbar) as their reference point. Thus 10^0 would refer to the power of a 1 dyne/cm^2 signal; 10^1 would be a signal of ten times the power of the 1 microbar standard; and 10^2 would describe a signal of 100 times the power of this reference level. Note again that because power increases as the square of the force, the hundredfold increase in power (10^2) is actually the result of a tenfold increase in pressure (from 1 microbar to 10 microbars, for example).

In auditory work, the commonly used reference level is 0.0002 dyne/cm^2, or 0.0002 microbar. This level has been chosen because it is the approximate absolute threshold for a young, healthy ear over the frequencies of maximum sensitivity.

The Decibel Scale. When you see an auditory signal referred to in print,

---

* Utilization of a logarithmic form of expression for sound has another basis. Many psychological dimensions of experience vary according to the logarithm of the stimulus rather than its absolute value. Hence a logarithmic nomenclature is more consistent with the experiential world.

it is not generally referred to as 10^8, 10^7, and so on. Rather, its power is generally expressed in terms of bels,* or more commonly decibels (abbreviated db). This is really just another way of expressing the power in logarithmic terms, simply omitting the base 10 expression and replacing it with the word *bel*. Thus a signal of 2 bels is one that is ten times as powerful as a signal of 1 bel and 100 times as powerful as one of 0 bels. Because the anchoring point is always identified as 0 bels, the comparative power of any signal expressed in bels can be readily calculated.

In practice, however, the distance encompassed by a bel is rather great. The average range of speech power, for example, at a distance of 3 ft from the speaker, might be something between 6 and 8 bels. We could, of course, indicate intermediate values in the form of 7.5 bels, 8.36 bels, and so on. In practice, the procedure is to express powers in terms of *decibels*, or tenths of bels. Thus a 6-bel level is almost universally referred to as 60 db.

Expressed in technical terms, a bel is the logarithm of the ratio between two powers:

$$\text{bels} = \log_{10} \frac{I_1}{I_2}$$

A decibel is defined† in similar terms:

$$\text{db} = 10 \log_{10} \frac{I_1}{I_2}$$

Whenever a power is expressed in bels or decibels it is essential that the reference level be known. When we say that one signal is 10 db more powerful than another, the reference is clearly implied. But when we say that a signal has a level of 20 db, it is imperative that we define 20 db with respect to a reference level. Therefore, decibel expressions are always written in the form 20 db re 0.0002 dyne/cm² or 20 db re 1 dyne/cm² for most auditory and electrical engineering uses, respectively.

Table 12–1 shows the relation between various power ratios and their respective value in decibels.

---

* Named after Alexander Graham Bell, one of the foremost workers in the early development of acoustics and sound research, as well as the inventor of the telephone.
† One may encounter the last formula in the form:

$$\text{db} = 20 \log_{10} \frac{P_1}{P_2}$$

In this case decibels are calculated as a function of the ratio of the two pressures or forces. In practice, the output of microphones, inputs to amplifiers, and so on, are normally expressed in volts, which are units of pressure. Hence the modified formula is necessary to go directly from pressure units to decibels without the need for calculating power.

TABLE 12-1
Relation of Power Ratios to Decibels

Power Ratio of Two Sounds I_1/I_2	Power or Intensity, db
0.001	−30
0.01	−20
0.10	−10
0.50	−3 (approx.)
1.00	0
2.00	3 (approx.)
4.00	6 (approx.)
10.00	10
100.00	20
1000.00	30
2000.00	33 (approx.)

The table can be read in this way: If a signal is 0.0001 as powerful as the reference signal (e.g., 0.002 dyne/cm²), it has a decibel rating of −30 db. Thus decibel values less than 1 simply mean that the sound in question is lower in power than the reference level. If a signal is equal to the reference signal, we say that it has a level of 0 db; if it is 1,000 times as powerful, it is 30 db. Note too that doubling (or halving) the power results in a change of approximately 3 db. To get such intermediate values as these, and for values of odd ratios such as 1.643 to 1, it is necessary to consult a table of decibel equivalents, found in most books dealing with acoustics and electrical phenomena. With slightly more difficulty, one could use tables of logarithms to achieve the same end.

If one must work with pressure or voltage ratios, a table such as Table 12–2 can be consulted. This table is an extension of Table 12–1, including both pressure or voltage ratios and power ratios. Most available tables do include both voltage and power ratios and are much more like Table 12–2 than Table 12–1.

If you have ever used a tape recorder with a VU (*volume-unit*) meter to maintain recording level, you have employed a decibel scale with a still different reference level. In a VU meter the 0 db you try to maintain (or at least not exceed) is simply some defined level, based on a specified voltage in a circuit of known characteristics. When you record at −6 db, your recording voltage is one-half the 0 db optimum; at −20 db your recording voltage is one-tenth the optimum 0 VU; and so on.

The Measurement of Sound

There are a number of ways in which the physical characteristics of sound can be specified and described. Let us look at several of them.

TABLE 12–2
Relation of Pressure, Power, and Decibels

Pressure Ratios P_1/P_2	Power Ratios I_1/I_2	Decibels (some are approx.)
0.01	0.0001	−40
0.1	0.01	−20
0.5	0.25	− 6
1.0	1.0	0
2.0	4.0	6
3.0	9.0	9.5
4.0	16.0	12
10.0	100.0	20
100.0	10,000.	40
1,000.0	1,000,000.	60

SOUND LEVEL MEASUREMENT

It should be rather obvious by now that the measurement of sound intensity involves the use of a microphone and the determination of its output as a result of an impinging sound level. A sound level meter, such as illustrated in Figure 12–3, measures the level of the sound at the surface of the microphone. A meter of this type measures the total sound-pressure level in decibels with reference to the conventional 0.0002 dyne/cm^2 standard. Thus if it reads 60 db, it indicates that the power is 60 db above the 0.0002 dyne/cm^2 reference level. Is it clear that, in this example, the pressure or force would be 0.2 dyne/cm^2 (that is, 0.0002 × 1000)? If it is not apparent look again at the last line of Table 12–2.

Sound level meters can tell us whether the levels are intense enough to interfere with speech or perhaps even damage the ear. Many tables and graphs have been worked out showing the effect on hearing and possible interference with speech as a function of the level and duration of intense sounds. The interested reader should consult the pertinent references at the end of the book. In Chapter 16 we will consider some applications of sound-measuring to problems of speech intelligibility, annoyance, and possible ear damage.

Most sound level meters do something else besides simply measure an overall energy level. Because we are interested in the intensity of sound as it affects the human listener, sound level meters are made so that they measure only those sound levels at the frequencies normally hard by humans. Thus most instruments have passbands from 20 to 20,000 Hz, filtering out frequencies beyond these limits. Also, because the ear's sensitivity is partly a function of the level of the overall sound, most meters have different scales for gross differences in level. Thus A, B, and C scales are often included to provide filtering-shaping capabilities to match the sensitivity curve of the human ear. Although sound level meters do not actually measure loudness (no instrument can do this, as we will see in a later chapter),

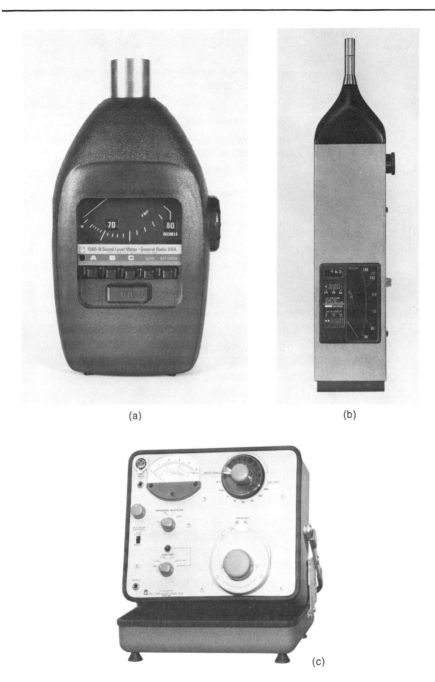

(a)

(b)

(c)

Figure 12–3
Sound-measuring equipment. (a) Type 1565-B Sound Level Meter, (b) Type 1982
Precision Sound Level Meter and Analyzer, and (c) Type 1568-A Wave Analyzer.
(Courtesy of Gen Rad, Inc.)

Level in db

db	
140	
	50 hp siren at a distance of 100 ft
	Jet fighter taking off—80 ft from tail
130	
	Boiler shop
	Air hammer—at position of operator
120	Rock and roll band
	Jet aircraft at 500 ft overhead
	Trumpet automobile horn at 3 ft
110	
	Crosscut saw at operator's position
100	Inside subway car
90	Train whistle at 500 ft
80	Inside automobile in city
70	Downtown city street (Chicago)
	Average traffic
60	
	Restaurant
50	Business office
	Classroom
40	Inside church
	Hospital room
30	Quiet bedroom
	Recording studio
20	
10	Threshold of hearing—young men

Figure 12-4

Typical sound levels in db re 0.0002 dyne/cm^2. Levels are only approximations and in many cases deviations of as much as 20 db might be expected.

their response in decibels *does* indeed approximate the human experience of loudness.

Figure 12–4 shows some typical sound levels in decibels as measured with a sound level meter. In this case the levels represent the total sound-pressure level over the 20 to 20,000-Hz frequency range.

FREQUENCY ANALYSIS

In addition to measuring the overall level of a complex sound, more often than not we are interested in its composition. The ear is not equally sensitive to the entire range from 20 to 20,000 Hz, and potential damage to the ear from excessive sound levels is much less serious for those frequencies far above normal speech frequencies. Intense frequencies at, say, 15,000 Hz might destroy your ability to hear subsequent tones at this frequency, but because most sounds such as speech and music are not concentrated at such high frequencies, you might never notice this loss of sensitivity. At least you would not be severely handicapped. But if you were to lose your sensitivity to a band of tones around 400 Hz, your ability to hear and recognize speech might be severely impaired. It is clear that a knowledge of the frequency characteristic of noise of interfering tones is of utmost importance.

Filtering devices known as octave-band and narrow-band analyzers are used to determine the power in different portions of the audio spectrum. The sound level meter and analyzer illustrated in Figure 12–3 actually combines the functions of level measurement and octave-band analysis. Octave-band analyzers determine the power in each of a number of octave bands, such as 37.5 to 75 Hz, 75 to 150 Hz, 150 to 300 Hz, all the way to 20,000 Hz. Figure 12–5 shows the octave-band composition of a sample of noise, that produced by a jet engine. This typical example has its maximum acoustic power in the 150- to 300- and 300- to 600-Hz bands, with a gradual falling off in power beyond these limits. Narrow-band analyzers, on the other hand, determine the total energy in each frequency, or at least in quite narrow bands, often specified as some percent of the total frequency.

When we know the overall levels and the relative power in the various bands or individual frequencies, we are better able to predict the results of the noise and take remedial steps to reduce the excessive levels if this is indicated.

PROBE MICROPHONES

Sound levels or sound intensities can be measured with other variations. Because we are generally interested in the sound level at the ear, or more precisely, at the human eardrum, might we not better measure the level right at that location? For many purposes, such as determining the results of amplitude variations with great precision, that is just what is done. For this purpose a probe microphone is used. A small, tubular arrangement is inserted in the ear canal until it is quite close to the eardrum,

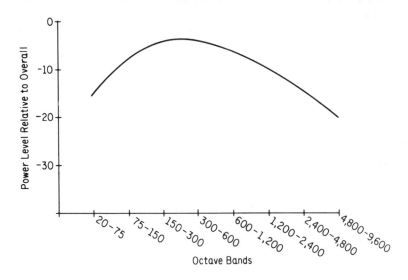

Figure 12–5

Typical audio spectrum for jet engine. This is a general curve, not representing any specific jet engine, but respresentative of all.

thus measuring the sound level at the drum itself. This technique requires a delicate touch and is not a method to be employed outside the laboratory. Note, however, that we can also take the output from the inserted microphone and run it through one of the analyzers mentioned earlier, thus determining the actual composition of the sound at the eardrum as well as its overall level.

COUPLER APPLICATION

A final measurement technique should be mentioned. We may wish to produce a sound-pressure level of known amplitude by means of a headphone. Or perhaps we might wish to know the level at the eardrum produced by a headphone. We could, of course, insert a probe microphone under the headphone and measure the level directly. More often, however, a device known as a *coupler* is used to calibrate the headphone, such that if the voltage of the signal at the phone is known, the sound-pressure level at the eardrum can be calculated. Figure 12–6 illustrates the use of a coupler in the calibration of a headphone.

To begin with, a calibrated microphone must be used, one for which we know the output in volts for various sound-pressure levels. In practice, an audio signal of a known voltage is fed into the phone and the output of the microphone is noted. Since the cavity in the coupler is designed to duplicate the volume of the external ear canal ($6\ cm^3$) the level impinging on the microphone will be essentially the same as that at the eardrum if the phone

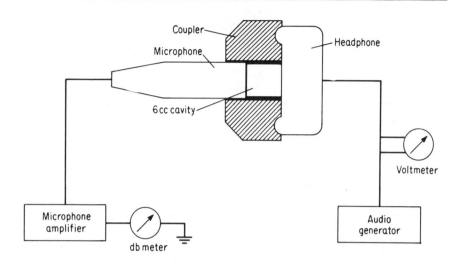

Figure 12-6
Calibration of head phone. Audio signal of known voltage is fed into headphone.
Calibrated microphone assembly indicates sound pressure level at eardrum.

were being worn. Thus when the calibrated headphone is worn, levels at the eardrum can be estimated quite precisely as a function of the voltage across the phone terminals.

In the case of insert phones, similar to the ones you get with small transistor radios, a coupler with a volume of 2 cm³ is used, thus duplicating the unoccupied portion of the external ear canal with this sort of transducer.

Control of Noise

Before leaving the realm of the physical nature of the phenomena that produce sound we should at least touch on the manner in which excessive or unwanted sound is controlled. The broad area of acoustic noise control is quite involved, and we can scarcely scratch the surface of this fascinating and highly technical profession.

DEFINITION OF NOISE

What is it we wish to control? What is this ubiquitous thing called noise? And why do we need to control it? Noise can be defined in either of two ways, not necessarily mutually exclusive.

1. It is complex sound of an inharmonious nature. Musical instruments are complex resonators; they produce complex sound containing many sinusoidal components or pure tones. But, as indicated earlier, their components have a simple mathematical relationship to each other and the

result (at least to a member of our Western culture) is music. When the components are not harmonically related, or are perhaps related in unfamiliar ways, the sound is not harmonious and we refer to it as noise.

2. Noise can also be defined as any unwanted sound. When you are trying to concentrate on studying, sounds that you might otherwise appreciate and perhaps call music are now noise. By this definition, noise is any acoustic activity that interferes in some way with ongoing behavior, or perhaps even results in damage to the subjected organism.

WHY CONTROL NOISE?

Excessive sound levels can damage the sensitive, delicate receptors in the inner ear. Persons working near jet aircraft engines frequently suffer hearing loss due to damage of the tiny hair cells in their inner ears. When this hearing loss is in the range normally required to understand speech, the result may be quite serious.

Noise also interferes with ongoing activity. Noise control techniques are employed in hospitals, schoolrooms, recording studios, and countless other places. One development of the acoustic engineers (and psychologists) is the concept of Speech-Interference Level (SIL). Based on the acoustic power in several specified octave bands, the SIL can predict the interference with speech of almost any complex sound if its composition is known. Thus acceptable levels for offices, churches, and similar locations can be determined and necessary control measures instituted to insure adequate speech communication.

NOISE REDUCTION

Controlling noise is not at all simple. One doesn't just install acoustic tile in the ceiling. All such a simplistic procedure does is to prevent (or reduce) reflection of the sound, thereby reducing potential echoes or reverberations. Any reduction in the actual level in the room rarely exceeds 2 or 3 db.

The ideal method to reduce noise is to control it at the source. Noisy engines can be equipped with mufflers and the volume on the radio can be turned down. In the long run, reducing noise level at the source is the only truly effective technique. Other techniques are merely treatments or ways of circumventing the problem.

Another method is to increase the distance between the noise source and the auditor. Because the sound waves spread out in all directions (not unlike the light rays from a candle), as one increases the distance between the source and the listener, the level at the listener's ear will decrease, not as the distance but as the *square* of the distance. Thus each doubling of the distance results in a 6-db drop in the experienced power. Mechanics working around jet engines, for example, are required to maintain some distance from the engine, unless specific and limited duties require greater proximity to the source of the noise.

A third possibility is the placing of a barrier between the source of the noise and the listener. One approach is to isolate the noise-producing source. Noisy machines, for example, are placed in enclosures surrounded by thick concrete or metal walls. Or, as another alternative, the place to be kept quiet can incorporate heavy walls and doors, as in recording studios. Such installations may even have double-layered windows and double doors to help keep out the noise.

A barrier may also be used right at the listener. Earplugs or (more effectively) heavy protectors covering the entire ear may be used to keep out much of the unwanted sound. Such devices have a limitation: even if all the sound is prevented from reaching the inner ear by way of the external ear and the auditory canal, one could still suffer irreparable damage to the inner ear as a result of sounds passing directly through the bone of the head. In fact, the transmission of the skull to the inner ear is only some 30 db poorer than that through the normal canal. Thus earplugs or pads can only reduce an intense sound by a maximum factor of 30 db. In practice, the reduction is usually much less.

Summary

In this chapter we considered briefly the nature of the physical changes in our environment that we identify as sound. We examined first the three principal variations in an acoustic signal, which we identified as frequency, purity, and amplitude. We suggested, with reference to later chapters, that the experiences of pitch, timbre, and loudness are related to these three physical variables. In the course of this discussion we examined concepts of force and power, and learned how the decibel system is employed in the measurement of physical quantity. We were also introduced to methods of measuring sound, involving such devices as microphones, couplers, sound level meters, and sound analyzers. Finally, we touched briefly on the methods used to control unwanted sound or noise.

Suggested Readings

1. A. P. G. Peterson and L. L. Beranek. *Handbook of Noise Measurement.* Concord, Mass.: GenRad, Inc., 1956. Later editions are of equal value. The second chapter of this manual to GenRad's sound-measuring equipment is one of the clearest and best descriptions of the decibel notation system. It is short (about four pages), lucid, and as complete as necessary for the beginner in acoustics and auditory measurements. Several of the remaining chapters should also prove of interest to the serious student, providing information on loudness, masking, thresholds, and other topics to be discussed in subsequent chapters.
2. From S. S. Stevens. *Handbook of Experimental Psychology.* New York: Wiley, 1951. Chapter 25, "Basic Correlates of the Auditory Stimulus," by J. C. R. Licklider, is an excellent description of the physical nature of sound and its

relation to the experiencing organism. The first 14 pages of this chapter are relevant to the material just covered, and the remaining pages are germane to the subsequent chapters on hearing in this book, and are recommended for the serious student.

3. A. T. Jones. *Sound.* New York: Van Nostrand, 1937. Although old and not available in all libraries, this book is one of the best sources for information on an introductory, highly readable level. It avoids highly technical terminology wherever possible, yet prepares the reader for more advanced study. The last sections on technical application are dated, but the remaining 360 pages are well worth selective reading by the serious student who has not yet mastered the highly technical area of sound and acoustics.

4. From W. A. Van Bergeijk, J. R. Pierce, and E. E. David, Jr. *Waves and the Ear.* Garden City, N.Y.: Doubleday, Anchor Books, 1960. The first 66 pages (chaps. I, II, and III) are concerned with the subject matter considered in this chapter. This reference is easy to read, interesting, and informative.

5. S. S. Stevens, F. Warshofsky, and the editors of *Life. Sound and Hearing.* New York: Time, Inc., 1965. This is another of the excellent little books (about 200 pages) in the *Life* Science Library series. It is beautifully illustrated, written for the intelligent layman, and of considerable value as an introductory survey of the field of sound and hearing.

6. From Bertram Scharf (ed.). *Experimental Sensory Psychology.* Glenview, Ill.: Scott, Foresman, 1975. Chapter 4 of this reference is quite complete and very readable. It is recommended as an additional source for much of the material covered in this chapter.

7. From H. R. Schiffman. *Sensation and Perception: An Integrated Approach.* New York: Wiley, 1976. Chapters 4, 5, and 6 may prove useful to the interested student. Chapter 4 is relevant to this and the following chapter, and chaps. 5 and 6 elaborate on the material covered in subsequent chapters. This is a good reference at about the level you have been reading.

8. L. L. Beranek. *Acoustic Measurement.* New York: Wiley, 1949.

9. L. L. Beranek. *Acoustics.* New York: McGraw-Hill, 1954. This and the preceding book, although relatively difficult reading, make a highly complex subject matter as simple and readable as is possible. As reference books, they are musts. Any person with a serious interest in acoustics as related to hearing requires access to these two books.

10. W. A. Yost and D. W. Nielsen. *Fundamentals of Hearing, An Introduction.* New York: Holt, Rinehart and Winston, 1977. This is one of the finest references for the entire area of auditory sensitivity. It is a new book, up-to-date, and relatively complete, yet consisting of only about 200 pages. It is so well written and illustrated that it should be of interest to any student and covers all the material in this and the next four chapters. This is as near to must reading as any reference I have suggested here.

13/the human ear

The development of the human ear makes for as interesting a tale as the development of the eye. In some respects they are quite similar. Sensitivity (irritability) to mechanical movement or vibratory activity is probably basic to all protoplasm. As in the case of sensitivity to electromagnetic waves, evolutionary development presumably resulted in the creation of specialized tissue and structures more ideally suited for mechanical sensitivity than the undifferentiated protoplasm.

An early example of specialization can be seen in the frog embryo. At a stage of development when one can scarcely tell which end of the embryo is which, a *lateral placode* begins to develop on the dorsolateral surface near the head end. This placode (remember the placode that eventually developed into the eye?) ultimately develops into the inner ear, and in many lower animals, especially fish, a remarkable structure known as the *lateral line* organ.

Most fish have a visible streak running along near the midline of the lateral surface. This is the visible portion of the lateral line organ, a string of sensitive hair cells imbedded in a gelatinous *cupula*. Any unusual movement of the water alongside the fish is sensed by the delicate sensory cells, and neural impulses transmitted to the central nervous system of the animal alert it to the untoward event.

Many animals phylogenetically lower than the fishes do not have such a well-developed sense as the lateral line organ provides. But many do have sensitive cells equipped with delicate hairlike processes that can respond to vibratory movement. In many worms these delicate hairlike transducers are located over a large portion of the body.

Unlike fish, which retain their lateral line organs while still developing rather complex inner ears, most higher animals such as birds and mammals do not develop lateral line organs. (Or at least they disappear before birth.) On the contrary, these higher animals develop quite sophisticated inner ears, as well as middle ears, and, in many of the highest-order animals, sophisticated outer or external ears.

Development of the Inner Ear

The development of the inner ear parallels the development of the eye in a disarmingly similar manner. The previously mentioned placode develops a dent or pit that becomes deeper and deeper until the surface ectoderm finally closes over it, leaving a little nodule or bubble of placode tissue. This bubble is called the *otic vesicle*. This description sounds like the development of the eye with its optic vesicle, does it not? But there is a difference! The optic placode and optic vesicle were composed of neural tissue; they developed from the wall of the forebrain. Indeed, the retina, which developed from the invagination of the forebrain, actually included several layers of neural tissue. The inner ear, like the lens of the eye, develops from the ectoderm layer of the embryo; hence it is not made up of neural tissue. As we shall see later, the inner ear does not have the multiple neural layers of the retina. Instead, impulses from the inner ear must travel some distance before reaching any ganglionic "switching station."

The otic vesicle, which is at first like a tiny fibrous tumor, continues to grow, becoming larger and more nearly spherical and generally filled with fluid. Rather suddenly, then, it begins to constrict in the center into a dumbbell shape, eventually into two cavities connected by a fine channel. These two halves of the structure develop into the major organs of the inner ear.

The upper of these two cavities develops into the organs of equilibrium or balance, consisting of three semicircular canals, lying in three distinct planes, and their associated structures. We return to the semicircular canals in a later chapter when we consider the sense of equilibrium.

The lower cavity develops into the inner ear in a manner much too complex to delineate at this time. It is so complex that much of the detailed development is not fully understood. Apparently hair cells, not entirely unlike those in the lateral line organs of the fish, develop in a membrane known as the *basilar membrane*, buried deeply in the bony, spiral structure called the *cochlea*. This latter structure is so named because it looks like a snail (Latin, *cochlea*). We shall look more deeply into the anatomical nature of the cochlea and its basilar membrane when we consider the ear in detail. In the meantime, let us pause a bit and examine the overall auditory organ, starting logically from the outside and working in.

Anatomy of the Ear

For purposes of description, the ear is commonly divided into three rather independent but still closely related parts: the outer ear, the middle ear, and

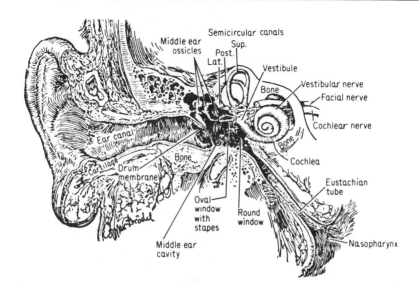

Figure 13-1

Cross section of the mammalian ear. (From *The Neurological Basis for Clinical Neurology*, 2nd ed., by T. L. Peale. Copyright 1961 by T. L. Peale. Used with permission of McGraw-Hill Book Company.)

the inner ear. Let us examine these three parts of the ear in detail with frequent reference to Figure 13–1.

THE OUTER EAR

This is the only part of the ear normally visible. It is totally lacking in many species and is probably the least critical part of the ear. It does have a function, however. The *pinna*, or external portion of the outer ear, works somewhat like a megaphone in reverse, or perhaps like the "snooper" or parabolic microphone the television networks use to pick up the quarterback's instructions in the huddle. Because of its larger area and particular shape, it tends to catch sound waves and "focus" them into the internal ear. Although the actual increase in level (amplification) is probably quite small at the inner boundary of the outer ear, the shape of the external ear does help provide information as to the direction of the sound source. Animals such as dogs improve their localization ability by moving or aiming their external ears. The directionality provided by man's pinna undoubtedly aids him in localizing the source of sounds as he moves his head about.

External Meatus. The second principal part of the outer ear is the *auditory canal*, or *external meatus*. This is simply a tube, about 1 in. long and with a volume of about 6 cm³, connecting the external ear with the eardrum. Many lower animals with no external pinnae likewise have no auditory canal; their eardrums are flush with the surface. It would appear that their hearing sensitivity should suffer from this lack.

The external meatus and its associated pinna probably provide some amplification because of their resonant frequency.* This canal is in effect an open pipe and presumably resonates according to well-established principles. With a resonant frequency of about 3,400 Hz and a maximum pressure point at the eardrum, this resonating device provides for an amplification of from 5 to 10 db, and, of great significance, largely in the frequency range most essential for hearing speech. Without this canal and its collecting devices—that is, if our eardrum were flush with the surface of the head —our hearing would be as much as 10 db less acute.

Tympanic Membrane. The eardrum, or tympanic membrane, which marks the boundary between the external ear and the middle ear, is a thin, membraneous tissue of a generally circular shape, anchored at its circumference. It is really quite similar to the head of a snare drum. Sound waves produce back-and-forth vibrations in this membrane, not entirely dissimilar to the vibrations in the diaphragm of a headphone, or perhaps the cone of a loudspeaker. At this point acoustical vibrations in the air are transformed into mechanical vibrations. Actually the vibratory movements of the eardrum, which must be transmitted to the inner ear by way of the middle-ear ossicles are incredibly small. For ordinary conversation, the displacement of the tympanic membrane is something like one one-hundred millionth (1/100,000,000) of a centimeter, or about equal to the diameter of a hydrogen molecule!

How important is this tympanic membrane? What happens if it is torn or punctured? When your doctor lances your ear because of a middle-ear infection, he simply makes a small, sharp cut through the tympanic membrane, thus allowing undesirable fluids to drain from the middle ear into the outer ear. When the infection is cleared up and the extra fluid has been absorbed, the clean slit in the drum heals with a minimum of scar tissue and your hearing is as good as before.

Even if the drum is slightly torn or punctured, hearing is usually not too severely damaged. Georg von Békésy, winner of the 1961 Nobel prize in medicine and physiology, and probably the foremost authority on the ear, showed that cats with perforations of about 1 mm, while losing hearing below 100 Hz, retained essentially normal hearing for those frequencies over 1,000 Hz (von Békésy, 1957). One millimeter is actually a rather large hole, especially for an animal as small as a cat. The resonant frequency may change somewhat as the result of membrane damage, and some amplification may be lost. In general, however, the drum can still vibrate and transmit most sound waves to the bones of the middle ear. If the damage is extensive, or if large portions of the tympanic membrane have been replaced by relatively stiff scar tissue, hearing may be impaired.

---

* We touched earlier on the resonant frequencies of musical instruments, which amplify some components of complex tones while suppressing other components.

Why then does a punctured eardrum keep a person out of the military service? The problem is due not so much to hearing loss as to the danger of middle-ear infection by way of the unsanitary opening into the middle ear. Dirt that is normally blocked off at the eardrum can now pass into the middle ear, greatly increasing the likelihood of infection. Indeed, when your punctured eardrum heals—if it does—you might find yourself again a likely prospect for military service.

It is also possible, under extreme conditions, to replace the tympanic membrane surgically if the remaining parts of the ear so warrant.

THE MIDDLE EAR

Many species of animals that do not have an outer ear do have a middle ear. The function of the middle ear seems to be to transform the mechanical vibrations of the tympanic membrane into vibrations in the liquid medium of the inner ear. Many fishes do not have a middle ear. The liquid-borne vibrations in their water milieu are transformed, with a minimum loss, to the liquid medium of their inner ears. In animals surrounded by air, however, the transformation of sound waves from acoustical vibration to mechanical vibration to vibrations in the liquid of the inner ear presents a much more formidable problem.

Without a middle ear the transformation of the airborne sound to vibrations in the liquid medium of the inner ear by way of the skull bones would result in a loss (drop in power) of nearly 30 db. This is roughly the figure we suggested as the theoretical maximum attenuation possible with ear protectors that block all of the sound at the opening of the ear canal. Notice too that the hearing loss in persons who have little or no functioning middle ear is frequently on the order of 30 db. That is, sounds are reduced by 30 db, or to a value of a thousandth of that of the normal ear.

Ossicles. Although all animals do not have such a complex system of bones or *ossicles*, most land-dwelling animals of reasonably high position in the phylogenetic scale do have some sort of amplification or impedance-matching device in the middle ear. Birds and some reptiles, for example, have a simple, elongated bone known as a *columella*, and some amphibians have an arrangement of two bones.

The origin of these middle-ear bones presents a fascinating example of evolutionary development. As you are probably aware, most vertebrates have the same number of skeletal bones. Some have atrophied to the point where they are barely discernible, and some have taken on rather unusual, even bizarre, forms. The long "finger" or "toe" of the horse is a case in point; the specialized wings of birds and the "wings" of bats are all examples of such modification and specialization. But basically the same structures exist in all. Primitive fishes have no middle ears, or at least no bones in their middle ears. They do have gills, however, each with a bony structure known as a *gill arch*. Through the process of evolution, these gill arches have decreased in number, having taken on various other forms, in many cases migrating to loci quite remote from the original gill location. Just as the horse walks on a single toe (cloven-hoofed animals walk on two toes), higher-order animals have developed uses for the no longer needed gill arches. Many of the bones of the face, for example, have been derived from the early gill arches. Of significance to us here is that the ossicles of the middle ear are direct descendants of portions of the early fishes' gill arches. Some success has been achieved in identifying those portions of the gill arches that evolved into the specific ossicular bones.

How the Ossicles Work. At higher levels of development most mammals have a leverlike arrangement of three bones arranged somewhat as shown in Figure 13–2. These three bones, or ossicles, called the hammer (*malleus*), anvil (*incus*), and stirrup (*stapes*) transfer the sound from the tympanic membrane to the inner ear by way of the *oval window*. As can be seen from this figure, back-and-forth movements of the tympanic membrane produce a movement in the malleus. The rocking movement of the loosely attached incus is then transmitted to the stapes, whose single point of contact with the oval window and pistonlike movement transforms the original acoutic vibrations into vibratory waves in the fluid of the inner ear (*perilymph*).

It has been estimated that the leverlike action of these three bones regains about 25.5 db of the 30-db loss that would prevail if sound had to go directly from the air medium into a liquid medium. As mentioned earlier, the pinna and meatus contribute some amplification, but the greater bulk of the improved impedance matching (from waves in an air medium to waves in a liquid medium) is provided by the design of the bones of the middle ear.

Amplification is accomplished in at least two ways. First, the lever action results in a smaller amplitude of movement at the output—that is, the oval window. Movements at the eardrum are reduced by a factor of from 1.3 to 3, thus resulting in a mechanical advantage at the oval window. Such a lever action is analogous to the familiar gear changes in an automobile or the lever action of a crowbar.

Second, the area of movement at the tympanic membrane (attachment of malleus is some 14 to 20 times greater than that at the oval window (stapes attachment. Thus a principle analogous to that employed in an hydraulic ram is built into middle-ear functioning. This latter amplification probably reduces the air-liquid transfer loss by as much as 23 db. With roughly 2.5-db gain by the lever functioning and some contribution of the external meatus resonance, the 30-db loss we referred to earlier is pretty well taken care of. The overall effect is to increase greatly the energy transfer from the light, compressible air to the dense, incompressible fluid of the inner ear—a remarkably well-designed system.

Birds, as suggested earlier, have a much simpler system. In addition to having no pinna, they have only a single columella in their middle ears. Hence they utilize only the areal ratio and hydraulic ram effect to counter-

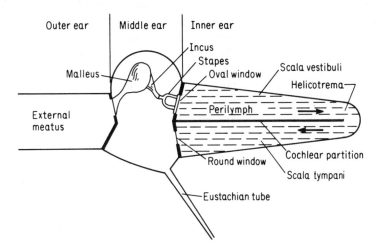

Figure 13-2
Schematic of ear. Note the direction of the wave movement, down the scala vestibuli, around the helicotrema, and back by way of the scala tympani. Note too that the cochlear partition is quite a complex structure as shown by Figures 13-4 and 13-5.

act the air-to-fluid transfer loss and still maintain excellent auditory sensitivity.

The ossicles of the middle ear also provide some protection to the inner ear from intense sounds. Under normal sound levels the ossicles vibrate in a manner to increase the energy at the oval window, as we have just seen. But when sounds are quite intense, the movement of the ossicles changes to an alternate mode; they vibrate differently, thus transmitting less of the energy to the inner ear.

Also, there are two muscles attached to the ossicles that may tend to damp their movement somewhat. Many persons question the efficacy of these slow-responding *tensor tympani* and *stapedius* muscles as means of protecting the inner ear from intense sounds. It would appear that their function may be analogous to the function of the iris, and its pupil—to set a resting tension to maximize sound transmission, rather than to protect the ear. The existence of autonomic nervous system ennervation of these muscles tends to support this view.

The Eustachian Tube. A small tube with an inside diameter roughly that of a pencil lead connects the middle-ear cavity with the back of the mouth. Although it plays a minor part in hearing, the *Eustachian tube* is of importance for the well-being of the middle ear. This tube drains undesirable fluids from the middle ear that might result in serious infections and damage to the delicate bones therein. In its normal, healthy state it also ensures that air pressures in the middle-ear cavity will be the same as those impinging on the outer surface of the tympanic membrane. You have all experienced the movement of air between the middle ear and the mouth concurrent with sudden changes in elevation, such as when you ascend or descend a mountain, or even in an elevator in a tall office building. For the proper functioning of the ear it is important that the normal resting pressures be the same on both sides of the eardrum.

If the Eustachian tube collapses from general systemic disorder or gets clogged up with a superabundance of fluids from the middle ear, serious problems may develop. It is even possible to clog the tube with germ-laden mucus as a result of a violent sneeze. This is why one should never completely block one nostril while blowing the other. Pressures building up in the middle ear can produce severe pain and the infectious material may damage the delicate contents of the middle ear. Lancing of the eardrum may be necessary in order to drain off excess fluid.

One semimedical organization that I once knew of attached particular importance to the functioning of the Eustachian tube. They believed that many cases of hearing loss can be attributed directly to a failure of the Eustachian tube to maintain a functional opening because of loss of muscular tonus in its walls. Their chiropracticlike treatment consisted of massaging the wall of the tube, first with a small tool inserted through the mouth and into the tube, later by actually massaging the interior of the tube with the finger. Can you imagine sticking your finger in your ear through your mouth? Apparently it can be done, for the walls of the Eustachian tube are quite flexible and stretchable. A healthy, well-defined Eustachian tube might be expected to perform its function better than a sickly, flabby one.

Round and Oval Windows. As can be seen from the schematic drawing of Figure 13–2, not one but two openings (covered by thin diaphragms) connect the middle ear with the cochlea of the inner ear. A portion of the stapes is attached to the *oval window*. Thus as the stapes rocks back and forth it imparts a wave motion to the fluid in the inner ear. The resultant pressure waves move along the path of the inner ear, crossing over a dividing septum at the *helicotrema* and returning to the round window. Without a flexible oval window the pressure waves could not move through the incompressible perilymph of the inner ear and stimulate the sensory elements located there. Thus both the oval window, to introduce the vibratory motion, and the round window, to permit compression of the liquid medium, are essential for hearing.

In a later section we discuss in more detail how the waves in the inner ear perilymph are converted into nervous impulses. However, when we get to that point we will be dealing somewhat in conjecture, because the nature of cochlear functioning is still not fully understood.

Disorders of the Middle Ear. Because the tiny precision-like bones of the middle ear are extremely delicate and yet must function as a complex mechanical device, problems with them might be expected. Indeed, much deafness, especially that found as an accompaniment of the aging process, can be attributed to malfunctions of the middle ear. Such disorders are referred to as *conduction deafness*, as distinguished from *nerve deafness*, which involves problems of the inner ear and the sensory organs located there. Fortunately, several methods for relieving deafness due to conduction or middle-ear malfunction are available, and no one should be truly deaf solely because of diseases of the middle ear.

The commonest defect of the middle ear is known as *otosclerosis*, which literally means, "auditory tissue turning to bone." It was once believed that the cartilaginous portions of the middle ear did indeed ossify, thus prohibiting their movement and the conduction of sound waves to the oval window. We now know differently. What does appear to happen as a concomitant of aging and the general systemic changes that accompany it is a depositing of hard, calceous material around the footplate of the stapes. Such a deposit prevents the free movement of this last link in the middle-ear chain, thus greatly reducing or even completely eliminating wave transfer through the oval window and to the inner ear.

Stapes Mobilization. One early approach to the treatment of otosclerosis was to go into the middle ear with a slender probe like a blunt needle and break the footplate loose from its calcified anchor. This was not a highly successful maneuver. Von Békésy suggests that success can be achieved in about 30 percent of the cases (von Békésy, 1957). He further adds, rather wryly, that he doubts that bone breaking can be improved to a standard procedure. Finding the obstreperous footplate and breaking it loose without damaging other delicate parts of the ear requires considerable skill. And even if the stapes is made free by the mobilization operation, continuing calcification ultimately interferes with its motion again, and deafness recurs.

Fenestration. A more successful surgical approach to the problem of conduction deafness is known as *fenestration*. As can be seen from Figure 13–2, the problem is to get the wave moving in that part of the cochlea known as the *scala vestibuli*. This can be accomplished by simply ignoring the normal conduction mode by way of the middle-ear bones and making a new opening (window, or *fenestra*) into the cochlea. The surgical technique involves boring a small hole (usually with a dental drill) into the scala vestibuli by way of the lateral canal of the *vestibular organ*.* When the hole is covered with a flap of skin, sound conduction from the middle ear into the inner ear is again achieved. The operation is straightforward, all steps are well under control, and prognosis, assuming the inner ear is functioning properly, is quite good. Because most of the amplification potential of the middle ear is lost, hearing, although much improved over the severe otosclerotic condition, is not as acute as that of the normal, healthy ear. A hearing aid in most cases makes up for the loss.

Artificial Ossicles. A still newer approach involves the replacement of the ossicles with a prosthetic device. This operation, made possible by the

---

* The vestibular organ is the nonauditory portion of the inner ear referred to earlier. Because of its primary involvement in equilibrium and balance, it is treated in a later chapter.

development of the binocular microscope and the perfection of micro-sur-
gical techniques, entails opening the ear drum, removing the damaged ossicles, and replacing them with a fine wire. This latter, when surgically
attached to the oval window and the replaced eardrum serves to conduct
sound waves to the inner ear. I understand the technique is quite successful
and rather widely employed.

Hearing Aids. The last approach alleviating conduction deafness we
shall mention is the use of a hearing aid. The old-fashioned ear trumpet
you may have seen in old pictures or museums was an example of a simple
hearing aid that did indeed work. The trumpet-shaped affair collected the
sound waves and focused them into the auditory canal, not entirely unlike
a convex lens that is used as a burning glass or the parabolic microphone
we referred to earlier.

Most conduction deafness, unless it has progressed to an extreme state,
is not the result of complete stapes immobilization. If the sound is intense
enough it can still force movements in the ossicles and subsequent conduction to the oval window. Modern hearing aids simply amplify the sound
electronically so that the reluctant ossicles are forced to conduct the sound
vibrations to the inner ear. Note, too, that electronic amplifying devices
have "tone" controls, amplifying those parts of the audio spectrum most
in need of amplification and not simply *all* sound frequencies equally irrespective of their importance to hearing and the unique nature of the hearing disorder.

If the ossicles are incapable of conducting any sound vibration at all, the
usual hearing aid will be of no value. Increasing air-conducted vibrations
to such a level that they can activate the oval window directly, without
the mediation of the middle-ear bones, may result in severe unpleasantness
and even pain. For extreme loss of middle-ear functioning where surgery
cannot be employed a bone-conduction device may be required.

It was suggested earlier that the difference in sensitivity between the
normal auditory mechanism and one without an external or middle ear
would be about 30 db. It should be apparent then that by amplifying the
sound some 30 db and introducing it into the inner ear directly by way of
the bones of the skull, hearing should approach normalcy. This is precisely
what is done in some cases of severe conduction deafness. A bone-conduction device is placed against the mastoid bone, behind the pinna, and sound
vibrations are conducted directly to the inner ear with no need for the
middle-ear involvement. There are problems inherent in such a technique.
Individual differences exist between heads and mastoid bones, and conduction of sound through bone is not the same as conduction through air.
Nevertheless, for the almost totally deaf individual who can adapt to it, a
bone-conduction hearing aid may be a great blessing.

If the deafness is due to inner-ear malfunction (discussed in the next
section), any hearing aid may be of little value. Von Békésy suggests that
an old test, often used by deaf musicians, was to touch one's teeth to a

vibrating musical instrument. If one cannot then hear the music, he knows he suffers from nerve deafness and there is no adequate treatment (von Békésy, 1957).

THE INNER EAR

As indicated at the beginning of this chapter, the portion of the inner ear involved in hearing is known as the cochlea. The human cochlea is a tube about 0.13 in. in diameter and perhaps 1.33 in. long. But it takes up somewhat less space than this because it is highly coiled, in the manner of a snail. The number of turns in the cochlea varies with the species: The guinea pig's cochlea, which is frequently studied in the laboratory, has about four and one-half turns; the human cochlea has about three and one-half turns.

Imbedded deep in the bones of the skull, it is a difficult organ to get at, and its function is not completely understood. For much of what we do know about the cochlea and its functioning we are indebted to the pioneering work of the aforementioned von Békésy. Perhaps no man has so dominated his field and achieved such wide recognition as has Georg von Békésy in the area of auditory functioning.

Scala Vestibuli and Scala Tympani. As can be seen from Figure 13–2, in which it has been "uncoiled," the cochlea is a two-chambered tube, being divided by a very complex structure identified as the *cochlear partition*. One chamber, the *scala vestibuli,* and the second parallel chamber, the *scala tympani,* are connected at the apex of the tube by the *helicotrema.*

Pistonlike movements of the stapes against the flexible oval window set the fluid (perilymph) in the inner ear into motion, reproducing the wave action of the original sound. These wavelike activities in the fluid proceed to travel the length of the scala vestibuli, through the helicotrema, and down the scala tympani, where they spend themselves against the flexible membrane of the round window. On their way through the entwined cochlea they presumably set up activity in the basilar membrane that serves as the stimulus for hearing.

Figure 13–3 shows a cross section taken through a cochlea. Note that several turns of the cochlea have been transected, exposing the interior of the tube in several places. Note too the helicotrema at the extreme left of the figure.

Basilar Membrane. Figure 13–4 shows a schematic drawing of a cross section taken at one point in the cochlear canal. As described earlier the cochlear canal is divided into two channels by a structure known, not unreasonably, as the cochlear partition. The functional portion of the cochlear partition is the basilar membrane, a tapered structure resting on a bony shelf at one side of the tube and apparently suspended from the other side by a ligamentlike contrivance. Although the overall width of the cochlear partition remains constant throughout its length, the basilar membrane is tapered. According to von Békésy, it has an average width of 0.04 mm at

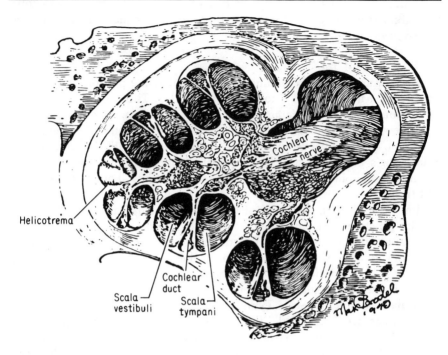

Helicotrema

Cochlear nerve

Scala vestibuli

Cochlear duct

Scala tympani

Figure 13–3

Cross section of the cochlea. Note the multiple cross sections due to the coiling of the organ. Notice too the three ducts and the helicotreama. (From the Otological Research Laboratory and the Department of Art in Medicine, Johns Hopkins University, *1940 Yearbook of the Eye, Ear, Nose and Throat*, drawn by Max Brodel. Copyright 1940 Yearbook Medical Publishers, Inc. Used by permission.)

the stapes and a width of 0.5 mm at the helicotrema (Stevens, 1951). Thus as the width of the membrane increases from the oval window to the helicotrema, the bony shelf on which it rests decreases in width.

Another thin membrane (*Reissner's membrane*) divides the cochlear canal and should be included as a part of the cochlear partition. Anchored near the base of the bony shelf at one side the presence of this membrane creates a third space or duct, known variously as the *cochlear duct, scala media,* or *endotic space.* It gets its last name from its containing endolymph, rather than perilymph. This basic cavity is continuous with structures of the nonauditory labyrinthe portions of the inner ear.

The basilar membrane, with its bony shelf and suspensory system, and Reissner's membrane team up in a remarkable manner to create a highly specialized chamber to house the delicate, sensitive organs of hearing, protected from external forces and bathed in the endolymphatic fluid.

Organ of Corti. The actual sensory unit in the ear is the organ of Corti, first demonstrated by Alfonso Corti in 1851 and pictured in Figures 13–4

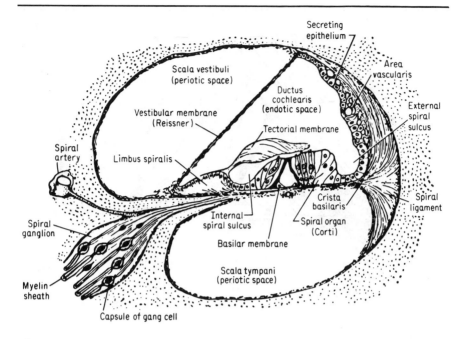

Figure 13–4
Cross secton of the cochlear canal. (From A. T. Rasmussen, *Outlines of Neuro-anatomy*, 3rd ed. Dubuque, Iowa: Wm. C. Brown Company, 1943.)

and 13–5. The organ of Corti is a collection of fleshy cells in the scala media, resting on the basilar membrane and the bony shelf of the cochlear partition. It is, indeed, a remarkable organ. You may recall that the lens of the eye has no blood vessels to interfere with the passage of light. Instead, any necessary interchange of nutrient and waste material is accomplished by direct interaction with the intraocular fluid. Although there are small blood vessels in the basilar membrane, the organ of Corti has no blood supply. If it had, as sensitive to movement as it is, one would be constantly hearing one's pulse. The amount of movement in even small blood vessels as a result of the pulse would probably be so great as to completely mask the infinitesimally small movements produced by sound stimuli. Remember that if the ear were any more sensitive you would be hearing the Brownian movement of air molecules. Instead of a vascular supply, the organ of Corti is bathed in the endolymph, a primitive highly nutritive embryological liquid, thus mitigating the need for any accessory blood supply.

The ultimate end organs in the organ of Corti are the *hair cells*, which are in turn supported by the *phalangeal cells*. There are two distinct groups of hair cells: the outer hair cells, numbering about 20,000, whose phalangeal cells rest on the flexible basilar membrane; and the inner hair cells,

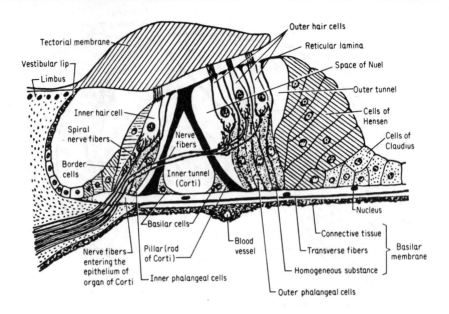

Figure 13–5
Cross section of the organ of Corti. (From A. T. Rasmussen, *Outlines of Neuro-anatomy*, 3rd ed. Dubuque, Iowa: Wm. C. Brown Company, 1943.)

numbering about 3,500, whose supporting cells rest on the bony edge of the cochlear partition. These hair cells pass through a perforated layer of cells known as the *reticular lamina* and terminate with their ends imbedded in the *tectorial membrane*. The hair cells are presumably activated as a result of a "shearing" action set up by motion of the fluid of the inner ear. It would appear that the tectorial membrane, the reticular lamina, and the organ of Corti slide with respect to each other, thus bending the hairs and setting off a neural discharge. Such a "shearing" action greatly amplifies the effects of the otherwise insignificant movements in the perilymph.

Von Békésy's efforts with an internal ear removed from a cadaver as well as his demonstrations with laboratory models were instrumental in our gaining an understanding of just how this remarkable organ of Corti performs its function.*

To complete the anatomical story, individual nerve fibers from the hair cells wend their way through the organ of Corti, meeting near the juncture of the basilar membrane and the bony ledge, from whence they proceed, by way of the VIIIth cranial nerve, to the brain.

Disorders of the Inner Ear. Hearing loss due to malfunction of the inner ear is indeed a serious problem. So-called nerve deafness, caused by atrophy

* We will return to the von Békésy explanation when we consider theories of hearing in a later chapter.

or disease of the hair cells and their associated neural connections, presents an irreversible condition. Once the neural connections are destroyed nothing can be done; a hearing aid cannot force a nonexistent end organ to fire.

In addition to general circulatory and systemic disease of old age, which may result in "death" of the organ of Corti cells, or the eighth nerve, at least one well-known drug, streptomycin, can produce nerve deafness. When taken to excess over long periods of time, this drug has resulted in numerous cases of deafness due to destruction of hair cells and/or nerve endings. But perhaps the situation is not as bad as suggested here. There may still be hope. At least one successful cochlear implantation of an electrode providing some hearing has been reported (*Newsweek*, 1974). The victim (of streptomycin) was able to recognize school bells, hands clapping, and the meowing of a cat. He could even carry on a very simple phone conversation. Dr. Michelson of the University of California at San Francisco, however, thinks much more work is needed before the technique can be widely used.

Another form of deafness attributable to the inner ear can be related to actual physical damage of the organ of Corti. If the basilar membrane is forced to vibrate violently by extremely intense acoustic stimulation, hair cells may be physically torn lose from their phalangeal cell roots. Such deafness presents an interesting opportunity, as well as a challenge, to the study of hearing. If the intense sound has a frequency of, say, 1,000 Hz, not all of the hair cells on the basilar membrane will be damaged. Only those in a narrowly circumscribed area will be destroyed. Thus the person will be deaf at only 1,000 Hz, and, of course, some distance on either side in a more or less graduated manner, depending on the intensity of the sound and the resultant spreading along the basilar membrane.

Such hearing losses are typified by *auditory scotoma*, or "blind" spots, in the auditory spectrum. Persons exposed to very intense narrow-band noises such as the compressor whine of a jet engine may lose their hearing over a relatively narrow range of frequencies. If the loss is at a frequency not critical for perceiving speech, the victim may not even know he has sustained inner-ear damage, or that he has a hearing loss.

A severe ringing sound or a whistling in the ear is a not too uncommon symptom and may or may not herald increasing deafness. Known as *tinnitus*, such symptoms are presumably the result of spontaneous activity, or perhaps hypersensitivity, of the delicate hair cells of the inner ear. There is normally a faint "background" noise anyone can hear if conditions are otherwise sufficiently quiet, but when the condition becomes severe some sort of degeneration is either in progress or has occurred.

As an example, subjection to intense sounds can produce a temporary tinnitus, apparently as a result of mechanical injury to the hair cells of the basilar membrane. It is significant too that the pitch of a tinnitus frequently corresponds to a pitch to which some sensitivity has been lost.

Tinnitus is frequently found in conjunction with Ménière's disease, the vertigo-producing disorder clearly attributable to damage or malfunction of the labyrinthine portion of the auditory nerve. Tumors or other mechanical damage to the auditory nerve also can result in tinnitus.

Auditory Nerve and Brain

We could continue on for many pages, tracing the auditory nerve into the lower brain levels such as the lateral geniculates, corpora quadrigemina, and all the way to the auditory cortex. But, as with our study of vision, space and time do not permit us to go beyond the receptor. However, much is known about the functioning of the brain in audition, and most of what we know is quite exciting. We know, for example, that there is an auditory area in the brain. Unlike the visual area, with its spatial distribution based on visual space, the cortical distribution for the auditory sense is related to the pitch or frequency of the sound. Moreover, the two cerebral hemispheres seem to play different roles: The left hemisphere, for example, seems to process speech, and the right hemisphere has a predilection for processing noise and other nonverbal material. See, for example, Cohn (1971) and also the chapters by Cherry, Woolsey, Neff, and Katsuki in Rosenblith (1962).

Summary

In this chapter we first discussed the general development of the ear, with emphasis on the inner ear and its possible evolution from the lateral line organs of lower animals. We then examined in some detail the three main divisions of the ear; the outer ear, the middle ear, and the inner ear. With respect to the outer ear we considered the pinna, external meatus, and tympanic membrane. For the middle ear we examined the ossicles and how they work; the round and oval windows; the Eustachian tube and its function; and potential disorders of the middle ear. We concluded this section with a discussion of hearing loss due to middle-ear malfunction and the corrective treatment indicated. With respect to the inner ear we described the scala vestibuli, scala tympani, and the interconnecting helicotrema. We described the cochlear partition in some detail, elaborating on the basilar membrane and its organs of Corti with their sensitive hair cells. We concluded the chapter with a discussion of inner-ear disorders and an even briefer mention of brain functioning in audition.

Suggested Readings

1. Georg von Békésy, "The Ear," *Scientific American,* August 1957. A short article of 10 pages, well worth reading. Professor Békésy points out some of the wonders of the auditory mechanism, describes the structure of the ear, and elaborates on a number of topics such as hearing pitch, hearing speech, vocal

feedback, auditory localization, and deafness. It is a short article that anyone can read, understand, and profit from. It is highly recommended.

2. Georg von Békésy and W. A. Rosenblith. "The Mechanical Properties of the Ear," in S. S. Stevens (ed.), *Handbook of Experimental Psychology*. New York: Wiley, 1951. These 38 pages are by far the best detailed descriptions of the human ear of which I am aware. Indeed, this chapter goes into fine detail to an extent not required for general understanding of the ear's functioning. However, for an advanced, complete understanding of the manner in which the ear functions, this chapter has no peer. Detailed reading is for the serious, advanced student.

3. From W. A. Van Bergeijk, J. R. Pierce, and E. E. David, Jr. *Waves and the Ear*. Garden City, N.Y.: Doubleday, 1960. Chapter V of this excellent little book is a fine, highly readable presentation of the development and structure of the mammalian ear. In addition, this chapter contains much of the information related to theories of hearing that we will cover in a later chapter. These 40 pages are well worth reading.

4. From C. C. Mueller. *Sensory Psychology*. Englewood Cliffs, N.J.: Prentice-Hall, 1965. Chapter 4 of this paperback is the shortest reference I have included for this chapter (8 pages). It is well worth reading, however, especially the treatment of cochlear partition activity and the neural response.

5. Various authors, from Békésy Commemorative Issue, *J. Acoust. Soc. Amer.* 34, (1962), 9 (Part 2). This is a complete issue of the journal dedicated to von Békésy to celebrate his winning of the Nobel prize in physiology and medicine. The original articles by pupils and contemporaries of von Békésy are of considerable value for the serious student.

6. Georg von Békésy. *Experiments in Hearing*, trans. E. G. Wever. New York: McGraw-Hill, 1960. This book of some 700 pages represents the collected works of Georg von Békésy. It is well worth reading if you are seriously interested in how the ear works. Chapters 1 through 6 (205 pages) are particularly germane to this chapter. Chapter 1 presents some fascinating historical perspective, while chaps. 1, 2, and 3 delve into the anatomy of the ear and the techniques, apparatus, etc., used for its investigation. Chapters 5 and 6 on middle-ear action and bone conduction are well worth reading. The last four chapters (11 to 14) provide, by far, the best description of cochlear action available. This is not an easy book. It is comprehensive, and for the serious student it is very important.

7. Hallowell Davis and S. Richard Silverman (eds.). *Hearing and Deafness*. New York: Holt, Rinehart and Winston, 1970. This is an excellent reference on most aspects of hearing, and is recommended for later chapters as well as this one. Being edited by a medical doctor, it does have a strong bias toward hearing loss and its correction. Chapters 3 to 6 are especially appropriate to our discussion in this chapter, and other chapters are more germane to our later material.

8. Clinton H. Woolsey. "Organization of Cortical Auditory System," from Walter A. Rosenblith (ed.), *Sensory Communication*. New York: Wiley, 1962. This is an excellent article on the auditory cortex and its functioning. It is not an easy article to read and understand, but it should prove of value for the student who has the background and interest to profit from it. Recommended for the serious, qualified student.

9. Douglas B. Webster. "Audition," from Edward C. Carterette and Morton P. Friedman (eds.), *Handbook of Perception, vol. III, Biology of Perceptual Systems.* New York: Academic Press, 1973. This is chap. 19 of an excellent book we have mentioned before. This reading presents the functioning of hair cells and describes the diversity of auditory mechanisms in submammalian species quite well. It is a surprisingly easy-to-read article for such an advanced collection of readings. It is well worth the average undergraduate's time.

14/auditory sensitivity and loudness

Some Terminology

Several terms are frequently encountered with respect to auditory stimulation that might best be clarified at this time. *Monaural* and *binaural* probably need no explanation; they simply refer to the use of one ear or two and are basically laymen's terms. *Stereophonic*, primarily a hi-fi term, refers to binaural listening in which differences in the signals to the two ears, normally experienced as a result of the location of the ears on the head, are simulated by means of separate speakers, separate headphones, or the like.

You may also encounter the terms *monotic, diotic,* and *dichotic*. Monotic simply means the stimulation of one ear and is essentially the same as monaural. Diotic and dichotic both refer to binaural stimulation, but they differ in that diotic refers to situations in which the stimulus signal is the same to both ears and dichotic refers to stimulation that is different to the two ears. If we stimulate both ears with a 300-Hz tone of the same sound-pressure level, we are employing diotic presentation, if we give a 300-Hz tone to one ear and a 500-Hz tone to the other, we are employing dichotic stimulation. For a relatively complete listing of terminology the pamphlet by Sonn (1969) is highly recommended.

The attribute of hearing, corresponding to the visual attribute of brightness is that of loudness. Like brightness, loudness is related to the intensity of the impinging stimulation, but like brightness, the relationship is not a simple monotonic function. Indeed, loudness is an experience; loudness is in the ear of the beholder. If the proverbial tree fell on the deserted island, there would be sound waves, but there would be no loudness. Before examining this psychological attribute of loudness, let us start at the beginning—the actual detection and recognition of intensity as a parameter of the auditory stimulus.

Threshold for Hearing

The absolute sensitivity of the ear is expressed in terms of absolute thresholds over a wide range of frequencies. Individual monaural determinations are made of the minimal sound pressure that can be detected for each of a number of pure tones, ranging from perhaps a low of 30 or 40 Hz to a high of 10,000 Hz or higher. When these individual thresholds, expressed in decibels re 0.0002 dyne/cm², are plotted, the result is a curve of sensitivity. (See the solid line of Figure 14–1 for a curve based on a "normal" ear.)* Any loss of hearing ability will show up as departures from the shape and location of the curve found for the normal or "ideal" individual.

Various psychophysical techniques may be employed in obtaining the data for plotting such a curve, or for clinical applications in which interest is focused on hearing loss, or departure from the "normal."

One common procedure for collecting such data involves a form of the method of limits, in which a signal below thresholds is gradually increased in intensity until the subject gives a positive response. Descending series can also be included to "bracket" the threshold or 50 percent detection point. (See Chapter 3, especially Figure 3–3.) The signal may be a continuous tone or be presented in discrete pulses of tone, with durations such as one second, for example.

As an alternative, a constant method may be employed in which numerous signals are presented in random order, some above the threshold and some below, the subject simply indicating where he hears the tone. In some cases a light may indicate when the subject should hear the tone. The absolute threshold is then determined in the manner described in Chapter 3 and illustrated by Figure 3–4.

One interesting technique eliminates the necessity of preselecting the values to be used in the constant method. In this method a computer is utilized to select stimulus values to be presented to the subject while the actual *audiometry* is in progress. If when a particular signal is presented, the person being tested cannot detect it, the next signal will be more intense three out of four times. If the signal is detected the reverse will obtain; that is, there is a 3 to 1 probability that the next signal will be of lower amplitude. Thus the subject cannot anticipate the next signal; it may be either more intense or less intense. Furthermore, an automatic form of bracketing is accomplished, with most of the stimuli being near the threshold and with a minimum of time being wasted on signals either too weak

---

* *Normal*, as used here, does not mean normal in the sense of the average. Rather, it is the "norm" for the ideal ear, based on young, healthy, almost perfect ears. As we will see later, few older persons exhibit hearing that meets this criterion.

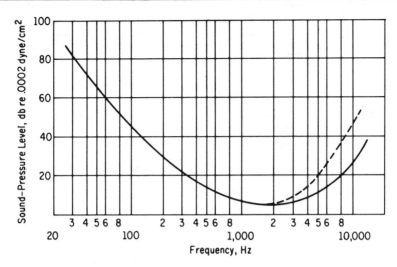

Figure 14-1

Sensitivity curve for the "normal" ear. This figure shows the absolute threshold as a standard for comparison. It is not the threshold curve for the average person; rather it is an accepted standard that only a few young persons attain.

to ever be detected or of such an amplitude that they are always detected. (The 3-to-1 probabilities could be replaced by 2 to 1, 3 to 2, or any other ratio desired.) Note too that the use of a computer to run the sensitivity check also involves automatic data collection, possibly with a printout of the threshold data in whatever form might be desired.

Finally, a production or adjustment method may be used. The testee physically adjusts the level of the tone until he can just hear it. Bracketing can also be employed in this method, with the subject alternately adjusting the output level up and down until he arrives at some arbitrary point he considers to be his threshold.

Equipment used to determine thresholds and ultimately plot sensitivity curves may vary widely. In one approach, loudspeakers driven by audio oscillators and associated amplifiers are used. More often calibrated headphones are employed, the tones being injected directly into the listener's ear. In Chapter 12 we learned how headphones are calibrated, utilizing couplers that simulate the external-ear cavity and inputs from audio signal generators.

The suggestion that methods employing either loudspeakers or headphones may be used may seem to imply that the choice is simply procedural and the same results will be obtained in either case. This is not so. Sensitivity curves obtained by the two methods are not directly comparable. We may examine briefly the differences between *minimum audible fields* (MAF), obtained by placing an individual in a previously calibrated sound field, and *minimum audible pressure* (MAP), obtained by measuring the actual level at the eardrum by means of a probe microphone or a coupler-calibrated headphone. Figure 14–2 shows four "standard" curves obtained by several experimenters, two by the MAF technique and two by the MAP procedure.

MINIMUM AUDIBLE FIELD

It might seem logical that the MAF technique would be most realistic, determining the sound level at a point in an open space and then placing the listener at this point. When this is done, the plot of thresholds is likely to resemble the two curves of Figure 14–2 identified as MAF measurements. Note that they are not smooth curves throughout their range. In the vicinity of 1,000 to 3,000 Hz they seem to have perturbations in their otherwise smooth functions. It is unlikely that the physiological response of the ear itself should show such discontinuities. When the head is placed in a free field of sound, the field is no longer a free field. The head (and the rest of the body, for that matter) have an influence on the field due to reflection and absorption that cannot be predicted precisely. Moreover, variations in the configuration of the external portion of the ear influence pure tones in a nonpredictable manner. In some cases this might be just the problem one wishes to investigate. For such purposes a free-field technique would be not only desirable, but necessary.

Note too that facilities for conducting minimum audible field measurements should ensure freedom from echoes and reverberations. A chamber designed to eliminate echoes and reverberations is known as an *anechoic* chamber. Such a room or chamber is a must for valid free-field measurements. As a result, free-field measurements are more of academic and scientific than of practical interest.

MINIMUM AUDIBLE PRESSURE

Thresholds for hearing and subsequent clinical audiograms are more commonly based on minimum audible pressures, in which the threshold level at the eardrum itself is determined. As described in Chapter 12, this can be accomplished by means of a probe microphone that actually measures the level at a point very close to the eardrum or by means of calibrated headphones the outputs of which have been determined precisely. Actual thresholds can be determined by any of the previously described psychophysical methods that are appropriate.

Perhaps "determined precisely" in the preceding paragraph is too strong a term. Microphones intended for use with couplers in the calibration of phones may be accurate to 0.1 db. Measurements of hearing sensitivity, however, rarely have precisions greater than 2 or 3 db. For practical purposes, and because of uncontrollable variables, any clinical audiogram that reports accuracies beyond 5 db is probably suspect. If you have a hearing loss of 20 db at some frequency this is really a loss in the range of 15 to 25 db. Sensitivity curves vary substantially from day to day and from test

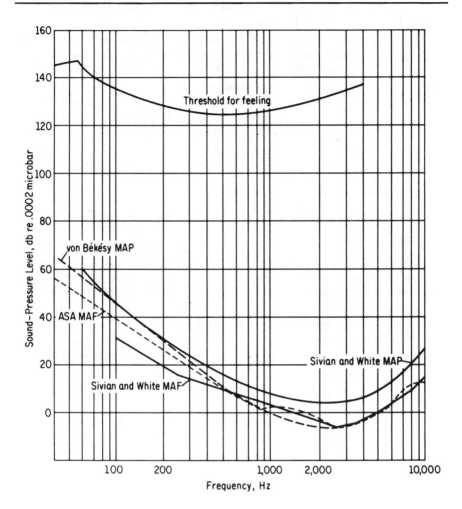

Figure 14-2

Representative sensitivity curves. Two threshold determinations by each method, minimum audible field and minimum audible pressure, are illustrated. In addition, the top curve is a representation of the approximate threshold for feeling based on several determinations. [Modified from S. S. Stevens (ed.), *Handbook of Experimental Psychology*, New York: John Wiley & Sons, Inc., 1951.]

method to test method, and any more precise statement should generally not be made. For practical purposes, differences of less than 10 db are not significant.

Audiometry

When the data are to be used for clinical purposes and the interest is in hearing loss, rather than sensitivity, they are not normally plotted in the form of Figure 14–1 or 14–2. Rather, they are plotted directly in decibels of hearing loss (see Figures 14–3 and 14–4).

The audiologist may use the equipments and techniques just described, but is more likely to employ a commercial audiometer that does much of the routine work automatically. Some, complete with calibrated headphones, vary intensity and frequency automatically, even plotting the final audiogram as a function of the patient's signals (e.g., key depressions). If you have your ears checked by a professional he will in all likelihood use some sort of automatic or semiautomatic audiometer, thus eliminating much of the tedium of manual calculations, frequency adjustments, and output level settings as well as the recording of responses and plotting the data.

MASKING NOISE

Frequently in the application of MAP techniques the audiologist may introduce a simultaneous masking signal in the ear opposite the one being tested. If the sensitivity of one ear is quite low, elevating a signal to the point where it is detectable may result in its being heard by the good ear by way of bone conduction. Because the listener cannot always be sure which ear is doing the hearing, determination of thresholds for relatively insensitive ears would be impossible. To avoid this problem, random or white noise may be introduced in the good ear while the test signal is injected into the less sensitive ear. One can utilize a masking signal for the opposite ear in all testing. Of course, the masking noise must not be so intense as to stimulate the ear being tested.

HEARING LOSS

The dotted line of Figure 14–1 shows an audiogram of a person with a mild hearing loss. The individual has normal* hearing for most of the audio spectrum, but at frequencies above about 2,000 Hz the threshold has been elevated. That is, sensitivity has been reduced. Although the normal individual can detect a 10,000-Hz tone of about 26 db, the ear identified by the broken line requires that a tone of 10,000 Hz be some 10 db more intense in order to be detected. Hearing loss such as this appears to be an inexorable result of the aging process and most individuals of 30 or 40 years of age may be expected to show a loss comparable to that of the broken line in Figure 14–1. With increasing age the loss can be expected to be greater, both in degree and in that it will spread to somewhat lower frequencies. A loss such as that shown here would not be of an great consequence, and the individual would in all likelihood not even be aware of it unless he or she were quite young and perhaps a musician.

If a sufficiently large number of points are plotted (measuring the threshold for more pure tones), the curve takes on a less regular form. There may be dips and humps, all indicating minor variations in the sensitivity curve.

* Recall our earlier definition of "normal."

If there are severe perturbations in the shape of the curve, indicating sharp losses of hearing sensitivity in relatively restricted frequency ranges, a more serious hearing loss may be indicated. If the curve at, say, 400 Hz suddenly rises to the 60-db level, then a loss of some 42-db for a 400-Hz tone is involved. Such uncommon instances are probably due to localized damage in the basilar membrane of the cochlea, rather than the simple conduction deficiencies leading to the broken line in the figure.

In practice, audiograms are generally plotted in terms of hearing *loss*, rather than sensitivity. Figure 14–3 is an example of how an actual hearing loss might be plotted. Notice that it is based on seven pure tones and that measurements are given only to the nearest 5 db, in keeping with our previous observations of precision of audiometric measurements. If more detailed analysis of the 30-db loss at 4,000 Hz were desired, additional pure tones could be employed for detailed exploration. Notice too that this individual has somewhat better than normal sensitivity at 1,000 Hz.

Figure 14–4 shows the manner in which hearing loss develops as a function of age. Included in this figure are differences due to sex. Are sex differences due to genetic characteristics or to the fact that men live somewhat different lives from those of women? Perhaps men are subjected to more severe noises in their work lives than are women, or perhaps the difference is due to biological factors. In Figure 14–4 it appears that even in the youngest group the males have less sensitivity at the higher frequencies than their female counterparts. At older ages this difference becomes more marked. It may be both genetic and environmental.

The data from which this figure was drawn were collected at the New York and San Francisco World's Fairs and might be considered to be representative of people in general. There has been some criticism of the procedures used, and the actual values may be more suggestive than definitive, but the curves are probably not too far from the truth. More recent but less extensive studies tend to bear out these earlier findings.

Additional Intensity Considerations

SUMMATION OVER FREQUENCY

Although most of what we have been considering involves single tones delivered to the ear (or ears), it should be recognized that under proper circumstances multiple tones can summate. For example, two tones at different frequencies are easier to detect than either one alone. Actually, each tone can be one-half as intense as either one alone in order to reach threshold. This statement is true only if the individual tones do not differ too much in frequency. This maximum difference within which summation can occur is known as the critical band (Scharf, 1970). Two tones separated by more than a critical band can be detected only when their levels are set as high as would be necessary for either one alone. Critical bands vary according to their frequency location: At about 500 Hz the critical band is

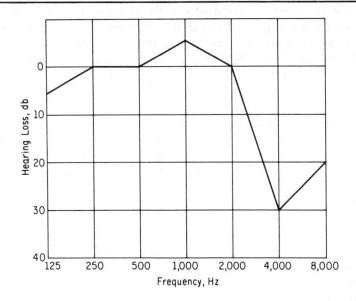

Figure 14-3
Typical audiogram with moderate hearing loss. Note that the loss of about 30 db is in the vicinity of 4,000 Hz with sensitivity to the 8,000 Hz tone being somewhat better.

approximately 100 Hz, whereas the critical band for tones on the order of 4,000 Hz is 700. The critical band concept is important for other aspects of hearing and will be referred to later in our discussion of the so-called mel scale and the subject of masking.

MONAURAL VERSUS BINAURAL THRESHOLDS

It has been recognized for some time that the absolute threshold for a pure tone is somewhat better—that is, lower—if two ears are employed rather than one. The normally encountered advantage for the binaural (diotic) condition is generally on the order of 2 to 4 db with 3 db as the average. It was natural to attribute such "binaural summation" to the central nervous system. However, recent contributions of those psychophysicists who espouse the signal-detection approach (see Chapter 4) offer a better explanation. The threshold for detecting a signal with one ear is defined as the 50 percent point, that signal which can be detected 50 percent of the time.* But look at what happens when you use two ears: At a given level (if the two ears have similar sensitivities) each ear will provide a 50-50 chance of detection. Hence the likelihood of a positive report is much greater when two ears are used, purely on a probability basis. It is really

---

* With some techniques, the threshold determination is based on a ratio other than 50/50 in order to allow for chance. Such procedures merely shift the calculated threshold; they do not eliminate the increased probability for two-ear detection.

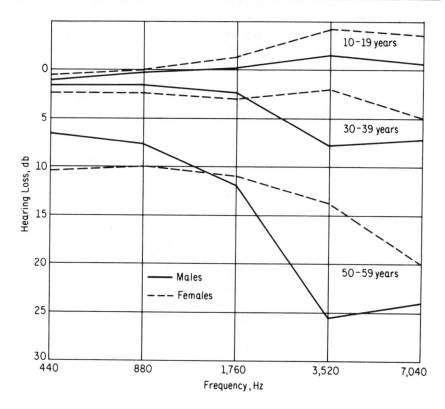

Figure 14-4

Hearing loss as a function of age and sex. Note the sharp falloff in the case of the 50 to 59 year group. Notice too that the losses for women tend to be somewhat less than those for men. [Adapted from J. C. Steinberg, H. C. Montgomery, and M. B. Gardner, *Bell System Tech. J.* 19 (October 1940), p. 538. Reprinted with permission from *The Bell System Technical Journal,* Copyright 1940, The American Telephone and Telegraph Company.]

not unlike tossing two coins at the same time. The probability of getting "heads" will be appreciably greater than if only one coin were tossed. The advantage of binaural over monaural detection is very nearly what would be predicted on the basis of the increased probability when two ears were used. A concept of binaural summation becomes unnecessary.

DIFFERENCE THRESHOLD FOR SOUND INTENSITY (DL)

One might assume that the determination of minimum detectable differences in the intensity (the experience of loudness) of two tones would be straightforward. In practice such a determination is not at all simple and straightforward. We know that DL's in general are influenced by the duration of the stimuli, their temporal separations, and various other experimentally controlled parameters. With sound amplitude and the resultant loudness experience, many of these changes may also change the physical nature of the sound waves. Hence any determination of difference thresholds for sound intensity is highly dependent on the technique employed, and various investigators may get highly divergent results.

Probably the most often cited research on DL's for intensity is the work of Riesz (1928). To avoid many of the pitfalls of induced transients, frequency changes, and the like, and having determined that the optimum rate for intensity change was three per second, Riesz produced intensity changes by a technique involving *beats*.* A pure tone of a given frequency was paired with a second tone differing from the first by precisely three cycles per second. Thus the two tones interacted, providing augmentation and partial cancellation at a rate of three cycles per second. The resultant experience is one of a tone changing in intensity (or beating) at a rate of three times per second. The difference in level between the partially canceled and the augmented component was the intensity difference being investigated. By changing the intensity levels of the paired tones while holding the frequency difference constant, the threshold for intensity was obtained. When the subject could just hear the beats, he was operating at the theshold for intensity change.

Some of Riesz's results are shown in Figure 14–5. The curve for the 4,000-Hz tone shows the highest discriminability. Had we included higher frequencies, their curves would have been similar to those for the lower frequencies, peak discriminabilities being in the 1,000 to 4,000-Hz range. Note too that for low levels such as 5 and 10 db, increments on the order of 3 db or higher are required for the subject to detect a difference. Recall that 3 db is a doubling of power. At a level of 15 db a 70-Hz tone must be doubled in power (3-db increase) to be recognized as being louder. At the other extreme, a 0.2-db increase, such as that required for a 4,000-Hz tone at 90-db sound pressure level, represents a ratio of 1.05 to 1.00.

TEMPORARY THRESHOLD SHIFTS (TTS)

When we studied the function of the eye and the retina we discovered the existence of remarkable adaptation effects that we likened to fatigue, based on reversible catabolic-anabolic chemical processes. Does the ear fatigue in the same way. The ear is basically a mechanical transducer rather than a chemical device, as was the case for the rods and cones; hence the same sort of adaptation would not be expected to occur, and indeed does not. There are, however, changes in sensitivity as a result of exposure to sound.

We have already indicated how permanent changes in sensitivity may result from damage to the inner ear as a result of its being subjected to intense sounds. We also indicated that, within limits, such damage to the ear is related to the duration and even lifetime exposure to inordinately

---

* The problem of beats is considered in more detail in the following chapter.

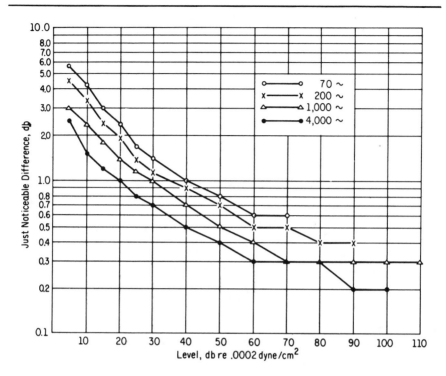

Figure 14-5

Difference thresholds for intensity of pure tones. Increments to various levels, shown on the abscissa, were obtained by a method of beats for four frequencies: 70, 200, 1,000, and 4,000 Hz. [Adapted from R. R. Riez, *Phys. Rev.* 31 (1928).]

intense sounds. In addition to these permanent shifts in threshold, exposure to sounds can also result in temporary changes in sensitivity—known, not unreasonably, as *temporary threshold shifts* (tts).

Figure 14–6 shows one example of the nature and magnitude of such shifts (Lüscher and Zwislocki, 1947). In this experiment the ear was stimulated by a very short, 0.4-second burst of a fatiguing or preconditioning tone, followed after an interval by a determination of the absolute threshold. The different curves in this figure are for various intensities of the preconditioning tone, expressed in conventional decibel units. For time intervals between the fatiguing stimulus and the test stimulus of a duration greater than perhaps 200 milliseconds, only a slight shift still remains, even for the more intense preconditioning tone.

Because of its implication for an understanding of the functioning of the ear, research on tts has been widespread in recent years. Frequencies, levels, and time intervals have been manipulated and a wealth of recent literature has resulted.

As an example of research on tts, Figure 14–7, based on the work of

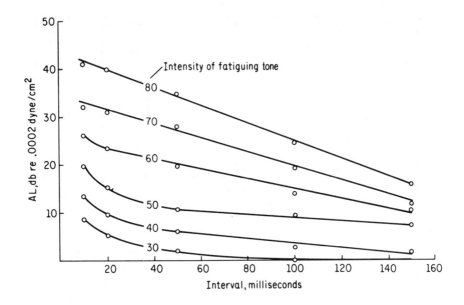

Figure 14-6

Temporary threshold shifts. The observed increases in absolute threshold were obtained as a result of a short preconditioning exposure to tones ranging from 30- to 80-db sensation level. [From J. J. Zwislocki, *Acta Otolaryng.* 35 (1947).]

Bell and Fairbanks (1963), indicates that some shift does indeed remain for an appreciable time, measurable in seconds rather than in the millisecond durations found by Lüscher and Zwislocki. The curve in this figure is based on a variety of low-level fatiguing conditions appreciably greater than the 0.4-second bursts explored by Lüscher and Zwislocki. Results shown for both these studies should only be considered as examples, and suggestive of the interest in tts. The interested serious student should consult the recent literature for developments in this fascinating area of auditory research.

Shifts in perceived pitch, as well as intensity thresholds, can result from prolonged pure-tone stimulation. Effects such as these will be considered in the next chapter when we examine the experience of pitch.

Loudness

Up to this point we have been dealing predominantly with the physical nature of sound and physiological ramifications, and only to a limited extent with the psychophysics of hearing. What about the last area? How is the experience of sound intensity, which we call loudness, related to the amplitude or intensity of the sound waves? We might surmise on the basis

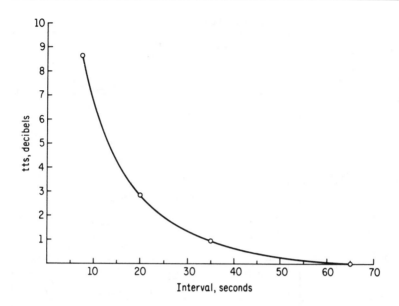

Figure 14-7
Temporary threshold shifts for low-level tones. The results are based on the pooling of several frequencies and levels. Note the relatively long time intervals and the lower amounts of tts as contrasted with Figure 14-6. [From D. W. Bell and G. Fairbanks, *J. Acoust. Soc. Amer.* 35 (1953).]

of our earlier experiences that the relationship would not be perfect. That is, doubling the intensity of a sound might not be expected to result in doubling of loudness. Let us examine the concept of loudness in some detail.

EQUAL-LOUDNESS CONTOURS AND PHONS

It is possible to determine various frequencies and intensities of tones that appear equally loud to a listener. Such a procedure is the basis for the development of the *equal-loudness contours* shown in Figures 14–8 and 14–9. The term *isophonic contours* is used interchangeably with equal-loudness contours and means exactly the same thing.

Determination of Isophonic Contours. The rationale for the computation of equal-loudness contours is straightforward. To begin with, before we can develop a mathematical scale of loudness having units that can be manipulated we need a scale of the basic psychophysical relations. The most obvious starting point for such a scale is the absolute threshold. And, because 1,000 Hz is a convenient even number and very close to the frequency of maximum sensitivity, what better point could be selected for the starting point of a loudness scale? A tone of 1,000 Hz at threshold was arbitrarily assigned the value of 1, or in the logarithmic scale 0. A level of 10 db above threshold would therefore be 10 db more intense, or have

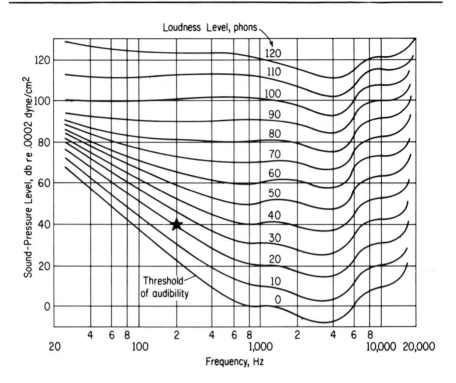

Figure 14–8
Equal-loudness contours (MAF). Note the loudness levels, in phons, from 0 to 120.
[From H. Fletcher, *Rev. Mod. Phys.* 12 (1940).]

a loudness level of 10 db. It was a relatively simple matter to determine just how much the intensity, in decibels above their absolute thresholds, of other frequencies would have to be raised to be equivalent in loudness to a 1,000-Hz tone of a specified level.

Let us look at Figure 14–8. Each contour line in this figure represents a single loudness level, with the lowermost contour, labeled 0, being the threshold of audibility. This line is the same line found as an average from Figure 14–2, and any point on this line will represent the threshold for that particular frequency. Let us examine additional contours—that labeled 40, for example. Any point on this line will have the same loudness level. A 1,000-Hz tone at an intensity level of 40 db has the same loudness level as an 80-Hz tone at an intensity level of about 65 db. Expressed in other words, an 80-Hz tone must be 25 db more intense than a 1,000-Hz tone to have the same loudness level, and a 10,000-Hz tone must be 12 db more intense to achieve the same loudness level.

Notice that each of the successive isophonic contours does indeed pass through the 1,000-Hz point with equal increments. That is, the contour

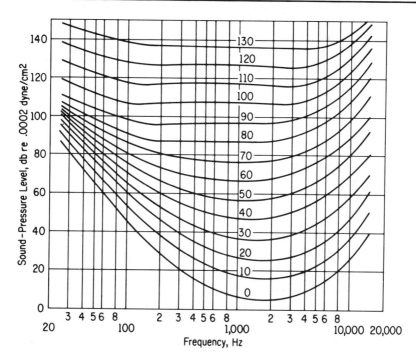

Figure 14–9

Equal-loudness contours (MAP). Note that the contour labeled 0 is the threshold for hearing for the normal subject. [From S. S. Stevens and H. Davis, *Hearing: Its Psychology and Physiology*, New York: John Wiley & Sons, Inc., 1938, and H. Fletcher and W. A. Munson, *J. Acoust. Soc. Amer.* 5 (1933).]

labeled 20 passes through the 1,000-Hz line at a level of 20 db, the contour labeled 30 passes through the 1,000-Hz point at a 30-db level, and so on, to the limit of the diagram. This is the basis for the identification and labeling of the contours: the loudness of a 1,000-Hz tone at a given sound-pressure level.

The contours are identified in terms of *phons*. Thus a 60-phon tone is one that has the same loudness level as a 1,000-Hz tone of 60-db sound-pressure level. A 100-Hz tone with a sound-pressure level of 71 db, a 400-Hz tone with a sound-pressure level of 61 db, and a 6,000-Hz tone with a level of 68 db would all have the same loudness level—60 phons.*

Figure 14–9, like Figure 14–8, also shows equal-loudness contours, but for minimum audible pressures rather than minimum audible fields. Most of

---

* Another term frequently encountered in conjunction with loudness level is *sensation level*. The sensation level of any sound is the pressure level of the sound in decibels above its absolute threshold. In Figure 14–8 a 100-Hz tone of 60 phons would have a sensation level of about 34 db—that is, a sound-pressure level of 72 db compared to the threshold level of 38 db (72 minus 38 equals 34) for the frequency under consideration.

what has been said concerning minimum audible fields also applies to minimum audible pressure measurements. Indeed, the curious shape of the equal-loudness contours for MAF measurements, especially at the high frequencies, might lead one to the conclusion that MAP techniques might better be employed to assign values for equal-loudness-level contours.

Practical Applications of Isophonic Contours. The concept of equal-loudness contours is of more than academic or scientific interest. It has very practical ramifications. Look at Figure 14–8 again. Suppose you are listening to music from your radio or hi-fi at a relatively high loudness level, say 90 phons. The appropriate curve indicates that your ear has about the same sensitivity throughout the audio spectrum, at least for the frequencies below several thousand hertz, where most musical tones are to be found. What happens if you reduce the volume of your amplifier by 50 db to provide background music, or to mollify complaining neighbors? If you do this a tone of 200 Hz will drop in loudness level from 90 phons to—not 40 phons, but 20 phons (the star in Figure 14–8). Considering the ambient noise in the room, the 200-Hz component of the music will in all likelihood be complete inaudible.

If you are a music lover and do not wish to lose the subtle components of the lower-register instruments, you may turn up the bass control of your amplifier, thus compensating for the frequency-sensitivity characteristics of your ear. As can be better seen in Figure 14–9, some loss of high-frequency components may also occur, but these are probably of less interest to you. You might, of course, increase your separate treble control to compensate for their loss.

Modern hi-fi amplifiers often have a separate control, commonly called a "loudness" control, that does this shaping of the audio output automatically. If your loudness control is in the "on" position, reducing the level simultaneously activates an electronic filtering-shaping circuit that results in less attenuation of the lower frequencies than those nearer the center of the spectrum. Thus a reduction in overall sound level does not result in loss of the lower-frequency components of the complex audio signal.

You may recall that references were made earlier to the existence of different modes, commonly called A, B, and C, for use of sound-pressure-level meters. These modes provide varying amounts of the shaping function for the differential sensitivities of the ear for different overall sound levels. The A-scale setting, for example, may be used for levels below 40-db sound pressure level. By utilizing these correction positions, readings on the instrument can be made to compare favorably with apparent sound levels sensed by the human ear.

SUBJECTIVE LOUDNESS AND SONES

As suggested in earlier chapters, the ultimate aim of any sensory-perceptual researcher is to relate the physical world to the world of experience. The system of phons does relate sound intensities to loudness level at the psychophysical level. But what about the subjective, experiential, psychological level? Can we develop a sensory scale that is indeed a ratio scale, a scale with units that can be added, subtracted, and otherwise manipulated mathematically, like dollars or apples? Expressed another way, can one sensation be twice as great as another? In the case of loudness, considerable progress has been made.

By means of some of the scaling techniques described in Chapter 4, such as single-stimulus estimation and fractionation methods, numerous investigators have attempted to develop ratio scales for loudness. The ratio scale developed by Fletcher and Munson in 1933, based largely on fractionation techniques, was a major milestone. Perhaps the greatest contribution was made by S. S. Stevens, who in 1936 gathered together and analyzed much of the diverse literature, including some of his own, developing a loudness scale with units he called *sones*.

A sone, as defined by Stevens, is the loudness of a 1,000-Hz tone 40 db above threshold (40 phons). The curve of Figure 14–10 shows subjective loudness in sones, plotted against loudness level in phons. Although this curve was based on the addition of two tones, there is evidence that the relation holds for combinations of more than two tones.*

Note that although a tone of 2 sones is twice as loud (subjectively) as a tone of 1 sone, an increase of about 9 db in loudness level is required to obtain this doubling of subjective loudness. This general relationship appears to hold for sounds of relatively high intensity, but at lower levels subjective loudness in sones increases somewhat more rapidly than loudness level in phons.

Subjective Attributes

The reader should be familiar with several other intensity related attributes of sound, if only to clarify layman-scientist differences in meanings.

Volume is an experience frequently alluded to when what we really mean is sound intensity, or perhaps loudness. As implied earlier, the volume control on your amplifier is not a volume control at all, but rather a sound intensity control, or a loudness control. To the psychophysicist, volume is a true attribute of sound, referring to the "size or extensity" of the sound. It is a subjective attribute in the truest sense of the word and may even be related to our knowledge of the source of the sound. The output of a tuba has more volume than that of a flute, and part of this difference may indeed be due to our knowledge of the appearance of the two instruments. Yet some researchers have been able to develop scales of volume,

---

* Addition of pure tones in this fashion assumes that the tones are of the same frequency and do not interact in any complex way. When combining tones of different frequencies (or the same frequency but differing phases), numerous complications such as beats, difference tones, or masking greatly complicate the results and simple additive characteristics do not obtain. Some of the complications encountered in combining tones with different parameters are considered in the next chapter.

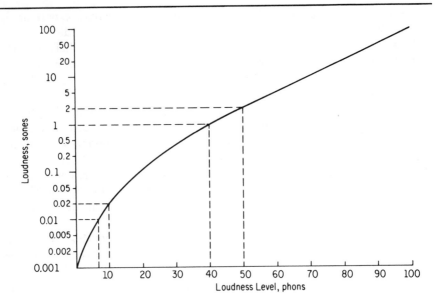

Figure 14–10

Subjective loudness in sones. Note the difference in the relationship between phons and sones for the two parts of the curve, as indicated by the dotted lines.

based on subjective judgments of listeners, that seem to be independent of simple loudness or pitch and are not dependent on the identification of specific tonal sources.

Other attributes that have been investigated include *density* and *brightness*. Independently of its pitch, loudness, and volume, a tone can be judged to be dense, compact, or hard. High-frequency loud sounds, for example, are judged to be more dense than low-frequency soft sounds. Brightness is a similar attribute, possibly the same (Sonn, 1969). Stevens (1944) was able to obtain contours for equal density and equal brightness as well as the better known equal-loudness contours. It is significant that a trained auditor can hold density constant while varying pitch, loudness, and volume. As with loudness, density appears to be a power function of sound pressure, and according to at least one formulation, loudness itself is a product of volume and density (Stevens et al., 1965).

An additional attribute, related more to pitch than to loudness, is that of *vocality*. Tones spaced at octave intervals are judged as more similar than tones closer in frequency. This quality of "C-ness" or "F-ness" is called vocality. It is not clear just why tones of 500, 1,000, and 2,000 Hz are judged more similar than tones of 500, 700, and 900 Hz. Although the cause may be related to harmonics generated in the ear, the effect is observed even with quite low-level tones, tones with levels so low that very few, if any, distortion-produced harmonics are observed. Whatever its physiological or psychological basis, vocality is an important phenomenon for music (Scharf, 1975).

Summary

In this chapter we have examined quantitative auditory experience as it relates to the physical world. We examined first the absolute threshold for hearing, describing techniques involving minimum audible fields and minimum audible pressures. We looked into audiometric procedures and the determination of hearing loss. We then considered several aspects of auditory sensitivity such as difference thresholds and shifts in sensitivity due to prior tonal subjection. Finally, we examined the overall area of loudness, describing the nature of equal-loudness contours and how they are derived, as well as the more subjective scales of loudness based on the unit of loudness, the sone. In addition to describing some applications of loudness data, we concluded with a cursory look at several additional subjective attributes related to the intensity of auditory stimuli.

Suggested Readings

1. From M. Lawrence. "Hearing," in M. Alpern, M. Lawrence, and D. Wolsk, Sensory Processes. Belmont, Calif.: Brooks/Cole, 1967. Pages 65 to 101 are concerned with hearing. This is a relatively easy reference and well worth reading in detail. The first 20 pages are particularly relevant to the material covered in our Chapter 14.
2. J. C. R. Licklider. "Basic Correlates of the Auditory Stimulus," in S. S. Stevens (ed.), *Handbook of Experimental Psychology*. New York: Wiley, 1951. These 50 pages present a thorough description of auditory sensory-perceptual processes. The material covers both this and the following chapter. The reader should read selectively, because the order of presentation differs from that of this book. The interested student should be familiar with Professor Licklider's excellent chapter in this handbook. It is well worth reading and is also invaluable for future reference.
3. I. J. Hirsh. *The Measurement of Hearing*. New York: McGraw-Hill, 1952. An excellent book, somewhat technical, perhaps, but ideal for the interested student. With its emphasis on clinical audiology and hearing loss, it is particularly relevant to the preceding chapter. This reference is recommended as a source book, rather than for general reading. Its wealth of informative material is useful when needed for a particular application.
4. S. S. Stevens. "A Scale for the Measurement of a Psychological Magnitude: Loudness," *Psychol. Rev.* 43 (1936), 405–416. This reference is included to give the reader a "feel" for the general area of scaling psychological attributes. This reading and the two to follow should provide enough background for the interested reader to pursue the problem of sensory scaling to any desired depth.
5. S. S. Stevens. "Calculating Loudness," *Noise Control* 3 (1957), 11–22 This is another description of the methods and results of work aimed at the establish-

ment of a "loudness" scale. It is somewhat less technical than other references and is recommended for the student interested in the area. It is aimed somewhat more at the "semiprofessional" or educated layman.

6. S. S. Stevens. "The Psychophysics of Sensory Function," in W. A. Rosenblith (ed.), *Sensory Communication*. New York: Wiley, 1961. This article summarizes the work of Stevens and is probably the most significant of the three Stevens references included. For the seriously interested student.

7. J. V. Tobias (ed.). *Foundations of Modern Auditory Theory*, vols. *I and II*. New York: Academic Press, 1970. This is an excellent reference, with numerous contributions by well-known authorities in the field. The typical undergraduate need not read the entire work, but should use it selectively for subjects of particular interest. This reference covers all our chapters on audition.

8. Bertram Scharff (ed.). *Experimental Sensory Psychology*. Glenview, Ill.: Scott, Foresman, 1975. I referred to this reference for an earlier chapter. It is also an excellent source for this and the following chapter. Chapter 4 is broad in coverage and yet thorough for the average undergraduate. A very highly recommended reading.

15/auditory sensitivity and pitch

Just as loudness is the psychological attitude for sound intensity, so is *pitch* the psychological attribute for tonal frequency. Pitch is related to the frequency of the sound waves much like hue is related to the wavelength (or frequency) of electromagnetic radiation. As can be seen from Figure 14–1, the human ear can hear sounds produced by mechanical waves from roughly 20 Hz to as rapid as 20,000 Hz, for the young, healthy ear. Some animals, like dogs and bats, are sensitive to sounds with frequencies above 20,000, but man can rarely hear sounds above this limit. Moreover, the bottom cutoff is not always clearly defined. At some low frequency, sound becomes vibration or perhaps pulsation, and the rough "sounds" below 30 Hz, when sensed, might better be called something other than sound. Indeed, they may owe their being sensed to something akin to a tactual vibratory sense, rather than hearing.

Scales of Pitch

There are two historic approaches to the scaling of pitch. The oldest and most widely accepted is the musical scale, which has existed in numerous forms since antiquity.

MUSICAL SCALE

The pitch scale with which we are most familiar is that of the musical scale, based on octaves or powers. Each "do" of the scale represents a doubling of the frequency. If middle C on the scale is assigned a frequency of 256 Hz, then C above middle C will have a frequency of 512 Hz, the C one octave higher will be 1,024 Hz, and so on. With a little practice we can detect a resemblance among the various C's, or any other selected note on the scale.

Aristotle recognized many years ago that the octave is probably "native," in that voices of different register tend to harmonize in octave separations (Boring, 1942). On the other hand, the (to our ears) curious musical scales developed by Oriental cultures and the subjective/physchophysical scale, described in the next section, do not completely support such a simple explanation.

In a book of this scope we cannot examine in any great detail the development of musical scales, nor indeed the voluminous history of music. The interested reader is directed to the many excellent descriptions and accounts of the history of musical development. As a starting point, Boring's chapter listed in the suggestive readings is recommended. If you are interested in historical perspective, Boring's references at the end of his chapter 9 are especially valuable.

THE MEL SCALE

Perhaps, as Licklider suggests (Stevens, 1952), there are two scales of frequency sensitivity: one based on the quality of tones, called *tone chroma* or *tonality*, and applicable to musical scales, the other based on psychophysical measurements and called *pitch*. It is the latter that concerns us in the following paragraphs.

Although we found loudness to be a function of both frequency and sound intensity, the experience of pitch appears to be somewhat more simple, with only slight dependence on intensity. We do know that pure tones below about 500 Hz sound lower in pitch when their intensities are increased, and pure tones above 3,000 Hz sound somewhat sharper when their intensities are increased. The differences are relatively slight, however, and for the middle frequencies of primary interest, pitch is to all intents and purposes a function of frequency.

In 1937 Stevens, Volkman, and Newman published their scale of pitch, with the unit of pitch being called a *mel*. As a result of additional data collection and refinement, the current form of the scale was published by the first two authors in 1940 (see Figure 15–1). For the purposes of the scale, the pitch of a 1,000-Hz tone, 40 db above threshold, was assigned the value of 1,000 mels and the remainder of the points were plotted as a result of many fractionations and bisections of subjective pitch. A frequency that sounded half as high in pitch was given the value 500 mels, and so on, until the entire range was encompassed.

Note that a tone of 400 Hz has a mel value of 500, whereas a 1,000-Hz tone is 1,000 mels. Thus a 1,000-Hz tone has a pitch twice as high as a 400-Hz tone, not a 500-Hz tone, as might be naively expected.

The controversy between the musical scale and the mel scale may not be entirely resolved, but there are some additional findings that appear

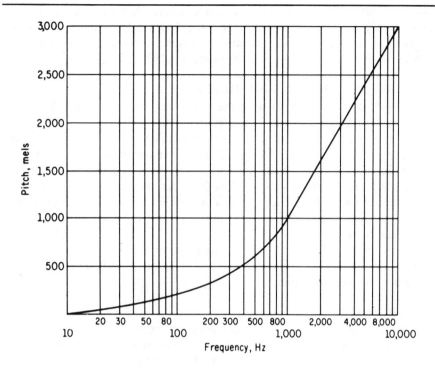

Figure 15-1
Relation of pitch (in mels) to frequency. (Based on data of S. S. Stevens and
J. Volkman, *Amer. J. Psych.* 53 (1940).

germane and seem to indicate that the mel scale is more than a strained
attempt to quantify something that cannot in fact be quantified. For example, the DL or just noticeable difference for pitch is almost always a
constant number of mels, actually about one-twentieth. In the preceding
chapter we alluded to the critical band, beyond which multiple tones fail
to summate. The width of these bands is about 1 mel. In addition, a critical
band for masking (to be considered later) is a constant number of mels
wide. Finally, frequency ranges that contribute equally to speech intelligibility are very nearly the same width in units of mels. As van Bergeijk et
al. (1960) point out, it is unlikly that such agreement is purely accidental.

Difference Thresholds for Pitch

When we suggested that the determination of DL's for intensity was difficult because of unpredictable changes in the tone as a result of temporal
manipulations, we were anticipating similar or even greater difficulties in
the determination of difference thresholds for frequency. In order to compare tones differing slightly in pitch or frequency, one must present suc-

cessive tones in some way. But any time one turns tones on and off rapidly or suddenly shifts an oscillator from, say 500 Hz to 503 Hz, an infinite number of transient frequencies and variations are produced that tend to confound any valid judgments with respect to pitch or frequency.

WORK OF SHOWER AND BIDDULPH

Despite or perhaps because of the difficulties involved, many investigators have tried various means to circumvent the switching difficulties and arrive at valid measures of difference thresholds. After trying numerous approaches, Shower and Biddulph (1931) suceeded in producing what are generally considered to be the most valid measures of difference threshold. They used a technique involving slow (two per second) sinusoidal changes from frequency to frequency. Their data are quite complex, because they varied not only frequency but also intensity and included monaural, binaural, and bone-conduction modes.

The curves of Figure 15–2 illustrate some of the Shower and Biddulph data. Note that for some frequencies, and at optimal levels, DL's approaching one cycle were obtained.

DIPLACUSIS

The clever reader might wonder why the early experimenters did not deliver one tone to one ear and the comparison tone to the other in order to determine a DL. Perhaps this method might be useful were it not for the existence of a little-studied phenomenon known as *diplacusis*. Persons with this condition hear different pitches in the two ears as a result of stimulation with the same frequency. For example, a 600-Hz tone may appear higher in pitch in the left ear than in the right. A moderate amount of such displacusis is probably quite common. Indeed, Licklider (1952) suggests that it is probably the rule rather than the exception.

Davis et al. (1944) showed experimentally induced diplacusis, using tones of 130 to 150 db as preconditioning or adapting stimuli. (Perhaps "deafening" would be more descriptive.) They obtained pitch shifts as great as one octave as a result of exposures to the fatiguing tone of several minutes. The "adaptation" effects of Davis et al. might indeed be likened to fatigue, a temporary theshold shift (tts) in pitch, rather than in sensitivity such as in the case of conventional tts investigations.

At the other extreme, the writer was able to induce diplacusis with pure tones at a moderate (85 db) level, for preconditioning durations of one minute or less, and in a predictable direction (Christman, 1954, 1963). Figure 15–3 shows the result of one experiment aimed at studying the decay effects of the shifts. In this experiment a 600-Hz tone in one ear was followed by a variable tone in the opposite ear and a match was made. The ear receiving the 600-Hz standard was preconditioned or "satiated" for one minute with either a 575- or 635-Hz tone of the same level as the subsequent test tones. After subjection to the preconditioning tone, the com-

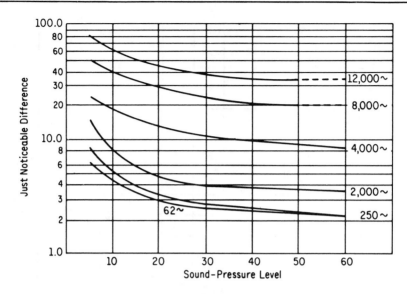

Figure 15–2
Difference thresholds for pitch. The curves have been smoothed to indicate the probable "true" function. [Based on the original data of E. G. Shower and R. Biddulph, *J. Acoust. Soc. Amer.* 3 (1931) but with considerable modification.]

parison was made. You can see from Figure 15–3 that with a time interval of one second between the preconditioning stimulus and the standard, the apparent pitch is shifted, in the case of 575 preconditioning tone to 608 Hz and for the 635-Hz satiation tone to about 596 Hz. Thus a fatiguing tone below the standard raised the pitch of the standard, whereas a fatiguing tone higher in frequency depressed the pitch of the standard. The remainder of Figure 15–3 simply shows the course of the effect as it decays with time (up to 30 seconds).

Simple Tonal Interaction

In the normal state of affairs one seldom hears pure tones. Rather, most sounds are complex combinations of many pure tones, varying in frequency as well as in temporal characteristics. Let us examine some of the available knowledge bearing on the experiences resulting from combinations of pure tones.

PAIRED TONES

Two pure tones of precisely the same frequency will, as indicated in Chapter 12, either reinforce or cancel each other, depending on the phase relationship of the two waves. If two waves of the same frequency are exactly in phase—that is, both waves have their peaks at precisely the same

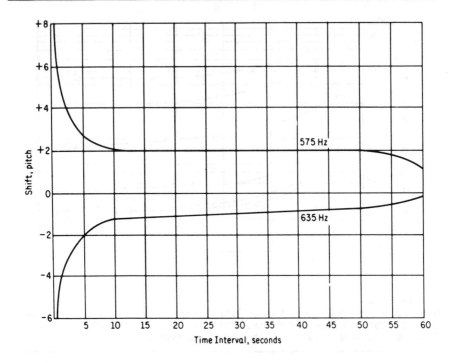

Figure 15–3
Experimentally induced diplacusis. The ordinate shows the amount and direction of pitch shift, as a result of preconditioning with either 575- or 635-Hz tones, for the time intervals shown on the abscissa. [From R. J. Christman and W. E. Williams, *J. Acoust. Soc. Amer.* 35 (1963).]

time—then the resultant overall wave amplitude will be the sum of the individual amplitudes. (See top drawing of Figure 15–4.) If the two waves are 180° out of phase (one leads the other by one-half wavelength) as shown in the second and third parts of Figure 15–4, then the resultant amplitude will be the difference between the individual amplitudes. With equal amplitudes, as shown in the second example in this figure, the two waves will subtract in such fashion as to cancel each other, and there will be in effect no sound. If the amplitudes are different, the result will be a tone represented by the difference between the two constituent tones, as shown in the bottom of the three figures.

Such reinforcement or cancellation effects are of serious consideration in the design of hi-fi audio reproduction equipment. If, for example, a speaker cabinet is so designed that internal reflections of the sound may differ by half-wavelength for a given frequency, then tones of this frequency may be canceled and the speaker system may in effect be "dead" to this frequency. At the other extreme, if strong reflections of pure tones tend to reinforce each other, there is a different problem. The system may

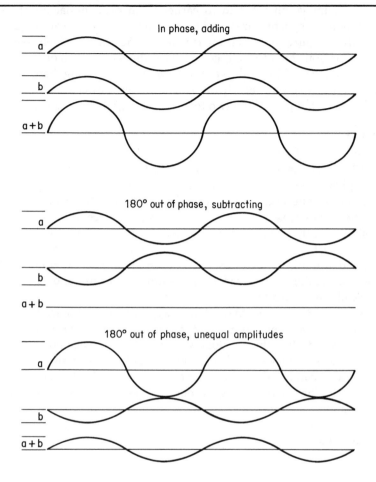

Figure 15-4
Combining tones of same frequency. The top drawing illustrates the addition of two tones, in phase. The middle drawing is the addition of two tones of equal amplitude, 180° out of phase; while the bottom drawing shows two tones of unequal amplitude, 180° out of phase. Note from the middle drawing, that if the phase difference were other than exactly 180°, the resultant tone would be greater than zero.

"boom," or even resonate at some particular frequency. In practice it is often some frequency near the bottom of the tonal register that is involved in such unwanted reinforcement or "booming." Expensive steps are taken to ensure that good speaker systems are "flat" and have outputs that truthfully reflect their input, avoiding both reinforcement and cancellation effects.

You may recall our referring in the last chapter to summation of tones within a critical band, resulting in increased loudness. The phenomenon discussed there is not the same as that mentioned in the preceding paragraph. The summation referred to earlier is an experiential effect, which does not require synchronization of frequencies or identical frequencies; such an effect requires only that the frequencies not be too widely separated. The result, as you should recall, is decreased thresholds and/or increases in perceived loudness. The additive effect we are addressing here is a true physical event; it can be seen if the two tones are displayed on an oscilloscope. But what happens if the two tones differ slightly in frequency?

BEATS

If pure tones of slightly differing frequency are paired, it is clear from Figure 15–4 that the simple addition or subtraction of amplitude will not occur. A phenomenon known as *beats* may result. If, for example, the two tones differ by one cycle per second (say 200 and 201 Hz), once every second the waves from the two tones will be in phase and reinforce each other; similarly, they will be out of phase, tending to cancel each other, at one instant each second. The result to the auditor will be a 200-Hz tone waxing and waning in loudness once per second. The experience of this waxing and waning is referred to as beating, or beats, and is illustrated schematically by Figure 15–5.

Notice from this figure that what is apparently experienced is an "envelope" of the two tones. If the difference between the two tones is two cycles per second, then the envelope will repeat itself twice per second, and two beats per second will be heard; with a difference of three cycles per second, three beats; and so on. Above six or seven beats per second the successive waxings and wanings produce something like a throbbing or pulsating auditory experience. At about 25 per second the throbbing experience tends to be replaced by something like a low "burr," or perhaps a low-pitched tone.

DICHOTIC BEATS

Although the effect has been known for more than 100 years, recent developments in sophisticated electronic equipment have intensified the study of *binaural beats* (Oster, 1973). Pure tones of slightly differing frequencies, presented dichotically, can result in an expenrience in some respects similar to the beats described in the preceding paragraph. A difference of 6 Hz can result in a beating phenomenon somewhat similar in experience to a vibrato, whereas more rapid beats, up to, say, 30 Hz, can result in an auditory roughness superimposed on the pure tone sound.

Binaural beats can be best heard when the tones used to produce them are of relatively low frequency (e.g., 450 Hz). With frequencies above 1,000 Hz, binaural beats cannot be produced. Such beats also appear to be localized in the head and are of a somewhat muffled nature as contrasted with conventional beats. For other differences between binaural and monaural beats, and possible physiological explanations, the interested reader is referred to Oster (1973).

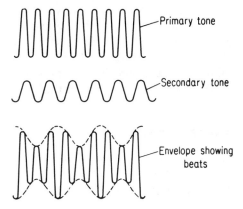

Figure 15–5
Production of beats. Combining the primary and secondary tones results in the envelope wave shown at the bottom.

COMBINATION TONES

Two tones with sufficient separation in frequency will, of course, be heard as two tones. A trained musician can indeed resolve not only two separate pitches, but often many pure tones within a complex pattern. He or she can detect the presence or absence of various instruments in the orchestra or the harmonically related frequencies produced by a single instrument.

Sometimes the combination of two tones may produce a third tone, and even additional harmonically related tones. Simultaneous presentation of a 600-Hz and an 800-Hz tone may result in the hearing of a 200-Hz tone and perhaps a 1,400-Hz tone, as well as various combinations of the harmonically related frequencies. Such effects are known as *combination tones.*

Although we can understand the production of beats as a simple phenomenon, reproducible, for example, on an oscilloscope, the situation with respect to combination tones is not that simple. Combination tones are not produced in nature unless there is some nonlinearity in the medium or mode of transmission. A linear system is one that reproduces its pure tone input with perfect fidelity A nonlinear system has an output that contains components not present in the input, consisting mainly of harmonic multiples of the input frequency. It has been demonstrated that the ear is nonlinear, particularly at relatively high sound levels; hence the nonlinearities in the ear mechanism are assumed to be responsible for the production of combination tones. At low sound levels, combination tones cannot be detected, and the ear *does* perform as an optimal analyzing device.

When the tone heard is the difference between the two frequencies, it is known as a *difference tone;* when it is the sum of the two combining frequencies, it is a *summation tone*. In practice, difference tones are much easier to produce and recognize and are probably of more significance than summation tones. If one activates two tuning forks of, say, 850 and 1,000 Hz of sufficient amplitude, the low, 150-Hz difference tone may be immediately apparent; the summation tone of 1,850 Hz may or may not be noticeable. Unless the levels are sufficient to produce nonlinearities, the summation tone of 1,850 may not exist at all for the listener.

Complex Tonal Interaction

In addition to the simple beats and combination tones, combining tones of different frequencies and intensities can produce varied results, results of particular importance in gaining an understanding of just how the auditory mechanism processes and recognizes tonal differences.

MASKING WITH PURE TONES

It has been implied that two different tones—different in frequency to an extent that beats are not distinguishable—will be heard as two tones, that the ear will analyze the aural components and sense each of them. In a sense, the ear will perform a Fourier analysis of the complex tone. Within limits this in indeed the case. However, when one tone is of sufficiently greater amplitude than the other, the weaker of the two tones may not be sensed; it may be masked by the louder tone. We can measure the extent of such masking by measuring the threshold of a tone, both by itself and in the presence of a masking tone—the threshold shift, then, being the measure of masking.

Probably the most extensive study of masking with pure tones was made many years ago by Wegel and Lane (1924). One example of their work is shown as Figure 15–6. In this figure the masking efficacy of a 1,200-Hz tone is shown as the shaded area. In this figure any combination of frequency and intensity found in the shaded area will be below the absolute threshold—it will not be heard. The curve itself shows the combination of frequency and sensation level that can just be detected in the presence of a 1,200-Hz masking tone at 80 db above threshold. Note, for example, that a 600-Hz tone need only be at about the 4-db sensation level in order to be detected, whereas a 1,000-Hz tone requires a sensation level of more than 36 db to be detected.

The nearer the tones are to each other, the greater the masking effect —that is, the more intense the masked tone must be in order to be detected. This phenomenon is known as the *spread of masking*. Masking spreads in both directions, the effect decreasing the farther one gets from the frequency of the masking tone.

You may also have noted that frequencies above the 1,200-Hz masking tone require greater intensities to be heard than do those below the mask-

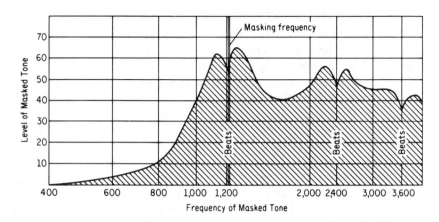

Figure 15–6
Masking of pure tones by 1,200-Hz tone at 80-db sensation level. Combinations of frequency and level in the shaded area are inaudible. [Adapted from R. L. Wegel and C. E. Lane, *Phys. Rev.* 23 (1924), and H. Fletcher, *Speech and Hearing*, New York: D. Van Nostrand Company, 1929.]

ing tone. In other words, spread of masking causes tones higher in pitch to be masked better than those lower in pitch. Even a pitch as high as 3,200 Hz requires a level of 45 db in order to be detected in the presence of an 80-db, 1,200-Hz masking tone.

When a 1,200-Hz tone is combined with other frequencies, several other phenomena may be observed. Note the presence of beats around the 1,200-Hz tones. Beats may also be observed in the immediate vicinity of the 2,400- and 3,600-Hz tones. In the former the 1,200-Hz masking tone is beating with the near-1,200-Hz secondary tone; in the latter the 2,400- and 3,600-Hz, second and third harmonics, respectively, are apparently beating with the near-2,400- and near-3,600-Hz tones.

On the basis of this and many other examples, several facts concerning masking with pure tones may be stated: (1) masking is greater for tones near the masking tone than for those farther away; (2) low-frequency tones mask higher-frequency tones better than the converse; and (3) the rate at which masking increases, as the intensity of the masking tone is increased, depends on the frequencies of the tones. The latter finding is based on many additional measurements by Wegel and Lane and cannot be deduced from the single example shown.

Wegel and Lane also establish that very little masking occurs if the two tones are applied to opposite ears (dichotic stimulation). Any masking that does occur appears to be a matter of sound leakage around the head. The basis of masking must therefore be found in the functioning of the inner ear. This is an important finding, bearing on the theoretical explanation of pitch discrimination to be discussed later.

MASKING WITH WHITE OR RANDOM NOISE

White noise contains all audible frequencies and should therefore have a profound effect on the detection of pure tones. Because it contains all of Wegel and Lane's pure tones, white noise should mask pure tones with considerable efficiency. Moreover, the masking effect should be less dependent on the pitch of the masked tone. Experimental evidence does indeed support these expectations. Figure 15–7 shows the threshold for pure tones presented in a background of white noise, based on the work of Hawkins and Stevens (1950). The various curves are for different levels of noise, expressed in decibels per cycle.* Notice from this figure that, except for quite low tones, and with respect to level per cycle, any pure tone must be from about 20 to 30 db more intense than the masking noise in order to be detected. If the masking noise is expressed in overall sound-pressure level instead of energy per cycle, the pure-tone signal must be no more than 10 to 20 db less intense than the masking level in order to be detected.

But what about masking with *bands* of noise, rather than the entire audible spectrum? Can we learn anything of value by making such comparisons? We surely can.

If we use two tones to mask a test tone, one on either side of the test tone, we can determine the distance we must move each tone from the test tone before the masking effect becomes negligible. We can get similar results by using narrow bands of noise centered on the frequency to be masked.

We find in this case that there is a point on either side of the masking band beyond which tones do not contribute equally to the masking effect. In other words, there is a *critical bandwidth* for masking. The situation in which tones close to a second tone produce greater masking effect appears not to be simply the result of a continuum, but to be rather a discrete locuslike effect.

Figure 15–8 shows critical bands for masking pure-tone signals. This curve tells us, for example: For a tone of 1,000 Hz, the critical band for masking is about 65 cycles. That is, individual frequencies within a band 65 cycles wide, centered at 1,000 Hz, summate to increase the effectiveness of the masking of a 1,000-Hz tone. Low-level tones that individually would not be intense enough to mask the test tone will summate in such a way that their total effect will be to mask the 1,000-Hz tone if they lie within this 65-cycle band. Frequencies outside of this 65-cycle band will not summate so as to contribute to the masking. Adding to the frequencies within the band would increase the masking effect in a proportional man-

---

* Decibels per cycle is a new way of expressing sound pressure or power. The overall sound pressure for a bandwidth of roughly 10,000 Hz would be 10,000 times that for each of the 10,000 components, assuming a flat spectrum. The overall sound pressure would therefore be 40 db greater $(10,000 = 10^4)$ than the level per cycle, as indicated on the curves of Figure 15–7.

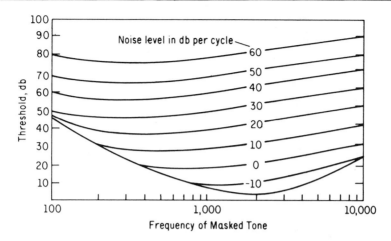

Figure 15–7
Masking pure tones with white noise. Note that the level of the masking noise is expressed in decibels per cycle. Expressed in overall sound-pressure level of the white masking noise, these values would be increased by about 40 db. [From J. E. Hawkins, Jr., and S. S. Stevens, *J. Acoust. Soc. Amer.* 22 (1950).]

ner; adding to frequencies beyond the critical band would contribute little to the overall masking effect.

The inclusion of such complex relationships in a book of this scope was not done to cause confusion. Rather, the purpose was first to point out the orderliness of the auditory sensory system, and second to provide the groundwork for later obtaining an understanding of auditory theory.

With respect to the former, note that critical band widths tend to increase with frequency, like the jnd's for pitch discrimination. It is significant that for frequencies above 100 Hz, the critical bandwidths for masking are almost exactly 20 times the smallest change in frequency (jnd) that can be noticed at that frequency (van Bergeijk, 1960). The implication is that there is a relationship between the frequency discrimination and the masking of one tone by other tones.

It is also worthy of note that the discrimination of speech seems to depend on the presence of bands of frequencies. The articulation index, considered in the next chapter, is based on 20 bands of frequencies, each contributing equally to speech intelligibility. Like critical bands for masking, the widths of each of these 20 bands increases with increasing frequency, and in a fashion not entirely unlike the bands for masking.

We referred in the last chapter to another form of critical band, critical bands for loudness summation. Pure tones, far removed from each other in frequency, summate in an orderly manner. That is, the loudness of two equally loud tones, widely separated in frequency, is twice the loudness of either of the tones alone. But two tones closer together in frequency,

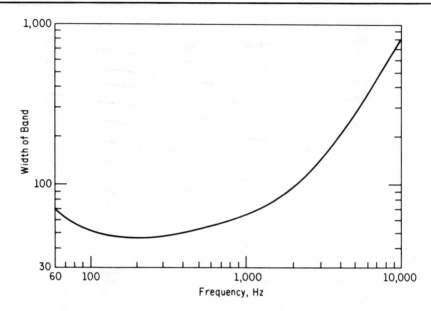

Figure 15–8

Critical bands for masking. The ordinate shows the width, in cps, of critical bands of noise for masking the frequencies shown on the abscissa. [Adapted from H. Fletcher, *Rev. Mod. Phys.* 12 (1940).]

within a so-called critical band for loudness, do not summate in such an orderly manner; their total loudness is not the sum of the loudness of the individual components. Although they may be based on similar physiological functions, critical bands for loudness summation are found to be some two and a half times as wide as critical bands for masking.

Findings such as the preceding are of great importance in gaining an understanding of how the auditory mechanism works. Any theory of hearing must account for such findings.

THE MISSING FUNDAMENTAL

There is yet another phenomenon, observable under rather unusual circumstances, that is worthy of mention. This is the case of the *missing fundamental* or *residue phenomenon*. If we listen to a complex tone made up of sinusoids with frequencies of 2,000, 2,100, 2,200, 2,300, . . . Hz we will hear a 100-Hz tone. Indeed, we will report the fundamental of the complex tone as being 100 Hz. Is this not simply a difference tone of 100 cps? Actually it appears to be other than a simple difference tone, as was shown by Schouten in 1940. If we listen to a tone made up of components of 300, 500, 700, 900, . . . Hz, we should, if a difference tone is the key, hear a fundamental of 200 Hz. What *is* heard, however, is a fundamental of 100 Hz. This frequency is the largest common denominator of the set of frequencies. The highest-frequency tone that could generate the 300, 500, . . . Hz components with simple harmonics is a 100-Hz tone. None of the frequencies is a multiple of 200 Hz, but all are multiples of 100 Hz. Hence 100 is the missing fundamental. Because it is generally true that the apparent pitch of any complex tone is the pitch of the fundamental, the perceived pitch of the combinations of 300, 500, 700, 900, . . . would be the pitch of a 100-Hz tone. Furthermore, this effect appears to be other than the result of difference tones, because it can be observed for quite weak tones. We pointed out earlier that normal difference tones require rather high levels to bring about their generation—presumably, levels high enough to induce nonlinear distortions in the auditory mechanism.

There is yet another clever bit of evidence militating against the difference-tone explanation. If the missing fundamental—for example, 200 Hz—exists in the ear as a result of distortion, it should be possible to mask it in the same way that any 200-Hz tone might be masked. The introduction of low-frequency random noise at a level that would mask a genuine 200-Hz tone does not mask the internally created missing fundamental of 200 Hz.

Another key to the nature of the missing fundamental, and its relation to auditory functioning, arose when many investigators were unable even to generate it. Moreover, some denied its existence. It was then discovered that all the elemental components of the complex tone must be in phase. If they are arranged randomly, the phenomenon disappears. It would appear from these results that the basis for the missing fundamental lies in the existence of an envelope of frequencies, not entirely unlike our illustration of Figure 15–5.

A final conclusion based on these and other data is that there are two pitch mechanisms. One is dependent on the existence of a sinusoidal component and a locus of activity on the basilar membrane (at least for high frequencies); the second is dependent on a rate of fluctuation and appears to be a less direct analysis of the envelope of the energy. With respect to the latter mechanism, even random noise, when alternated at low frequencies, such as 200 cps, will appear to have the pitch of the repetition rate.

Theories of pitch perception, discussed in the next section, must account for these phenomena.

How Pitch Is Perceived

Man has long wondered how he is able to perceive pitch—how different frequencies could be heard as different pitches. Even today we do not understand fully just what happens in the inner ear to allow for such fine discriminations and such a range of possible tones and combinations of tones that can be sensed. There have, however, been numerous attempts to make some sense out of the chaos. Let us look at some of the early thinking and trace the development of theories of pitch perception up to the present time. We will have to be highly selective and can hit only the high spots of auditory theory. The reader who wishes really to delve into the matter should consult references at the end of the chapter and in the bibliography.

RESONANCE THEORIES

Resonance theories fall into two general categories: place-resonance theories and pattern-resonance theories. The best example and indeed the most thoroughly worked-out place-resonance theory was that of Helmholtz.

Resonance Theory of Helmholtz. According to E. G. Weaver, "The year 1857 marks the beginning of modern auditory theory" (Wever, 1949). In that year Hermann von Helmholtz offered the first version of his resonance theory. Six years later his classic *Die Lehre von don Tonempfindungen* appeared, elaborating on his theory, but now quite complete and documented with considerable care.* In effect, Helmholtz tied together current developments involving Ohm's law of auditory analysis, Mueller's doctrine of specific energy of nerves, and the brilliant anatomical work of Corti.

Helmholtz's theory was not entirely original. Many persons anticipated and contributed materially to the development of resonance theories. For example, Du Verney, in 1683, not knowing of the inner-ear fluids, thought that the nerve fibers were spread out on the bony part of the inner ear and that resonant vibrations of the bony organs (i.e., to airborne variations) produced the nerve impulses. Du Verney thought that because the bony shelf (spiral lamina) is wider at the base of the cochlea, this portion must resonate for lower frequencies, and the narrow shelf at the apical end must resonate for higher frequencies. This is just the opposite of the situation as we understand it today. The bony shelf *is* wider at the basal end, but this means simply that the flexible basilar membrane, which occupies the space not taken up by the bony shelf, is narrow at the basal end of the cochlea and wide at the apical end.

Helmholtz proposed that there are specific resonators that are tuned for the various audible frequencies and that respond in a highly selective manner. Presumably resonators (organs of Corti?) located near the basal end of the basilar membrane respond to high-frequency tones, whereas resonators near the apical end must be tuned to lower frequencies.

There may be and probably is a resonance effect at work in the inner ear, but it is not as simple as Helmholtz's rather naive theory would indicate. Anatomical evidence does not disclose organs capable of resonating in the manner his theory would require. Furthermore, we know that any sharply tuned resonating body (and Helmholtz's hypothesized resonators would have to be rather sharply tuned) tends to continue resonating after

---

* The English version of this book, Ellis's translation in 1885 of the 1870 third edition and called by Ellis *Sensations of Tone*, is a true classic in every sense of the word. It has been reprinted right up to the present time, one edition being as recent as 1930.

the inducing force had been removed. The ear simply does not act in this manner. If it were indeed highly enough damped so as to eliminate post-stimulus resonances, then it would not be as sharply tuned as it clearly is.

To be sure, many aspects of auditory experience seem to fit in quite nicely with a resonance theory. The specific localization of damage as a result of high-intensity, pure-frequency, or narrow-band noise might lead one to accept a resonance theory. We showed earlier how a single frequency at extreme levels or long durations can be found to produce highly localized lesions in the basilar membrane, with higher frequencies producing physical damage nearer the basal end of the basilar membrane and lower frequencies tearing hair cells away at points nearer the apical end. Furthermore, results of masking experiments can be quite nicely explained in terms of a physical spreading effect, especially if one allows for somewhat less than maximal sharpness in the tuning of the resonators. Finally, other recent investigators, such as Fletcher and von Békésy, have indeed shown that many frequencies *can* be located along the basilar membrane. Helmholtz was not far wrong, but he erred in oversimplifying the effect—in attributing pitch perception to rigidly tuned entities, resonating in response to physical vibrations of the sound.

Pattern-Resonance Theories. Several early theories followed, either based on or in opposition to the resonance theory of Helmholtz. These theories emphasized the pressure-pattern response of the basilar membrane, rather than the discrete resonances Helmholtz's theory required. Ewald, for example, around 1900, developed a "standing wave" theory. Using a membrane in which standing waves were set up by acoustic stimuli, he photographed from this model patterns of loops and nodes, thus demonstrating (at least for his model) a sort of pattern-resonance effect, and thereby providing evidence against Helmholtz's theory.

Ewald and others like him were anticipating modern traveling-wave theories and the generally accepted explanations of Békésy today.

Before examining what is currently thought to be the true state of affairs, let us look into some additional historical landmarks.

FREQUENCY THEORIES

A number of earlier theories that placed the analyzing function in the brain might be lumped under the title of "frequency theories."

Rutherford's Telephone Theory. In 1886 W. Rutherford suggested that the ear works like a telephone, merely transmitting simple and compound frequencies, by way of the auditory nerve to the brain. According to Rutherford, the brain then serves as the analyzing instrument to perform, in effect, a Fourier analysis of the compound waveform. Apparently the recency of the invention of the telephone (1877) served to convince Rutherford that known limitations in the rate of firing of neurons were not effective in determining the maximum frequencies that could be transmitted by way of the auditory nerve.

The Volley Theory. Rutherford did indeed overestimate the maximum rate of firing of individual neurons, which is accepted as 1,000 per second, and even that rate for very few fibers. One possible solution to Rutherford's dilemma was proposed by Wever and Bray in 1930. They expounded a "volley theory." They suggested that, although individual fibers could not fire at a rate adequate to account for high-frequency tones, there might be a condition wherein fibers would drop out and other fibers would pick up, so that the volleying of fibers with the same or different time constants could cause the auditory nerve, as a whole, to carry the actual frequency of the stimulating tone. Such an effect was proposed, at least for frequencies too high for individual neuron response.

Wever-Bray Effect. One reason perhaps for believing that the auditory nerve could indeed carry the complex, high-frequency signals to the brain for analysis was based on early electrical recordings. It was found that when electrodes were inserted into the auditory nerve, the same signal that entered the ear could be recorded from the nerve. One could, for example, talk into a cat's ear, take the recordings from its auditory nerve, amplify them, and hear the output from a loudspeaker. It looked like the nerve was, indeed, carrying the complex, high-frequency signals to the brain. Later investigators showed, however, that what was being picked up and amplified was not the neural impulses at all, but an alternating electrical field, arising not in the auditory nerve, but in the cochlea itself. It was shown that there are two types of electrical energy that can be recorded: (1) that arising from the hair cells of the basilar membrane, mirroring the acoustical input, and (2) that from the neurons that is indeed like all other neuron impulses, with the same chemical-physical constraints of any neural response. Variations in neural response indicate magnitude, with intense stimuli forcing the neuron to fire more rapidly, and probably bringing in additional neurons with higher thresholds. Frequency, on the other hand, must be determined by *which* fiber is activated, not *how* it is activated.

Another scientific "error" bites the dust! The auditory nerve cannot carry a replica of the impinging stimulation, only discrete coded pulses. But in spite of our superior understanding, workers in the field have continued to record electrical responses from neural pathways that are excellent reproductions of the waveform and frequency of the sound stimulus! A frequency-following response (FFR) has been observed at frequencies well beyond the limits of individual neural units, and under conditions where accidental pickup of the cochlear microphonic has been ruled out (Marsh, 1970). Why this should be is not at all clear. It is impossible, but it happens. We certainly lack many answers to questions concerning the functioning of the auditory mechanism.

MODERN THEORY

All the phenomena we have mentioned to this point must be accounted for by any theory worthy of wide acceptance. But most classical theory finds instances wherein it falls somewhat short of this ideal. Modern theory was greatly influenced by the need to explain the various phenomena we have been discussing. Indeed, knowledge of such phenomena as masking, critical bands, the mel scale, and psychophysical parameters was instrumental in the development of modern auditory theory. For example, if one looks at the pattern of excitation along the basilar membrane, one can find correlates for jnd's, the mel scale, and critical bands. Lindsay and Norman (1972) point out these approximate relationships:

1 critical band	1,300 neurons;	108 mels;	25 jnd's
1 jnd	52 neurons;	4.3 mels;	0.04 critical bands
1 mel	12 neurons;	23 jnd's;	0.009 critical bands

Modern theory, really an elaboration of the early traveling-wave theories, might properly be called the von Békésy theory. In 1928 Georg von Békésy pointed out that the essential difference among the various theories lay in their assumptions concerning the nature of the basilar membrane, its elasticity, friction, mass, and so on. He constructed and worked with countless models of the inner ear, all based on anatomical and histological examination of living ears. In 1956 he was able to review the entire history of auditory theory and show that by manipulating only two variables of the basilar membrane—the absolute stiffness and the coupling of adjacent parts—he could produce all the necessary vibratory patterns to account for the physical data. In fact, he did such a good job that in 1961 he was awarded the Nobel prize in medicine and physiology.*

Békésy showed the existence of traveling-wave patterns on the basilar membranes of various animals and demonstrated that resonance was not the requisite factor. Thus location on the basilar membrane à la Helmholtz was indeed the key, but the resonances of Helmholtz was contraindicated.

There is also, as indicated earlier in this chapter, a possible second basis for pitch perception. The sensing of pitch for low-frequency tones appears to be a matter of the direct analysis of the fluctuations or the envelope of the pattern, as distinguished from the basilar membrane involvement for higher frequencies. The entire question of how the ear produces the experience of pitch has not yet been completely resolved.

Moreover, there is yet another paradox to be accounted for: Discriminations as good as 1 to 3 cps can be made. The traveling-wave theory of von Békésy is not entirely up to resolving this question. With respect to this limitation of the traveling-wave theory, he *has* suggested a function, called

---

* The interested reader is highly encouraged to read the short (about 8 pages) description of von Békésy's experiments from the Lawrence reference at the end of the chapter. Note too the special supplement to the *Journal of the Acoustical Society of America* listed in the Suggested Readings.

funneling, in which the broad response of the basilar membrane is narrowed down by means of the individual fibers leading to the brain. It has been shown, for example, that recordings from individual fibers show sharper tuning as one progresses from the cochlea to the cortex. A cell in the medial geniculate shows a narrower, sharper response than a cell in the cochlear nucleus. That is, it responds to a narrower range of frequencies than a comparable cell in the cochlear nucleus. Do you recall the inhibitory effects postulated for the retina that presumably result in greatly enhanced contrast? One example of such an effect was demonstrated by Mach bands (see Chapter 7) and generally attributed to the retinal bipolar cells. There are indeed cells in the auditory chain that resemble the retinal bipolar cells and could conceivably produce such an effect of gradient enhancement, increasing auditory contrast rather than brightness contrast.

Summary

In this chapter we examined the perception of pitch, the experiential correlate of frequency. First we considered scales of pitch, namely, musical scales and the psychological mel scale. We then examined knowledge concerning differential thresholds for pitch and the nature of diplacusis. Both simple and complex tonal interactions were considered, including such phenomena as beats, summation tones, difference tones, and the result of combinations whose effect includes the masking of other tones. We discussed masking with pure tones, broad-band white noise, and bands of noise. Concepts of critical masking band and the elusive missing fundamental were described. Finally, we described past and present theories of pitch perception, beginning with the early Helmholtz resonance theory, progressing through telephone theories, and concluding with an all to brief account of von Békésy's traveling-wave theory.

Suggested Readings

There are not many available readings that limit themselves specifically to the material covered in this chapter. Most of the readings suggested for Chapter 14 are also applicable to this chapter. Furthermore, although several have been included that appear more appropriate for the material covered in this chapter, most of the following readings contain material appropriate for both the preceding and following chapters.

1. From E. G. Boring. *Sensation and Perception in the History of Experimental Psychology.* New York: Appleton, 1942. Chapter 9, consisting of 39 easy-to-read pages, is recommended for its historical value. The first nine pages present one of the best, short histories of the development of musical scales. The excellent bibliography at the end of the chapter is particularly recommended. Chapter 11 is also recommended. In 32 pages Professor Boring presents an excellent summary of the history of auditory theory. The serious student will

want to go beyond the history of Boring and learn of the more recent investigators, such as von Békésy and Rosenblith. For early history, however, this chapter from Boring is excellent.

2. J. C. R. Licklider. "Basic Correlates of the Auditory Stimulus," in S. S. Stevens (ed.). *Handbook of Experimental Psychology*. New York: Wiley, 1951. This reference is applicable to the area of pitch and frequency effects. Very important for general use.

3. E. G. Wever. *Theory of Hearing*. New York: Wiley, 1949. The serious student should be familiar with this book. It is somewhat old and more recent data pertaining to auditory theory does exist, but it is still a highly complete treatment of auditory theory. The early chapters are of particular interest for historical perspective.

4. J. C. R. Licklider. "Three Auditory Theories," in S. Koch (ed.), *Psychology: A Study of Science*, vol. I, *Sensory, Perceptual, and Physiological Formulations*. New York: McGraw-Hill, 1959. This chapter by Professor Licklider is well worth reading. The three theories he describes are those of signal detection, which we touched on in Chapter 4; speech intelligibility, which will be considered in the next chapter; and pitch perception, considered in the present chapter. The roughly 35 pages devoted to theory of pitch perception is certainly worth reading, but it is a technical presentation and requires concentration. For the student interested in current thinking on the matter, the chapter is required reading.

5. M. Lawrence. "Hearing," in M. Alpern, M. Lawrence, and D. Wolsk, *Sensory Processes*. Belmont, Calif.: Brooks/Cole, 1967. I have recommended this publication before, both for vision, and for the chapter on sound intensity. Pages 91–98 are especially pertinent to the theoretical explanation of pitch perception and are highly recommended.

6. Gerald Oster. "Auditory Beats in the Brain," *Scientific American*, October 1973. This is an interesting and informative article, well illustrated and easy to read. For the student with some interest in high-level processing of the auditory signal, it is highly recommended.

7. B. Scharf. "Critical Bands," from J. V. Tobias (ed.), *Foundations of Modern Auditory Theory*, vol. I. New York: Academic Press, 1970. This is one of the best references on the subject. It is comparatively difficult to read and understand, but it is worth the effort.

8. Békésy Commemorative Issue, *J. Acoust. Soc. Amer.*, Supplement, 34 (1962): 1319–1534. This special supplement is dedicated to von Békésy in honor of his being awarded the Nobel Prize. It is a collection of invited papers written by some 20 authors, all of which are, in some way, related to the monumental work of von Békésy.

16/complex auditory processes

In this chapter we examine several auditory functions that do not quite fit into the previous topics of intensity and frequency, or loudness and pitch. Some of these topics might be considered more akin to perception than to sensory processes. Because of their apparently fundamental nature, however, and their simple dependence on the auditory sense, we consider them together at this time.

Auditory Space Perception

INTRODUCTORY COMMENTS

People have two ears, one on either side of their head. As a result of this rather fortunate circumstance, sounds at the two ears are not quite the same. One ear is often farther away from the source of the sound, and the head blocks off (partially, at least) some of the sound from one side. Obviously, the two ears do not "hear" exactly the same thing. It is this difference in the stimuli to the two ears that makes localization of sound sources possible. To be sure, vision probably plays the most important role in determining where a sound is coming from. But even with no visual clues we can still judge the location of a sound source with surprising accuracy.

In the next few pages we refer to "cues" for direction. Do not conclude that we sense these interaural differences and then interpret them as direction. The direction of an auditory source is probably sensed as directly as is visual space. We did not conclude that a person learns to interpret disparate visual images as three-dimensional. Neither is it likely that we learn to interpret our auditory cues as spatial localization. The word *cue* is used not to indicate an experience that the listener interprets as auditory space but simply as a convenient term to indicate possible physical characteristics that lead automatically and unconsciously to the sensation of directionality.

Learning does play some part in auditory space perception. We probably learn that a human voice of low amplitude is coming from a speaker at a distance, whereas a loud voice indicates a speaker somewhat closer. Judging the direction of a sound source, however, is not based on such a simple comparison. What are the cues for sound direction? How do we know, for example, that a sound is coming from the left?

Cues for Direction. There are perhaps four differences in the signals to the two ears that can be experienced in terms of direction of the source of a sound. First, sounds, unless they lie directly in the sagittal plane, reach one ear before the other. Particularly in the case of clicks or similar transients, simple time of arrival may be a clue to direction. Second, because of these time differences, pure tones or near-pure-tone frequencies are in different phase at the two ears, which may serve as a cue for direction. Third, a sound appears louder to the closer ear. Finally, sounds made up of complex combinations of high and low frequencies (such as speech) arrive at the two ears with differing amounts of distortion because of the differences in absorption and reflection and bending patterns of the high and low frequencies.

Methods for Studying Cues. Before examining cues for distance and direction in more detail, let us consider briefly the manner in which they are studied. An equipment often used for studying the perception of direction of auditory signals is a sound cage. As shown in Figure 16–1, a sound cage is a device that permits the precise positioning of a loudspeaker in various orientations with respect to the listener's ears. One can study the ability of an individual to localize a single sound as a function of amplitude, frequency, tonal complexity, and other variables.

Another, more analytical approach is to use a pair of headphones, manipulating the dichotic sounds to the two ears. One can thus simulate three-dimensional or stereophonic hearing. By varying differences in loudness, phase and so on, these cues can be analyzed individually or in combination with each other.

A simpler technique, in vogue before the use of electronic headphones became commonplace, involved tubes to the two ears, with the sound source being placed at varying locations within the tube. One could thus change the time relations to the two ears by changing the relative lengths of the left and right segments of the tube.

Let us now examine the manner in which differences in the signals to the two ears are sensed as direction of the source.

TEMPORAL DIFFERENCES

In 1920, Klemm and other experimenters who followed him were able to show that two clicks, presented dichotically to the ears with a time dif-

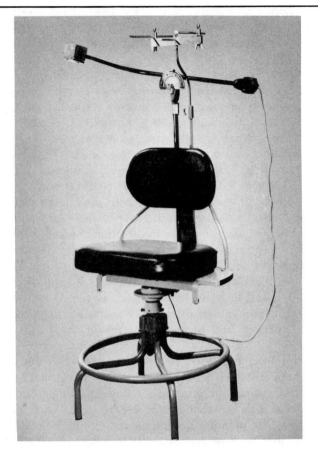

Figure 16–1
Sound cage. Used for studying auditory cues for localization. (Courtesy of Marietta Apparatus Company.

ferential as small as 0.03 millisecond, were heard as a single click, localized to one side of the median or saggital plane. It was further demonstrated that as the time between clicks is increased, the apparent source moves away from the medial plane, until with a temporal difference of about 0.65 millisecond, the click appears at a 90° angle, or directly to the side of the head; that is, opposite the ear that has the leading click. If the time difference is increased, the click remains at the leading ear until a difference of about 2.5 milliseconds results in the hearing of two separate clicks, one in each ear.

That the important cue in the early, rather crude experiments was time and not loudness was demonstrated by von Hornbostel and Wertheimer (1920). They showed that even with differences in loudness favoring the ear getting the delayed click, the sound was still perceived as coming from the side receiving the leading click. Only when the loudness of the delayed click was very much greater than that of the leading click could the perceived direction be reversed. Thus it was demonstrated that a small time difference would prevail over an appreciable, opposing intensity difference.

It is rewarding to notice how closely the phenomenal data of Klemm and his followers agree with the physical times based on distance the sound must travel for various binaural aspects. Figure 16–2 shows the physical time differences required for sound transmission for various angles from the sagittal plane to a point opposite one ear.

According to the curve in this figure, it requires about 0.65 additional millisecond for a sound to reach the distant ear when it originates from the side of the head (90° point). This was precisely the experimental delay required for a sound to be localized directly opposite the ear. At the other end of the curve, it may be seen that a time difference of 0.027 millisecond should result from a source 3° from the sagittal plane. Early workers, as we mentioned, found the smallest temporal difference that could be interpreted as directionally to be about 0.03 millisecond, and remarkably, the minimum angle of a source from the median plane that can be reliably discriminated is something on the order of 3°. The experimental data do indeed agree astonishingly well with the physics of the situation. Zwislocki and Feldman (1956), incidentally, found interaural time differences as small as 0.01 millisecond to be detectable.

PHASE DIFFERENCES

Temporal differences, as described in the preceding paragraphs, relate to the onset of a sound and are particularly effective for complex waves, such as clicks, and those with relatively sudden or steep onsets. In the case of pure-tone stimulation, localization is possible without the sudden onset and the transients of clicks. Time differences for the two ears may arise as a result of differences in phase of the sounds reaching the two ears. In practice, for research purposes, pure tones of the same frequency and amplitude are delivered to the two ears, but with a slight delay for one ear, thus resulting in the corresponding sinusoids being out of phase. When this is done it appears that the necessary and sufficient condition for the sensation of direction is the temporal relationship of corresponding points on the tone's compression waves. In other words, the ear does not recognize phase directly; rather, the points of maximum pressure of the two waves, for example, arrive at the two ears with the delays corresponding to the phase differences. It is the delay that is important, not the phase differences.

Nevertheless, the question of whether one detects phase differences directly or simply utilizes the temporal differences of the waves has bothered numerous investigators, and the question is not entirely settled at the present writing. Shaxby and Gage (1932), for example, showed that in order to counteract a localization cue for intensity, the critical factor was

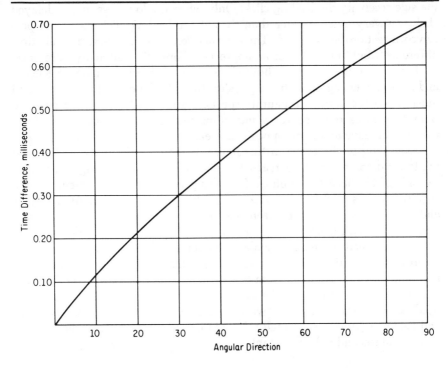

Figure 16-2
Temporal differences to the two ears as a function of direction of sound. This figure indicates that a sound from an angle 50° from the sagittal plane arrives at the distant ear about 0.45 milliseconds later than at the nearer ear.

not the degree of phase shift, but the actual temporal delay. They found that for different frequencies the amount of delay was constant, not in terms of degrees phase shift but in terms of delay time or time of arrival to the separate ears.

Whether there is a sensitivity to phase differences or simply a sensitivity to time differences is perhaps academic. Within limits the ears *can* utilize such cues to localize the source of sounds. One limit to localization as a function of temporal or phase differences is that of the frequency of the signal. The auditory response, like all other physiological functions, occurs in time. Just as we indicated a lower limit for the discrimination of temporal differences for clicks (about 0.03 millisecond), there is a temporal limit for continuous tones. Translated in terms of the frequencies of the signals, this appears to be on the order of 1,500 Hz. Frequencies higher than this figure cannot be localized with the same precision as lower frequencies, at least not by temporal or phase differences. It would appear that dichotic differences other than phase or time must be important for the localization of higher-frequency tones.

INTENSITY DIFFERENCE

The fact that sounds are louder in the nearer ear than in the other appears to be the basis for considerable localization ability. Because a sound has farther to travel (as much as 10 in.) to get to the opposite ear, it will be less loud at that ear. Note, however, that intensity or power decreases only 6 db for each doubling of distance. A sound arising 100 ft away will not be much weaker as a result of traveling an additional 10 in.—probably not enough differential to even be noticed. How, then, can intensity be a cue for direction if distance per se is so insignificant?

The answer lies in the nature of sound wave transmission. Long sound waves, like waves of the ocean, bend around obstacles in their path. A 100-Hz tone, with a wavelength on the order of 11 ft, is not blocked off by the head. It reaches the opposite ear with the same amplitude as the closer ear. Higher-frequency tones, however, do not bend around the head in the same manner. They tend to be blocked off, reflected, or absorbed by the head. Sivian and White (1933) calculated the loss in intensity at the distant ear for an angle of incidence 15°. Their calculations show, for a 300-Hz tone, a loss of less than 1 db, for a 4,000-Hz tone a loss of 5 db, and a difference of 10 db for a 15,000-Hz tone. Such data explain why intensity differences serve as cues, primarily for the tones of relatively high frequency.

Probably the most nearly complete recent research on the relation between temporal and intensity cues for direction is that of Mills (1958). Mills showed that from 250 to 1,400 Hz, localization depends primarily on temporal differences; on the other hand, for frequencies with wavelengths greater than the distance between the two ears, intensity differences are of importance. According to Mills, interaural intensity differences as small as 0.5 db can serve as cues for direction.

When cues are in conflict—that is, when temporal factors indicate one direction and loudness the opposite direction—the temporal factors seem to have priority. Perhaps if most of our listening involved only high-frequency tones, this would not be true.

TIMBRE AS A CUE FOR DIRECTION

Complex sounds should sound differently to the two ears. They should differ in timbre, or as we described it earlier, the complexity of the wave pattern. Timbre, to be sure, is the composite result of the three variables just described, so that it is perhaps not an independent cue. On the other hand, there may be a characteristic of timbre that is unique and goes beyond the three cues listed previously. Perhaps with timbre we have a learning factor at work, just as with such secondary cues for visual depth as shadows and aerial perspective. The sound of an orchestra will be different in the right ear from that in the left ear, unless it originates directly in the sagittal plane of the auditor. The near ear will tend to hear more of the

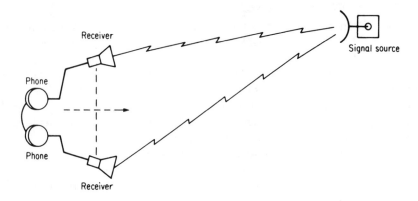

Figure 16–3
Passive detection radio receivers. Receiver antenna horns are worn on head, thus picking up radar signals from approaching aircraft. Pulse repetition frequency of airborne radar is heard by listener.

higher-frequency overtones, which will be somewhat more attenuated in the opposite ear. Similarly, the complex sounds of speech will be differentially attenuated, so that the resulting sounds to the two ears will be different. Our excellent ability to locate a speaker may be partially due to learning, to interpreting the differing timbres to the two ears as spatial localization. With quite complex sounds we may indeed learn to interpret cues.

PRACTICAL APPLICATIONS

In addition to the rather obvious stereo recording of music—with two spatially separated microphones and subsequent reproduction with separate speakers or headphones—numerous, less prosaic applications of auditory space perception data might be described.

Direction Cues for Passive Detection. Your author once assisted in the development of a passive detection device to be used by Civil Defense personnel (1956). The proposed apparatus consisted of a hard hat with two radio receivers on its top and individual antennae pointed in divergent directions (see Figure 16–3). The receivers were tuned for air-borne search radar, the idea being that the listener could hear the pulse repetition frequency (prf) of an approaching aircraft's radar before visible contact could be made. With the left-divergent antenna horn feeding a radio receiver for the left ear and the right horn feeding a receiver for the right ear, the hope was that the wearer could "hear" the direction of an approaching aircraft and could, by unconsciously matching the signals to the two ears, search in the correct direction. He might say, "I cannot see it yet, but it sounds like it's in *that* direction."

Recognizing that temporal differences are probably of more importance than loudness differences, we performed a series of experiments utilizing

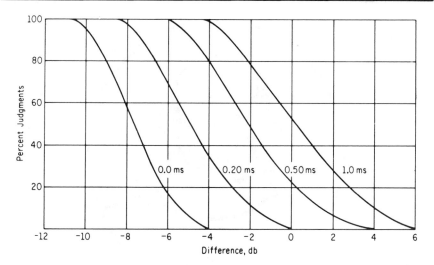

Figure 16–4
Combinations of time delay and loudness differences to produce auditory localization. Stimulus material was trains of pulses with a prf of 400 rather than the conventional sinusoidal frequencies.

signals to simulate the airborne radar's prf and general auditory characteristics. In addition, we manipulated both temporal delays and intensity differences to the two ears. Figure 16–4 shows the results of some of these data. In this figure four delays, from 0 to 1.0 millisecond, were employed. The abscissa of the figure shows the intensity differences necessary to produce the percent correct directional judgments shown on the ordinate. The figure shows, for example, that with a zero delay, a difference in loudness of about 8 db is required to produce 80 percent correct judgments as to direction. But with a delay of 1.0 millisecond, the leading tone would need to be only slightly over 2 db more intense for 80 percent correct direction identification. The figures on the ordinate to the right of the zero are cases where the leading tone is lower in amplitude than the delayed tone. For instance, a tone with a delay of 1.0 millisecond can be localized accurately 40 percent of the time, even though the delayed tone is 1 db louder than the leading tone.

There were problems in the application of the technique. Judgments were not as good as might be hoped for. For one thing, signals were not optimum, being trains of pulses rather than sine waves, and of higher than ideal frequency. Second, time delays would have had to have been produced artificially, because for all practical purposes, radio waves reach the two ears at the same time. Although the perfected article never reached the production stage, it was an interesting exercise in the application of psychophysical data.

Person-to-Person Communication in an Atmosphere-free Environment.

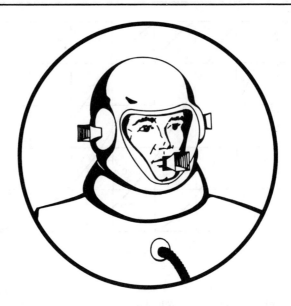

Figure 16–5
Pictorial version of person-to-person communications for an atmosphere-free environment. The three hornlike devices are microwave guides for transmitting and receiving antennae.

Figure 16–5 is a schematic drawing of a portion of a highly sophisticated communication system once recommended for our space program (1960).*
As everyone is aware, the normal conversation we take for granted in our everyday life is unattainable on, say, the moon or some other planet, or for deep-sea divers walking on the bottom of the sea. Direct aural contact is simply not attainable in an atmosphere-free environment. Except when they are in sealed, pressurized cabins, such persons must wear helmets with conventional walkie-talkie radios. There is no provision for "Hey, Joe look here, see what I found," with Joe recognizing instantly where the speaker is. To be sure, our astronauts on the moon were able to converse together, but direct recognition of the source of the speaker was not attainable, either with respect to direction or distance. The device illustrated in Figure 16–5 was meant to bring back "normal" conversation to persons working in an environment restricted to radio or similar electronic communications.

The hornlike affair at the man's mouth is indeed a horn, but a microwave horn that provides directionality to the microwave transmission. The

* Although no criticism of the system was ever made, it was never employed. In light of other, more pressing and critical considerations, the capability of recognizing just where a speaker's voice is coming from was not thought to be of sufficient importance to warrant development of the actual hardware.

horns at the ears are directional receiving antennae that feed signals to separate receivers for the two ears. With a properly designed horn configuration and judicial selection of frequencies, appropriate amplitude differences at the ears could result from directional differences and could be made to truly simulate amplitude differences for airborne sound and God-given ears. Furthermore, temporal differences, to reinforce the amplitude differences, could be produced electronically by means of variable delay circuits. It was further suggested that the loudness of the auditory signal be made consistent with distance, so that conversational-level signals could be heard for distances no greater than those encountered in airborne vocal communication. For long-distance communications conventional radio equipment would be retained, but for general person-to-person conversation everything possible should be done to reproduce the acoustic and auditory milieu of terrestrial man.

Although our first astronauts on the moon did not utilize such a sophisticated simulation of natural speech, something like this will probably be done when the man on the moon becomes hundreds of men (and women too) on the moon.

Speech Intelligibility and Noise Criteria

A problem long of interest to psychologists and of particular importance to those associated with the military and military communications is that of speech intelligibility. Under conditions of noise and signal loss, speech clearly becomes less intelligible. Can we understand the effects of noise on speech and do something to mitigate the deleterious effects. The basic problem is to determine just how intelligible speech might be when subjected to various noise backgrounds, and under various conditions of filtering, clipping, or time-sharing.

USE OF TEST MATERIAL

Early work in the study of speech intelligibility involved the use of actual speech material, either recorded by a trained speaker and played back to a listener or delivered live over the system to be tested. In some cases face-to-face presentations of test material were employed. The writer once tested Air Force single-side-band communications equipment by providing aircraft and ground stations with prerecorded test tapes that could be transmitted over the air-ground and ground-air link, recorded at the receiving end, and later analyzed for intelligibility.

Test material to be used might be phonetic sounds, nonsense syllables, short monosyllabic words, or meaningful sentences. The percentage of the material heard correctly would differ widely, depending on the nature of the test material; phonetic sounds or nonsense syllables would be much more difficult to identify correctly than meaningful words, or at the easiest extreme, connected discourse. Figure 16–6 shows some approximations of

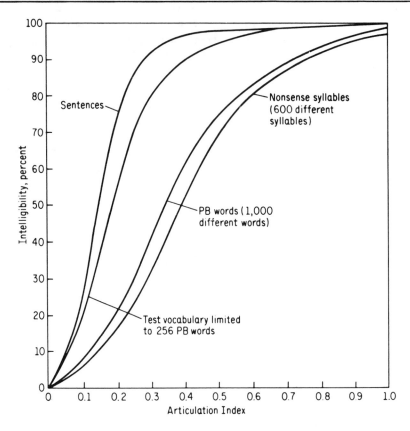

Figure 16–6

Comparison of different intelligibility test material. The values given must be considered as approximations, since such factors as the skill of the speakers and listeners, the methods used, and so on, all tend to influence the results. [Adapted from *Human Engineering Guide to Equipment Design* by C. T. Morgan, J. S. Cook III, A. Chapanis, and M. W. Lund (eds.). Copyright 1963. Used with permission of McGraw-Hill Book Company.]

speech intelligibility in percent as a function of several different test materials. The abscissa for this figure is the Articulation Index (AI), a construct to be discussed in the next section. For purposes of understanding this figure, AI is simply a measure of the "goodness" of the speech, with 1.0 representing the ideal, broad-band no-noise condition and 0.0 being the hopeless extreme.

Note from this figure that syllables at an AI of 0.5 are 70 percent intelligible, PB (phonetically balanced) words are about 84 percent intelligible, and sentences are almost 100 percent intelligible. An individual using any of these test materials would have to generalize carefully in order to predict for the operational situation.

PB Word Lists. The test material that probably received the most attention and therefore achieved the highest degree of sophistication and standardization was that of the PB or phonetically balanced word lists. Egan (1949) and his associates at the Harvard Psycho-Acoustic Laboratory developed twenty lists of 50 words each that were said to be phonetically balanced (see, for example, Table 16–1). That is, each of the lists contained the same number of phonetic sounds, and the frequencies of occurrence of different sounds was presumably the same as the frequency of occurrence in general speech. The lists were therefore representative of speech in general and quite comparable, one to the other. A sample of one of the lists is shown in the table. In use it was customary to randomize the order of presentation of the individual words. Thus, unless learning was too great, the same list might be used more than once for the same listener.

In practice the speaker reads the words, each in a carrier sentence, and the listener writes down what he or she hears. It should go without saying that careful attention to the speaker's output level, enunciation, and pronunciation must be maintained at all times. Curiously enough, the carrier sentence is rather important. One might say quite naturally, "You will write *smile*." If you try this you will notice the position of your tongue at the end of the word *write* is not in a natural position to form the first consonant of the test word. The last sound preceding the test word should ideally be a neutral vowel, one not requiring tongue or lip movement. The carrier sentence we used was "You will tra *smile*" with a vowel sound like the "a" in "art," enabling the speaker to move effortlessly from the carrier sentence to the test word. In addition, a vowel sound preceding the test word made it possible for the speaker, by means of a decible meter, to monitor his speech level somewhat more precisely. With respect to this last, the speaker could see the results of his entire carrier sentence in the swing of the meter's needle. If he concentrated on the test word's level, he would have trouble, because various *phonemes* (phonetic sounds) differ dramatically in their acoustic power. (Moreover, his reading of the meter would be after the fact if he concentrated on the test word.) If the speaker tried to

TABLE 16–1
Phonetically Balanced (PB) Word List 1

1. smile	11. there	21. rub	31. hive	41. folk
2. strife	12. then	22. slip	32. bask	42. bar
3. pest	13. fern	23. use (yews)	33. plush	43. dike
4. end	14. box	24. is	34. rag	44. such
5. toe	15. deed	25. not	35. ford	45. wheat
6. heap	16. feast	26. pile	36. rise	46. nook
7. hid	17. bunt	27. are	37. dish	47. pan
8. rat	18. grove	28. cleanse	38. fraud	48. death
9. creed	19. bad	29. clove	39. ride	49. pants
10. no	20. image	30. crash	40. fuss	50. cane

speak an *s* sound with as much power as a vowel such as *a,* he would probably have clogged his microphone with spit! What was required was a constant, normal level of overall speech effort, so that *sit* would indeed have less acoustical power than *bar.* The use of a word like *tra* preceding the test word solved the problem.

After the word lists are read to the subject, the results are simply stated in terms of percent of words reproduced correctly. Naturally, because this is a test of intelligibility only, any spelling of the word is accepted. *Their* for *there,* for example, is a perfectly legitimate spelling, or *kat* for *cat* is also perfectly acceptable.

It should be apparent to the reader that much more sophisticated research is possible utilizing PB words. Knowing the relative frequency of different sounds in the lists, one can determine, for example, just what sounds are most interfered with by a particular noise or filtering process. In addition, because the individual sounds can be analyzed for their spectral content, in some cases one could evaluate the hearing ability of a listener in a much more analytical fashion than is possible with simple audiometry.

ARTICULATION INDEX

An experimentally developed construct, known as the *Articulation Index,* is particularly useful for predicting the effect of various noises and bandwidth restrictions on the intelligibility of speech. Such a technique is particularly useful in the case of electronic transmission, where bandwidths and background noise levels can be ascertained in advance. It has been determined, largely by French and Steinberg (1947) and by Beranek (1947) and his co-workers, that the auditory spectrum from 200 to 1,600 Hz can be divided into 20 bands, each of which contributes equally to the intelligibility of speech. The upper and lower limits and the widths of these 20 bands are shown in Table 16–2 (Beranek, 1947).

In utilizing the Articulation Index technique a chart such as that shown in Figure 16–7 is employed. The bottom curve of this figure shows the threshold of audibility for continuous-spectrum sounds, at least those within the frequency range of importance for the perception of speech. The useful range of speech sounds, then, lies above this threshold curve and within the general limits set by the other curves: speech minima, average levels, and levels of speech peaks. These curves refer to a man talking in a raised voice, measured 1 m directly in front of him. According to the originators of the technique, if the spectrum levels of the speech lie above the threshold curve and above any ambient noise, and also below some maximum (overload) level not shown on the curve, speech intelligibility will be nearly perfect. On the other hand, loss of any frequencies by masking or attenuation will result in some loss of intelligibility, which can be stated in terms of the Articulation Index. This index is determined by adding up the individual contributions of each of the 20 bands, each based on

TABLE 16–2
Frequency Bands that Contribute Equally to Intelligibility

Band No.	Lower Frequency	Middle Frequency	Upper Frequency	Bandwidth
1	200	270	330	130
2	330	380	430	100
3	430	490	560	130
4	560	630	700	140
5	700	770	840	140
6	840	920	1,000	160
7	1,000	1,070	1,150	150
8	1,150	1,230	1,310	160
9	1,310	1,400	1,480	170
10	1,480	1,570	1,660	180
11	1,660	1,740	1,830	170
12	1,830	1,920	2,020	190
13	2,020	2,130	2,240	220
14	2,240	2,370	2,500	260
15	2,500	2,660	2,820	320
16	2,820	2,900	3,200	380
17	3,200	3,400	3,650	450
18	3,650	3,950	4,250	600
19	4,250	4,650	5,050	800
20	5,050	5,600	6,100	1,050

the amount of signal above the threshold and not masked by noise in that particular band.

In order to predict the efficiency of a transmission system, it is necessary to determine (1) the energy shape of the output and (2) the amount of noise in each of the 20 bands. When these are known it is a relatively simple matter to calculate an Articulation Index by summating the contribution of each of the 20 bands.

It is also possible to "shape" the transmitted speech in such a manner that all (or a maximum) the components lie above the noise, yet below the overload limit. Frequency-modulated radio uses a "shaping" system at the transmitter end, greatly amplifying high-frequency components before transmission. The receiver then reshapes the audio signal to provide a realistic reproduction of the original sounds. The purpose of this procedure is to ensure that all signal components are well above the level of the noise in the system.

Figure 16–6 has the Articulation Index as its abscissa. With this and similar curves one can go from Articulation Index to prediction of speech intelligibility, and it matters not whether the departure from perfect intelligibility is due to the addition of noise in the system or to the removal of important speech frequencies. There are some problems when the interfering noise is not continuous but made up essentially of pure-tone components or, even worse, such complex elements as impact noises or clicks.

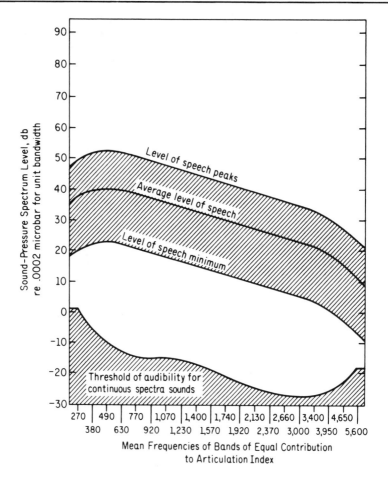

Figure 16–7

Figure for computing articulation index. The 20 bands contributing equally to intelligibility are shown on the abscissa (not in scale); the ordinate is the sound-pressure level in db re 0.0002 dyne/cm². Since unit bandwidths are employed, levels below −20 db per cycle are possible for threshold. Also shown are levels of speech minima, peaks, and average level of speech for the condition shown (raised voice, 69 db at 1 meter distance). [From L. L. Beranek, *Proc. Inst. Radio Engrs.* 35 (1947).]

However, progress is being made in the prediction of the amount of interference produced by such special conditions.

SPEECH-INTERFERENCE LEVEL

The computation of the Articulation Index is rather time-consuming and, because of inaccuracies and uncontrollable variables in its measurement, often not warranted for practical applications. In this case a simplified procedure, resulting in a measure known as the *Speech-Interference*

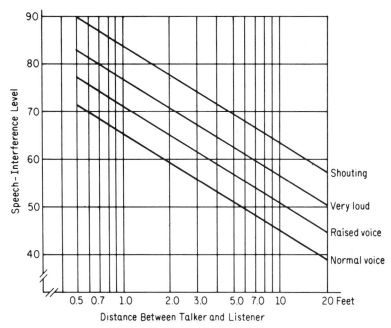

Figure 16–8

Speech-interference level for reliable (75 percent PB words) conversation at four-voice levels. Data should be considered as approximations, since many variables, such as nature of speaker, listener, etc. would work to determine precise values. [Based on data from Beranek, 1954; adapted from *Human Engineering Guide to Equipment Design* by C. T. Morgan, J. S. Cook III, A. Chapanis, and M. W. Lund (eds.). Copyright 1963. Used with permission of McGraw-Hill Book Company.]

Level (SIL) is often resorted to. The SIL is simply the arithmetic average of the sound-pressure levels in the three bands: 600 to 1,200, 1,200 to 2,400, and 2,400 to 4,8000 Hz. If the level in the 300- to 600-Hz band is 10 db or more greater than the level in the 600- to 1,200-Hz band, then all four bands are employed in the calculation of the SIL.

In some modern application three octave bands with centers at 500, 1,000, and 2,000 Hz are used. The SIL is especially useful in predicting intelligibility in noisy environments, such as offices and schoolrooms. Furthermore, because most measuring equipment provides octave-band levels rather than the 20-band units, the SIL is more easily obtained than the Articulation Index.

Figure 16–8 shows the relation between Speech-Interference Level and distance between speaker and listener for several arbitrary levels of speech. These curves indicate the various combinations of distance and Speech-Interference Level permitting reliable conversation, that is, 75 percent PB word intelligibility.

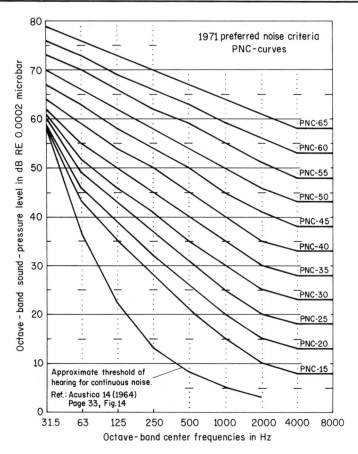

Figure 16–9
Preferred noise criterion (PNC) curves. [From L. L. Beranek, W. E. Blazier, and J.J. Figwer, *J. Acoust. Soc. Amer.* 50 (1971).]

NOISE CRITERIA

A final measure of noise effects to be mentioned in passing is that of the Preferred Noise Criterion (PNC) curves, developed by Leo Beranek (see Figure 16–9). These curves consider the entire gamut of effects produced by noise, such as damage and annoyance as well as interference with speech. These curves are basically maximum-tolerance levels for various conditions and are of interest primarily to acousticians involved in reducing or minimizing the effects of noisy equipment, workplaces, and similar industrial and domestic situations. Figure 16–9 illustrates the PNC curves.

Some of the criteria (limits) for specific applications are shown in Table 16–3 (Beranek, 1957). This table applies primarily to person-to-person voice communication and telephone communication. Additional tables are available for various other applications.

TABLE 16–3
Recommended Noise Criteria Range (Steady Background Noise for Various Areas and Functons)

Type of Space and Function	PNC Curve
Concert halls, recital halls (for listening to faint musical sounds)	10 to 20
Broadcast and recording studios	10 to 25
Bedrooms, hospitals, residences, hotels	25 to 40
Private or semiprivate offices, small conference rooms, libraries	30 to 40
Large offices, reception areas, retail stores, cafeterias	35 to 45
Lobbies, laboratory work spaces, drafting rooms	40 to 50
Light maintenance shops, kitchens, laundries	45 to 55
Shops, garages, power-plant control rooms	50 to 60
Work spaces where speech or telephone communication is not required, but where there must be no risk of hearing damage	60 to 75

Adapted from L. L. Beranek, W. E. Blazier, and J. J. Figwer, *J. Acoust. Soc. Amer.* 50 (1971).

Summary

Two major topics were considered in this chapter: (1) the ability to localize sounds in space and (2) the prediction of speech intelligibility in noise. With respect to the former, we consider four possible "cues" for direction: loudness differences, temporal differences, phase difference, and differences in timbre of the sounds of the two ears. We recognized that these cues might not be mutually exclusive, because timbre is really the result of all the other cues. We also suggested that phase differences might better be considered as temporal differences, at least so far as the ear is concerned. We recognized the complex interaction among the cues and presented two specific applications wherein a knowledge of auditory cues for localization might be applied.

In the last half of the chapter we examined four approaches to the specification of speech intelligibility and the influence of noise. We considered first the direct assessment approach, utilizing syllables, nonsense words, and meaningful material; second, we considered prediction by means of the Articulation Index; the third approach involved the Speech-Interference Level; and finally we presented the noise-criterion approach, including the annoyance factor of noise as well as intelligibility of speech.

Suggested Readings

1. From R. S. Woodworth and H. Schlosberg. *Experimental Psychology*, rev. ed. New York: Holt, Rinehart and Winston, 1954. Pages 349 to 361 present a very good description of how one senses space by means of the auditory mechanism.

Both direction and distance are considered and numerous tables and figures make the presentation both interesting and informative.

2. From Gerald M. Murch. *Visual and Auditory Perception.* Indianapolis: Bobbs-Merrill, 1973. Pages 205 to 214 of this book, which was also recommended for its coverage of visual space perception, provide additional material on auditory space perception. This reference is easy to read and makes an excellent contribution for the undergraduate student.

3. Cherry, Colin. "Two Ears—But One World," in Walter A. Rosenblith (ed.), *Sensory Communication.* New York: Wiley, 1962. Unlike the preceding reference, this article is in no way elementary or particularly easy to read and comprehend. It does, however, make a valuable contribution and is well worth reading.

4. G. A. Miller. *Language and Communication.* New York: McGraw-Hill, 1951. This entire book is recommended for the student who is especially interested in the subject matter. It is a rather advanced book, ideal for the graduate student. Pages 47 to 49 are particularly appropriate for an understanding of speech perception. One should be aware of this book for possible later reference.

5. J. P. Egan. "Articulation Testing Methods," *Laryngoscope* 58 (1948), 955–991. Probably the best of the early descriptions of articulation testing methods. Although it is more difficult to obtain than most of the suggested readings, for the really interested reader the effort may indeed be worthwhile. This article has good historical perspective and detailed descriptions of "why" and "how." Much of the material in this article may also be found in several technical reports: OSRD Report 3802, 1944, from the Psycho-Acoustical Lab., Harvard University and PNR-36 of the Office of Naval Research, 1947, also from the Psycho-Acoustical Lab.

6. From L. L. Beranek. *Acoustics.* New York: McGraw-Hill, 1954. An excellent book. For a generally readable and informative book on acoustics it has no peers. Of particular interest to this chapter, however, is the 26-page material of parts XXXI and XXXII, Speech Intelligibility and Psychoacoustic Criteria. Incidentally, part XXX of this book also presents a very readable and relatively complete description of much of the material we have included in the preceding two chapters.

7. From C. T. Morgan, J. S. Cook III, A. Chapanis, and M. W. Lund (eds.), *Human Engineering Guide to Equipment Design.* New York: McGraw-Hill, 1963. Chapter 4 of this rather unlikely sounding reference presents an excellent description of speech communications. Section 4.1 (eight pages) is an excellent short summary of the nature of speech, which we did not cover in this chapter; Section 4.2 considers speech intelligibility in excellent detail with examples of test material and methodology. These 13 pages are especially recommended. The balance of the chapter is concerned with noise criteria, component selection, and systems requirements.

8. Karl D. Kryter. *The Effect of Noise on Man.* New York: Academic Press, 1970. This is a formidable book, but it does contain a wealth of material, and should be kept in mind for the solution of specific problems.

17/chemoreception: general background

It may seem strange to the reader that we have waited until this late point in the book to consider the most primitive, elemental senses of all, the chemical senses. They are perhaps the bases for all the other senses and might very well have been considered first. Despite their evolutionary primacy (or perhaps because of it), they are the least understood of all our sensory capabilities. There is even a question about what the physical stimuli are in some cases! Had we disclosed our lack of knowledge concerning such significant organism-environment relations in Chapter 5, many readers might have turned away, appalled by our apparent ignorance.

From a historical point of view, we need make no apologies for our chemical senses. Attempts at satisfying their unique whims have literally shaped the destiny of mankind. Early ocean navigators blazed trails to find new sources of spices and scents. The exploits of Christopher Columbus might never have occurred had there not been a demand for a safer route to the spice-rich Orient. Note also the Biblical tale of the gifts presented by the Magi in Bethlehem. In the days before daily bathing and modern cooking, people had practical reasons for using perfumes and incense, and they needed strong spices to mask the unpalatable odors and to preserve food that otherwise would have spoiled without refrigeration.

Today Madison Avenue never lets us forget the need for deodorants, perfumes, and good-tasting food. Foods and drinks are not often advertised for their nutritional value, but because they taste or smell good. Our chemical senses may no longer be as important to individual survival as they once were, but for the survival of our modern economic system, they are probably critical.

What Is Chemosensitivity?

In this chapter, the first of three devoted to the chemical senses, we examine the general nature of chemoreception, its development in lower animals, and its importance in the world of survival. We examine *chemotaxis*, that is, basic, unlearned behavior involving selective attraction to or repulsion from specific chemical compounds. Are there specific chemoreceptors? If so, how many? Do they behave like the conventional receptors we considered in earlier chapters of this book? What is their significance for higher animals such as man? We may not answer all these questions, but at least we can consider them.

We will discover the world of *pheromones*, those chemical attractants and repellants of such importance for the behavior of insects and other organisms of similar phylogenetic status. We will consider the importance of pheromones as communication devices for many species and their possible importance for animals as high in the scale as man.

Also to be considered in this chapter is the problem of *aversions*. How can an organism as low as a single-celled bacterium "know" not to ingest a particular substance that may be noxious? An understanding of such aversions in lower organisms might lead to a better understanding of taste and smell preferences and aversions in man.

Before proceeding to the specifics of taste and smell in man we will briefly touch on a possible third chemical sense, the *common chemical sense*. Is it a true chemical sense, a combination of both taste and smell, or simply a particular manifestation of the tactual or skin senses?

Chemical Sensitivity and Chemotaxis

Chemical sensitivity is apparently basic to all living matter. The basic animate functions, such as growth, reproduction, or assimilation, are all mediated by chemical means and organisms that lack sensitivity to such environmental influences as light and sound but that still respond to chemical influences. In the processes of evolution the simple (?) chemical sensitivity of protoplasm has apparently developed profoundly, culminating in the establishment of receptors whose sole function appears to be the response to chemical stimulation.

Some of the most promising of current research on chemical sensitivity involves the study of chemotaxis in quite low forms of life. As early as 1880 chemotaxis had been demonstrated by exposing a suspension of bacteria to an attractant solution in a capillary tube and observing their behavior microscopically. The organisms accumulated at the mouth of the tube and eventually inside. More recently, considerable interest has been devoted to *Escherichia coli*, a common bacterium found in the human digestive tract. Adler (1969) discovered that this organism has at least five different *chemoreceptors*. That is, it behaves differently (for example, different thresholds) to at least that number of attractants. The five principal chemoreceptors described by Adler are those for *galactose, glucose, ribose, aspartate,* and *serines.* Other possible receptors are those for *fructose, maltose,* and *trehalose.* In addition, there are probably other substances that are noxious and therefore serve as repellants rather than attractants. Also, oxygen is an attractant, so there may be a receptor for it. To complicate the matter further, it is known that some bacteria have a sensitivity (and therefore receptors!) to detect light (*phototaxis*), gravity (*geotaxis*), and temperature (*thermotaxis*), because these stimuli may elicit responses.

How do these very primitive receptors work? Adler asks whether the organism compares the differences in concentration of the substances at its two ends or whether there is a "memory," so that changes in the substance's concentration are sensed. This latter suggestion is consistent with our knowledge of more complex receptors in higher animals and has been demonstrated in the case of phototaxis for bacteria. Nevertheless, we do not know exactly how chemotaxis works. In some manner the chemical or physical gradient affects the receptor, and this in turn results in activity of the cilia and/or flagella that propel the creature. Beyond this we can only conjecture.

Although our ignorance of how chemotaxis works may indeed be profound, continued effort at understanding the process is indicated. An understanding of permeability characteristics, electrical responses, and so on, may eventually cast considerable light on the more practical questions involving the human chemical senses. An example of such a question was given recently when Deutsch and Wang (1977) demonstrated the existence of chemical sensors in the stomach of a rat. Their data indicate that the stomach alone can recognize some components of food and signal their arrival rapidly to the central nervous system. I doubt that such receptors should be called taste receptors, because the animal in no way tastes the food. But, they are indeed some sort of chemical sensor or receptor.

Olfaction or Gustation?

The distinction between *olfaction* (sense of smell) and *gustation* (sense of taste) is not always clear. Indeed, in a later chapter we will employ the word *flavor* to indicate those experiences that presumably include both smell and taste, as well perhaps, as other tactual and thermal senses. It would appear that substances to be tasted by higher animals must be in liquid form, or at least in solution, whereas odors can be sensed only in gaseous form. It has been suggested that odor-producing molecules must first be dissolved in the olfactory epithelial mucus before they can be detected. But, as Pfaffman (1951) points out, "efforts to stimulate the olfactory receptors of man by stimulus solutions introduced directly into the nostrils have not been conclusive." However, with water-inhabiting vertebrates, olfactory stimulation by substances dissolved in the water must surely occur. In the preceding paragraphs on chemical sensitivity and chemotaxis we did not attempt to distinguish between olfaction and gustation. Do the bacteria taste the glucose or do they smell it? The question may be academic. Perhaps true olfaction and gustation are features of only higher animals, a result of evolutionary specialization, and the inability of human nostrils to smell odorants dissolved in liquids may be a product of this evolutionary development.

In the next section we examine the nature of chemoreception in insects. Insects provide valuable information on chemical sensitivity, midway between the chemotaxes of bacteria and the highly specialized chemical senses of the vertebrates.

Chemoreception in Insects

The study of chemoreception in insects might help us in gaining an understanding of the more advanced structure and function in higher animals. A thorough knowledge of insect chemical sensitivity might also help us in controlling their numbers, perhaps without the use of conventional pesticides. Insects have, to be sure, a gustatory sense. Some insects taste with hair cells on their *labellae*. Dethier (1962) points out that the fly has taste receptors in the sensitive hairs of its feet. If the substance it is walking on is edible and the fly is hungry, the proboscis is extended and the fly proceeds to dine. When a fly walks across your table it is sampling the remains of your meal to see if it is good to eat!

Nevertheless, it would appear that the most important chemosense for insects is that of olfaction. The complex behavior of insects is determined to a great extent by olfactory stimuli (Kaissling, 1971). Although species sensitivity may be restricted to a few odors, the list of substances sensed by insects in general is quite extensive. Many substances that, for example, are odorless to man can obstensibly be perceived by insects. Water vapor and carbon dioxide are two examples of gaseous substances odorless to man but within many insects' range of sensitivity. Some complex compounds that are odorless to man can be detected by insects at extremely low levels of concentration. Moths, for example, have a more sensitive sense of smell than dogs (Kaissling, 1971).

Odors are important to insects as guides to food sources, in initiating mating behavior, for protection, and in communication.

MORPHOLOGY OF INSECT OLFACTORY ORGANS

Insects generally perceive odors or scents with their paired "feelers" or *antennae*. These antennae are equipped with muscles in the lower segments that permit limited movement of the more distal portions that bear the sensitive cells for olfaction. Notice in Figure 17–1 the wide variety of antennae forms in several common insects.

It should be pointed out that in addition to olfactory sensitivity and

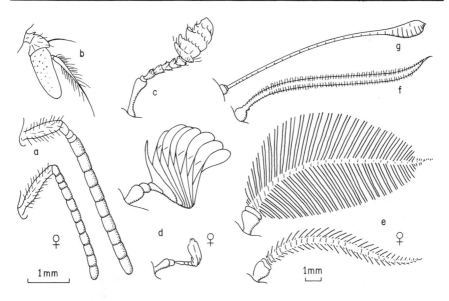

Figure 17-1
Antennae of male and female (♀) insects with well-developed olfactory sense. (a)
Honeybee; (b) flesh fly; (c) carrion beetle; (d) scarabeid beetle; (e) saturniid moth;
(f) hawkmoth; (g) butterfly. Notice extreme differences in size and complexity; notice,
too, differences between sexes of the same species. [From L. M. Beidler (ed.),
Handbook of Sensory Physiology, Vol. IV, Berlin: Springer-Verlag, 1971.]

sensitivity to carbon dioxide and humidity, the highly versatile antenna
may also include organs for such modalities as touch, air movement, sound,
temperature, and taste. An insect's antenna serves other functions, such
as facilitating optical signaling, mechanical or acoustical signaling, and
flying and hovering (Wheeler, 1960). It is, indeed, a very versatile organ.
Schneider (1969) points out that the giant antenna of the male Polyphemus
moth bears about 60,000 *sensilla* containing 150,000 cells. From 60 to 70
percent of these cells are specialized receptors for the female sex attractant.
Twenty percent respond to other odors, and the remainder serve modalities
other than olfaction.

Studies have been conducted to determine the relative efficiency of
various antenna configurations. Indeed, a "filter coefficient," based on
several characteristics of the antenna, including primarily the external
geometry of the antenna itself, has been worked out. Taking into consideration the efficiency of the antenna, in addition to such factors as air
movement (e.g., fast-flying insects versus relatively sedentary ones), one
can determine the effectiveness of various antennae as "catchers" of olfactory molecules. Notice, for example, that the size of the antenna is a
function of sex for many species. One sex may be better at olfactory re-

ception than the other. The member with the better sense of smell locates its mate by using that sense.

The olfactory cells on the insect's antenna are the primary sense cells. The actual cell body is part of the epithelial layer and has a direct connection to the creature's central nervous system by way of its axon. One or more dendrites of the olfactory cell lie within a thin-walled protrusion, the olfactory hair. The entire complex, which may involve more than one sensory dendrite per hair, and including several additional supportive and accessory cells, is known as the *sensillum*. This, the true sensory organ, is quite complex, involving a finely detailed structure of the hair-wall, complete with pores and other structural details. Figure 17–2 is a highly schematized sketch of a typical sensillum. Note that this example has two dendrites within the thin-walled protrusion. Actually, like neurons we considered before, sensilla are found in extremely diverse variety from species to species.

Detailed studies of the sensilla of insects should prove to be of extreme value in gaining an understanding of the human olfactory sense, wherein similar hair cells are surely involved. Indeed, the location of the soma and the projection of the dendritic processes in mammals does seem to be amazingly similar to that of the lowly insects.

PSYCHOPHYSICS OF INSECT OLFACTION

Perhaps psychophysics is not the correct term to use when dealing with insects, because we really do not know what the insect experience is. However, a study of apparent thresholds, discriminability, adaptation, and so on, with respect to insects' chemical sensitivity might help us in better understanding the olfactory psychophysics of higher animals. Although we cannot ask the insect what its experience is, we can study its behavior under controlled conditions of chemical stimulation. We can study activity behavior, approach-avoidance behavior, and simple conditioning as well as the underlying neural activity.

Electrophysiological Studies. Electrophysiological studies have been conducted involving receptor potentials as well as true neural impulses. It has been demonstrated, for instance, that the reaction time from the beginning of the stimulus to the onset of the nerve impulse can vary from 10 milliseconds to 100 milliseconds, depending on the strength of the stimulation, and that the impulse frequency can be as high as 200 or more per second. Interestingly, in some instances temporal patterns of spike frequency may differ, depending on the odor quality. It is also worth mentioning that such phenomena as adaptation and fatigue, not entirely unlike those described for mammals in earlier chapters, can be demonstrated. Inhibition and facilitation, surprisingly similar to that which we described for vision, are also characteristic of insect receptors.

Thresholds. Very precise measurements of behavior thresholds have been determined for some insects, particularly the honeybee. Using a con-

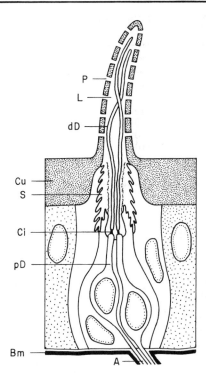

Figure 17-2
Schematc diagram of insect sensillum in longitudinal section. P, pores; L, sensillen-liquor; dD, distal segement of dendrite; Ci, ciliary segment of dendrite; PD, proximal segment of dendrite; Cu, cuticle, S, dendrite sheath; Bm, basal membrane; A, axon. Additional cells shown with gray nuclei are supportive and formative cells (From R. A. Steinbrecht, "Comparative Morphology of Olfactory Receptors." Article appears in Carl Pfaffman (ed.) *Olfaction and Taste,* Proceedings of the Third International Symposium, 1969, Rockefeller University Press.)

ditioning method developed by Frisch and a precision *olfactometer* that measured the evaporation rate of an odorant, Schwarz (1955) determined honeybee absolute thresholds for numerous organic odorants with considerable precision. Threshold concentrations for odorants are usually expressed as number of molecules per cm^3 of air. Schwarz found concentrations as low as 2×10^9 molecules/cm^3 for some flower odorants. In the case of one particular ant species, Moser et al. (1968) found concentrations of one odorant as low as 2.7×10^7 molecules/cm^3 to be effective in eliciting an alarm response. Table 17-1 shows several interesting comparisons of olfactory thresholds for man and the honeybee.

Receptor Specificity. It is possible to study relative sensitivity of individual receptors (or groups of receptors) to specific odorants. Evidence indicates that some receptors are indeed selectively sensitive. Many authors

TABLE 17–1
Olfactory Thresholds for Man and Honeybee in
Molecules per cm³ of Air

Odor	Man	Honeybee
Phenyl propyl alcohol	6.5×10^9	2.2×10^9
Ethyl undecylate	1.4×10^{10}	1.8×10^{10}
Ethyl pelargonate	3.1×10^{10}	3.7×10^{10}
Ethyl caproate	1.3×10^{11}	3.8×10^{11}
Caproic acid	2.0×10^{11}	2.2×10^{11}
Citral	4.0×10^{11}	6.0×10^{11}
Proprionic-acid	4.2×10^{11}	4.3×10^{11}
Eugenol	8.5×10^{11}	2.0×10^{10}

propose the existence of two primary categories of chemical receptors: (1) the "specialists"—such as those for sexual attraction, alarm functions, the carbon dioxide and humidity receptors, and some food receptors—and (2) the "generalists," with overlapping sensitivity to such stimuli as the aromatic and flowery odorants.

I suspect that increased knowledge about insect olfaction could help us in understanding the nature of human olfaction. The search for primary olfactory qualities, analogous to those identified for vision and hearing, may prove impossible. Perhaps olfactory attributes analogous to hue and pitch, for example, do not exist. Only additional research can answer these questions.

Pheromones

Olfactory stimuli are frequently associated with emotional experiences; perfumes and deodorants, for example, are evidence of our recognition that our lives are profoundly influenced by odors. Advertisers tell us about body odor, halitosis, and the amazing effects of perfumes and scented soaps. Much of ancient commerce involved spices and odorants to be used on the body and in religious rites. (Do you remember the gifts brought to the baby Jesus?) Whether we like it or not, we do indeed communicate with the aid of our "smells" and our olfactory sensitivity.

INSECT PHEROMONES

For subhuman animals olfactory communication appears to have considerable importance for survival. Olfactory communication has been extensively studied, especially for insects. The chemical substances involved in intraspecies communication are called *pheromones*. Such chemical substances are secreted to the external environment from specialized glands near the surface of the body and exchanged among members of the same species. Sometimes especially among higher organisms, such secretions as urine may bear pheromones.

You have probably read some of the memorable work on honeybee behavior by Karl von Frisch: how bees communicate among themselves by means of their "dance," telling other bees the location and even the distance of nectar-bearing blossoms. Today there is some question concerning the importance of the "dance" as a communication medium (Davenport, 1974, and Wilson, 1965). It may be that pheromones secreted by the returning worker bees are the true bearers of the good news. In fact, the scent released by the worker honeybees has even been identified as *geraniol* and *citral*. Many other investigators, too numerous to to identify here, have presented examples of insect communication by means of pheromones. As an example, Möglich et al. (1974) described the basis for so-called tandem calling, wherein an ant who has discovered a new source of food returns to the colony and "recruits" another ant to go along back to the food source with him. This communication is made possible by virtue of the second ant touching a secretion from the first ant's poison gland. Hölldobler and Haskins (1977) have shown that in at least one species of ant, the virgin female attracts the male by means of a pheromone released from a hitherto unrecognized gland located between two abdominal segments. Indeed, both Wilson (1965) and Hölldobler and Wilson (1977) suggest that much of insect society may be under the close influence of pheromones.

Although pheromones often demonstrate a high order of specificity, this is not always the case; in some instances female pheromones (e.g., those from moths) may attract males of other related species. Presumably, other chemical properties prevent undue promiscuity on the part of such species.

The operation of pheromones may take one of two broad forms. Some pheromones are *releasers;* they produce (release?) an immediate, direct effect. The female sex attractant is an example of a releaser. Other pheromones fall into the category of *primers.* They may, for example, influence the estrus cycle. They seem to trigger the endocrine system rather than overt behavior. Is this a fortuitous analog to the functioning of the autonomic and skeletal nervous systems in higher animals?

Although the study of pheromonal activity in insects may be of inestimable value in helping us gain an understanding of chemosensitivity in general, it has other, more immediate and practical applications. Insect control is made possible in many instances without the ecological damage of pesticides. Use of synthetic female pheromones for example, can attract male insects of the same species in large numbers to places where no actual females exist. Thus, in theory at least, the males cannot mate with the females and the harmful progeny do not come into the world in their normal overabundance. As a further advantage over pesticides, pheromonal attractants can be synthetized with much greater specificity, thus eliminating or greatly reducing harmful species but not killing such useful insects as honeybees or those insects that normally feed on their harmful relatives.

Pheromones may, in addition to serving as attractants, function as warning or alarm signals. Wasserman and Jenner (1969), for example, demonstrated that the odor trace of a rat undergoing experimental extinction can disrupt the performance of other, nonextinguished rats. The pheromonal activity of fish, both in the area of warning signals and in such social behavior as colonization, is well documented (see, for example, Atema et al., 1969).

PHEROMONES IN HIGHER ANIMALS

We have just mentioned one instance of pheromonal activity in rats. Is this capability rare or common in higher animals? Although we all recognize the importance of olfaction for female dogs in heat, as an example, the role of pheromones is probably of much greater importance in animal behavior than one might think. When they are separated from their mothers, infant rats reduce their activity in response to maternal odors (Schapiro and Sales, 1970). A frightened fish emits a pheromone that releases escape behavior in nearby fish of the same species. Bardach and Todd (1970) point out, "Many fish probably have evolved pheromones as a means whereby individuality and status can be communicated irrespective of water transparency or time of day and, thus, they have taken a step in the subsequent evolution of complex social behavior."

Olfactory bulb removal in various rodent species has been shown to have profound effects on mating behavior (Brown, 1975). Both maternal behavior and nest building are said to be eliminated as a result of olfactory bulb removal (Gandelman et al., 1971). Similar olfactory bulb removal was found to eliminate mating behavior in hamsters (Murphy and Schneider, 1970). Michael et al. (1971) not only have demonstrated that sexual excitation and activity of the male rhesus monkey can be induced by a pheromone of vaginal origin, but have actually isolated and identified the chemical substance.

To be sure, the role of pheromones in human behavior is not well recognized, although it probably does exist. McClintock (1971), for example, reported a study purporting to show that the menstrual cycles of women who were close friends and roommates tended to become somewhat synchronized. The critical factor producing such temporal synchrony was that the individuals interact and be in close proximity to each other. One explanation for such synchrony would be pheromonal influences.

Aversions

Although we discuss taste and olfactory preferences in man in the two following chapters, some mention of the manner in which lower animals avoid noxious and nonneeded chemical substances should be made. The term used to describe an animal's avoidance of such substances is *aversion*, which is the opposite of *preference*. In general, most studies of aversions refer to taste or flavor aversions, but the introduction of such a basic subject in this chapter would serve to remind the reader that the distinction between gustation and olfaction is not always clear, especially where lower animals are concerned.

There is little we can add to our earlier discussion of chemotaxis in the case of lower organisms such as *Escherichia coli*. Bacteria do indeed react to chemical stimuli; they are attracted to some, repelled by others. How this is accomplished is not known. Fortunately, they do not always discriminate in a manner most favorable to their continued existence. Our fight against disease would be hopeless if they were clever enough to avoid all poisons and harmful substances.

For animals higher than the lowly bacteria somewhat more information is available, although the basic chemical reason for preferences and aversions is still not known.

Two categories of aversions and preferences can be described: first, the long-term, genetically and deeply rooted aversions and preferences, frequently species and even sexually specific; second, those determined by temporary special conditions, such as metabolic imbalances. With respect to the former, the taste of sweetness is almost always appealing, whereas the bitter taste is almost universally rejected. Have you ever noticed that dogs seem to like candy but that cats are not especially turned on by sweets of any kind? What about rotten, decaying food? Most animals eschew such odors, but carrion eaters are obviously attracted by the odor of decaying flesh. Some animals prefer a diet restricted to vegetation; others eat meat exclusively. Some animals restrict their diets to nuts, and one very particular creature can live only on Eucalyptus leaves. Because of biological and anatomical limitations, some animals must restrict their diets to grass, for instance, whereas other creatures cannot eat it at all. Still other animals, such as man, prefer a varied diet. Dethier (1962) has shown that although male and virgin female flies prefer sweet substances, pregnant females prefer protein-rich foods. (Most of the flies around your garbage can may be pregnant females.)

But the problem goes deeper than this. Most animals prefer the foods they eat; alternative foods, equivalent in nutritive value, are often refused. It is fairly well established that taste and smell are the keys to most food selection. Artificially flavored, nonnutritive foods are often eaten with gusto even though such food has no survival value to the animal.

In 1942 C. P. Richter reported his now classic studies on self-selection of foodstuffs by rats. This study demonstrated the ability of the animals to compensate for various nutritive, endocrine, and vitamin deficiencies by altering their feeding patterns. Although normal rats tend to prefer a weak solution of salt to pure water, it was shown that adrenalectomized rats show such an increased preference for salt as to ingest voluntarily enough of the mineral to counteract the normally fatal adrenal insufficiency.

It was once believed that the animals deficient in salt had a lowered threshold, so that they could detect the presence of salt in much weaker solutions than could be detected with a deficiency. Pfaffman and Bare (1949) showed that the threshold for detecting salt is the same whether the animal is deprived or not. The change is apparently not one of sensitivity of the taste buds, but rather a higher-order, inexplicable hunger for the needed substance.

It has also been shown that insulin injection, which results in increased sugar consumption, does not change absolute thresholds for sweet, at least when electrical recordings of taste-bud response are employed as the dependent variable. Mayer-Gross and Walker (1946), however, found a reduced supraliminal sensitivity for sugar following insulin injection. Reduction of blood-sugar level below 50 mg per 100 cm^3 resulted in an animal's preferring a 30 percent sucrose solution, which would, under normal blood-sugar levels, have been rejected as too sweet.

It would appear that internal factors do not increase absolute sensitivities to weak concentrations of a needed substance. Internal changes, however, seem to produce "hungers," causing the animal to eat more of the needed substance "because it tastes good." An animal deprived for some time of salt may spend hours licking from a salt block. And animals in need of sugar can be fed quantities of food with artificial sweeteners such as saccharine, which supply none of the needed nutrient. Apparently, in some manner we do not understand, the need for a specific substance simply heightens the pleasure experienced from eating it.

Perhaps the last mentioned use of sensory information discussed in Chapter 2 is the key, the creation of pleasure. Lloyd Morgan's canon notwithstanding, animals do seem to get pleasure from eating and drinking. Indeed, investigation of the *limbic* system of the brain has even isolated the neural locus of such pleasure. It would appear that the long process of evolution has resulted in the development of a pleasure experience. Food preferences and aversions are the result of this evolutionary process.

Many aversions and preferences, of course, are of the long-standing, species-determined sort we have been discussing, but others of a quite specific nature can be learned, apparently by simple conditioning. If rats are nonlethally poisoned by a direct injection of lithium chloride, coupled with eating or drinking some specific substance, they will show a subsequent aversion to the substance. However, if the substance is placed directly into the stomach so that its taste is denied, no subsequent aversion develops (Smith, 1970).

Aversions are not limited to gustatory and olfactory experiences. Visual cues can also be linked to aversions. Wilcoxon et al. (1971) showed that whereas induced aversions in rats are mediated almost exclusively by taste and smell, Bobwhite quail can learn in one trial not to drink a liquid darkened by harmless vegetable dye. Hence the appearance of some otherwise edible substance *can* make us sick! For an interesting, informative discussion of aversions and their relation with learning the reader should consult Wallace (1976).

Common Chemical Sense

In addition to the simple (?) chemosensitivity of lower animals and the relatively distinct gustation and olfaction of higher animals, there is yet another generally recognized chemical sensitivity. Known as a *common chemical sense*, its nature and even its existence are not at all apparent. For example, there is a common chemical sense such as that found on mucous membranes like the eyeball, nasal and oral cavities, and presumably the skin surface of many organisms, especially those inhabiting the water. The free nerve endings mediating such a sense are less sensitive, provide far less discriminability, and are among the most general in their response of all the senses. Although their response may be to stimuli similar to those eliciting conventional gustation, olfaction, and tactual experiences, common chemical sensitivity is said to be distinct from the other, more specific senses (Crozier, 1916).

As an example, two classes of receptors have long been recognized in the nasal passages. In addition to the true olfactory nerve endings that are able in some way to discriminate different odors, there is a common chemical sense, mediated by simple endings of the trigeminal nerve. Being sensitive to irritating vapors, for example, stimulation of these receptors may cause discomfort or pain, often leading to reflexive sneezing, crying, or coughing. Allen (1929) showed, by surgical removal, that only mild agents, such as oil of cloves, extract of orange, and so on, stimulated the sense of smell alone, whereas such agents as acetic acid or ammonia stimulate both conventional olfactory receptors and free nerve endings. There is some evidence to indicate that pain sensitivity and common chemical sensitivity may be mediated by the same nerve endings.

Parker and Stabler, in 1913, determined sensitivities of the common chemical sense, contrasted with the gustation and olfactory senses. Using alcohol, which is an adequate stimulus for all three, they showed that a concentration of from 5 to 10 mol* was required to evoke the common chemical sense, whereas the taste response could be evoked at a concentration of 3 mol and an odor response could result from a concentration of only 0.000125 mol.

I suspect when we use the term *flavor*, we are admitting the existence of a common chemical sense as well as taste and smell. In addition, flavor probably also includes tactual and temperature experiences.

---

* Mol is the abbreviation for molar concentration. The number of grams of a solute, divided by its molecular weight equals the gram-molecular weight. A molar concentration of 1.0 is a solution containing one gram-molecular weight in 1 liter of solution.

Although common chemical sensitivity is fascinating, it will be left to the researchers and not considered further in this book. Rather, let us turn to the remaining two classes of chemoreceptors, those responsible for mediating taste and olfaction.

Summary

In this chapter we addressed ourselves to some of the basics of the chemical senses. We examined what is meant by chemosensitivity and chemoreception. The subject of chemotaxis in lower organisms was discussed briefly. We posed a question concerning the distinction between olfaction and gustation. Chemoreception by insects was discussed with a progression into the interesting subject of pheromones. The discussion of pheromones led into a short section on aversions and preferences. Our last topic of discussion was the suggestion of a common chemical sense, neither taste nor smell but of major importance for understanding flavor, the combination of several sensory experiences.

Suggested Readings

1. J. Adler. "Chemoreception in Bacteria," *Science,* 166 (1969):1588–1597. This is a rather difficult reading, but for the student interested in the basics of chemical sensitivity it is certainly worthwhile. Some knowledge of chemistry is a necessity for complete understanding of the material.
2. Karl-Ernst Kaissling. "Insect Olfaction," chap. 14, in Lloyd M. Beidler (ed.), *Handbook of Sensory Physiology,* vol. IV, *Chemical Senses, Part 1, Olfaction.* Berlin: Springer-Verlag, 1971. This chapter includes over 80 pages and is, therefore, quite thorough in its coverage of morphology and function. For the student who is interested in insect olfaction, I know of no better single source of information. Like the remainder of this book, this article is rather advanced and in no way like reading an elementary text.
3. Carl Pfaffman (ed.). *Olfaction and Taste: Proceedings of the Third International Symposium.* New York: The Rockefeller University Press, 1969. This is a large volume, much too extensive to be read in its entirety by the average student. It does include, however, numerous articles that might be of interest and prove to be highly informative. The comparative approach (insects, fish, frogs, birds, and animals) should be appreciated by many readers. The first section, containing articles on receptor mechanisms, is quite good and applicable to this as well as the two succeeding chapters. Chapters written by Priesner, Whitten, Schultze-Westrum, and Wenzel et al. should be read by the student interested in pheromones. A very good collection of readings to be read selectively and as interest dictates.
4. Bernice M. Wenzel. "Chemoreception," chap. 9, and "Tasting and Smelling," chap. 10, in Edward C. Carterette and Morton P. Friedman (eds.), *Handbook of Perception,* vol. III, *Biology of Perceptual Systems.* New York: Academic Press, 1973. These two chapters have information on just about everything covered in Chapter 17. These references are well written, easy to follow, and

well worth your time. Material pertinent to the next two chapters of this book is also covered. Good reading and an excellent source of primary references.

5. Lloyd M. Beidler. "Mechanisms of Gustatory and Olfactory Receptor Stimulation," in Walter A. Rosenblith (ed.), *Sensory Communication*. New York: Wiley, 1962. This is a fine reference, providing basic information on taste and smell. It examines the nature of the stimuli and the subsequent behavior of the receptor, including chemical and electrical behavior of each. A good reading for those interested in the electrochemistry of the process who do not require extreme depth of presentation.

6. Patricia Wallace. "Animal Behavior: The Puzzle of Flavor Aversion," *Science* 193 (1976):989–991. This is a short, easy-to-read discussion of aversions with emphasis on learning and learning theory. It is highly recommended as an introduction to this interesting subject.

18/olfaction
in man

The sense of olfaction retains a primitive nature, similar to that for the sense of taste. It lacks most of the discriminative capabilities, spatial characteristics, and high level of development of the visual and auditory senses. In the case of man, it might even be considered a somewhat degenerated or at least degenerating sense. The proportion of the brain, for example, devoted to the chemical senses in lower animals is much greater than that for man. The highly developed olfactory lobes found in fishes are not even detectable in man, at least not with an olfactory function.

The olfactory sense is rather obviously of extreme importance for many lower species. In the animal world both predators and prey require a keen sense of smell in order to survive. As we suggested in the preceding chapter, mating behavior of many lower species cannot occur without olfactory involvement.

Although the olfactory sense may have lost much of its survival value for man, it is still of considerable importance. Miners must use canaries to detect the presence of minute amounts of poisonous gases to which the human nostril is inadequately sensitive, and hunters must resort to the employment of dogs to trail game. Nevertheless, the perception of odors does have some survival value. Note that noxious substances frequently have rather unpleasant odors, just as they frequently have bitter tastes. The formation of harmful bacteria in decaying foodstuffs and body wastes is often accompanied by very unpleasant, putrid odors, thus serving as a warning to the potential eater. Many lower animals disdain eating food with a putrid or rotten smell.

To modern man the matter of esthetics, cleanliness, and so on, as discussed in the last chapter, probably play a much more important role in his interest in olfaction. As previously indicated, flavor is made up of both taste and smell, and the latter is probably of no less importance than the former. Olfaction probably plays a more important role in flavor than does taste.

A critical problem in olfaction, as indeed in all the senses, is the specification of the stimulus. Although we will discuss this matter in some detail in the pages to follow, some general statements may be made at this time. As with taste, odorous materials must be in chemical form and must be soluble in water, at least to some extent. In addition, it would appear that in order to be detected by the olfactory mechanism, a substance must be volatile; it must be in the form of airborne particles. Finally, it would appear that odorous materials must be soluble in lipids (fatty substances) in order to penetrate through the lipid layer that forms the surface membrane of the sensory cells.

Before examining the nature of substances that can produce the experience of odor, or smell, it will help to examine the physiological and anatomical mechanism involved.

Olfactory Anatomy

In the human, olfactory receptors are found exclusively in a pair of small patches located in the two nasal cavities, the area of each of these patches being about 2.5 cm^2, or somewhat less than 0.5 in.^{2} The patches are found on the medial wall of the *superior concha* and the adjacent lateral wall of the *nasal septum* and can be identified by the presence of a yellowish brown mucous membrane (see Figure 18–1). This coloration is said to be due to the presence of pigment localized in supporting cells and *Bowman's gland* cells. The importance of this coloration for optimal olfactory functioning has been stressed by many writers. Yet today, in spite of its almost universal presence, its function is not understood and even its chemical composition is not clear. Much of the evidence linking olfactory pigment with olfactory sensitivity can be traced back to Darwin. Other persons also stress the association of *anosmia* (lack or partial lack of olfactory sensitivity) and albinism. Actually, the linking of albinism and anosmia seems to be fortuitous, if it exists at all. For the reader interested in the function of the olfactory pigment, the chapter by Moulton (1971) is suggested as a starting point.

The olfactory mucosa of adult vertebrates contains numerous structures of both a sensory and nonsensory nature, such as the neuroepithelium that contains the olfactory neurons, a basal lamina, and the tubular glands known as Bowman's glands, whose function is not at all clear (see the lower portion of Figures 18–1 and 18–2). There are also supportive cells and general sensory fibers from the trigeminal nerve. (For the common chemical sense referred to in the preceding chapter?)

The olfactory receptor is a typical primary sensory neuron. It tends to be flask shaped, its length proportional to the thickness of the epithelium,

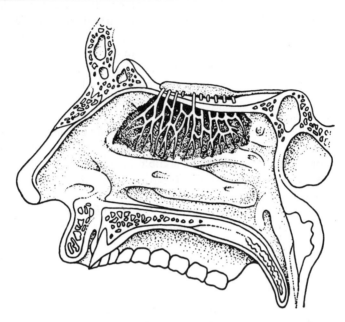

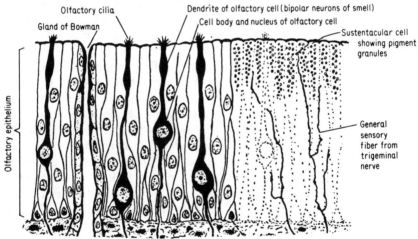

Figure 18–1
Olfactory sensory system. [(*Top*) From "Smell and Taste," A. J. Haagen-Smit. Copyright © 1952 by Scientific American, Inc. All rights reserved. (*Bottom*) Modified from A. T. Rasmussen, *Outlines of Neuro-anatomy,* 3rd ed. Dubuque, Iowa: Wm. C. Brown Company, 1943.]

which can vary from as little as 30 μ in moles to perhaps 200 μ in frogs. The olfactory *vesicle*, the bare part of the dendrite that may protrude from the epithelial surface, has a thickness of 1 to 3 μ, tapering into a cell body of 5 to 8 μ, and thence to an unmyelinated 0.2 to 0.3 axon that remains constant in diameter all the way to the olfactory bulb of the brain.

It is highly significant that, unlike most sensory cells, the sense cells for olfaction perform both the primary reception and the conduction functions. Their fine unmyelinated axonal fibers, as small as 0.2 mμ in diameter, leave the nasal cavity by way of fine perforations in the bony *cribriform plate*. This combining of both sensory and conduction in the same cell is similar to that found in the primary senses of insects, and in the case of higher-order animals is unique to the olfactory sense. Such an arrangement probably contributes to the enhanced sensitivity of the olfactory mechanism through the elimination of one synapse. The axon of the bipolar olfactory cell simply synapses with a second-order neuron that transmits the olfactory impulse directly to higher-order olfactory centers.

Still another observation seems to set olfactory neurons apart from the conventional neurons of the central nervous system: Graziadei and Metcalf (1971) are two of a number of investigators who point out that olfactory neurons can be regenerated. Indeed, their evidence indicates that olfactory neurons are continually being replaced from cells once described as nonnervous basal cells.

In spite of the rather restricted anatomical area of the sensitive surface, the functional area for olfactory reception is incredibly large. The densely packed sensory cells number some 100,000 per square millimeter, for a total in the hundreds of millions, perhaps a number even greater than the number of visual rods and cones as described in an earlier chapter. But that is not all that contributes to olfactory sensitivity.

Note from Figure 18–2 that each individual cell terminates in numerous fingerlike processes or *cilia*. It has been estimated that a single sensory cell may have as many as 1,000 of these processes. These numerous tendrils, ranging in length from 1 to 100 mμ, greatly increase the receptive area of the dendritic end of the receptor cell, so that the 2.5-cm^2 surface becomes, in effect, as great as an area of 600 cm^2 or more. Such an areal magnification probably plays an important role in the extreme sensitivity of the olfactory sense.* Notice the similarity between the processes of Figure 18–1 (lower illustration) and Figure 18–2 and the structure described for insects and similar lower species in Chapter 17. The similarity is probably more than superficial. The evolutionary process has not changed the fundamental receptor mechanisms appreciably.

There is yet an additional morphological situation that might contribute

---

* There is some question whether the cilia really play such an important role in increasing the effective area of the sensitive surface. Some animals do not have cilia on their olfactory neurons, yet their olfactory sense does not appear to be restricted or limited.

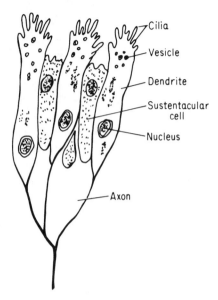

Figure 18–2
Olfactory receptor cells

to extreme sensivity. In the olfactory bulb (first brain level), thousands of receptor cell axons synapse with only about 100 second-order neurons, which then transmit their impulses to higher centers. In the rabbit about 26,000 axonal processes synapse with 100 second-order neurons, for a ratio of 260 to 1. Another reference suggests that the ratio should be 1,000 to 1. Whichever figure we take as the truth, such a summative process should greatly increase the sensitivity of the overall system. The entire olfactory system seems to utilize a summation effect that, in the case of vision, is largely restricted to the relatively peripheral rods. If there are olfactory fibers that maintain the relative one-to-one direct pathways of foveal cones, they have not been disclosed. But olfaction does indeed play a rather crude survival role and does not provide the perceptual experiences analogous to form perception in vision, or the speech analysis function of audition.

Sensitivity

Although we might expect, on the basis of the preceding anatomical description, that the olfactory sense would show a high degree of sensitivity, the observed facts are almost beyond belief. The amount of an odorant necessary to produce an olfactory experience is almost infinitesimal. The amount of odorous material deposited by a rabbit as it leaves its trail for the pursuing beagle must be exceedingly slight; detection of a cow in heat, perhaps a mile away, must be the result of an unbelievably small amount of the chemical substance reaching sensitive areas of the bull's nasal cavity. With respect to the small amount of substance necessary to elicit an olfactory response, Wolsk (1967) suggests, for example, that if the active ingredient of musk, originally obtained from the anal scent gland of the musk deer, were to be spread on a surface exposed to a continuous breeze, in 1 million years it would lose only about 1 percent of its potency as an odorant. The rapid disappearance of perfume from the opened bottle, on the other hand, is due to the rapid evaporation of the volatile vehicle, not to the direct loss of any great amount of odorant per se.

DeVries and Stuiver (1961) have considered the extreme sensitivity of olfaction. They calculated that in mercaptans, such as those involved in skunk smell, thresholds can be achieved with as few as one molecule for every two receptor cells. They further suggested that the threshold for stimulating a single olfactory cell is at most eight molecules of the odorant substance.

METHODS FOR STUDYING

Although it is possible to study insect olfaction with considerable precision, delivering known amounts of odorous material to the animal's olfactory organ, the situation with respect to the human is not nearly as simple. As was pointed out earlier, the human sense of smell is dependent on receptors located well within the bony portion of the nose. It is very difficult to deliver precisely measured concentrations of olfactory stimuli to narrowly defined areas of the olfactory system. Note too that in order to measure such things as absolute thresholds it is necessary to start out with no stimuli at all. This is of course difficult, if for no other reason than the presence of physical nooks and crannies in the olfactory structure that can retain small quantities of gaseous material for long durations.

Boring (1942) suggests that the first determination of the absolute threshold for olfaction was made by Fischer and Penzoldt in 1886. These experimentors released known amounts of various chemical stimuli into a chamber of standard size. Subjects in the chamber could then report on the minimum concentration required for detection.

Although some progress has been made, equipment used to study olfactory sensitivity does not differ greatly today from that designed some years ago by Zwaardemaker and Elsberg and illustrated in Figure 18–3. The top drawing shows schematically the Olfactometer of Zwaardemaker (1895); the bottom drawing depicts the more recent blast-injection device of Elsberg (1935). Some modern devices meter the odorant with greater precision, and many devices are capable of mixing various odorants in relatively known quantities, but the basic principles of these two devices remain the tools of today's researcher.

In Zwaardemaker's Olfactometer, the odorant lines the outside tube. As the inner tube is moved back and forth, the amount of odorant exposed

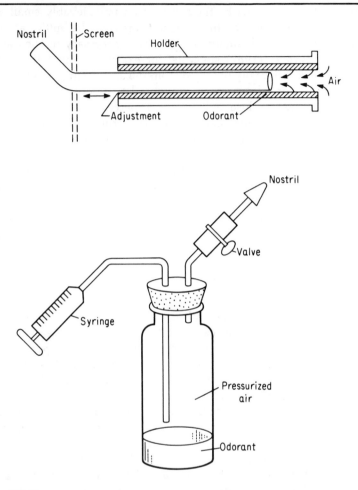

Figure 18–3
Olfactometer of Zwaardemaker and blast-injection device of Elsberg. See text for explanation.

to air, and hence subject to being sniffed by the subject, is varied. A standard unit of odorant sometimes employed is the length, in centimeters, of the odorant that must be exposed in order to achieve threshold. The amount of odorant exposure needed for threshold detection is called an *olfactie*. One olfactie of India rubber equals 0.7 cm, at least for a tube with the dimensions employed by Zwaardemaker. Less odorous substances might require more than 0.7 cm of exposure in order to be detected, whereas a highly odorous substance such as the mercaptans might be detected with an exposed area of appreciably less than 0.7 cm.

It should be obvious to the reader that such a measure is not very precise, because such uncontrollable variables as the strength of the subject's sniffing or inhalation would markedly affect the amount of air passing over the exposed adorant, and therefore the threshold. Indeed, the method developed by Zwaardemaker is little used today; the olfactie as a measure of olfactory sensitivity has only historical significance.

The second device pictured, Elsberg's blast-injection device, does remove the variable of sniffing, but at the same time provides a less realistic perceptual or sensory task. In this case a measured amount of air is forced under pressure into a bottle by means of a small syringe or pump. When the exhaust valve is opened, a known amount of the odorant-laden air is forced into the nostril or nostrils of the subject.* By using more than one bottle at the same time, it is possible to mix odorants in relatively known amounts, or to deliver one odorant to one nostril and a different odorant to the other.

More recently, we have the *olfactorium*, a much improved version of the earlier Fischer and Penzoldt approach. Developed by Foster, Schofield, and Dallenbach (1950), this is a room and anteroom made of glass and stainless steel, which can be steam cleaned to guarantee absolute cleanliness and freedom from all undesired odors. Subjects must wear plastic garments that can also be made odor-free. In practice, appropriately warmed, washed, and humidified air is forced into the chamber along with known amounts of olfactory stimuli. The system can be employed for the determination of absolute thresholds, difference thresholds, and similar psychophysical and/or esthetic applications.

THRESHOLDS

Determination of olfactory thresholds, both absolute and difference, is indeed a complex, difficult task. There are so many variables involved that even if the concentration of the odorant could be specified with precision, results would still be highly imprecise. The complex physical nature of the nasal cavities makes an understanding of the aerodynamic character of the space surrounding the sensory patches almost impossible. Probably no two people have olfactory cavities of precisely the same size and shape. Thus the amount of odorant actually reaching the sensitive receptor surface must be largely a matter of conjecture. Also, such factors as temperature and humidity influence thresholds for odors, largely because they influence the volatility of the odorant.

Absolute Thresholds. It has been suggested that olfaction is by far the more sensitive of the chemical senses. Moncrief (1967) puts the sensitivity ratio of olfaction and gustation at 10,000 to 1. He asserts that 1 mg of *skatol*, which produces an unpleasant fecal odor, will, if placed in a room

---

* While the drawings picture a single output for one nostril, more often than not, both nostrils are stimulated simultaneously. In the former case, *monorhinic* stimulation is said to be employed; *dirhinic* stimulation refers to simultaneous stimulation of both nostrils, and hence both olfactory areas, by means of a simple bifurcation of the exhaust tube.

500 m long by 100 m wide by 50 m high, result in a decidedly unpleasant odor! When we recognize that only about 2 percent of the odorant molecules entering the nose ever reach the olfactory epithelium, this sensitivity is even more remarkable. Incidentally, Mozell (1971) points out that the olfactory system is more sensitive than most laboratory detection systems.

When monorhinic stimulation is employed, thresholds for detection are higher than when dirhinic stimulation is employed. Perhaps this difference can be explained in the same way as the differences between monaural and binaural auditory thresholds—in terms of probability rather than any hypothesized neural summation. The still primitive, crude nature of olfactory research, and the general dearth of knowledge, however, militate against any firm conclusion on the matter.

We can make some crude comparisons among various odorant materials and at least get a vague feeling for the relative sensitivity of the olfactory mechanism to different substances. Although many different measures of the concentration of an odorant might be used, such as mols or molecules per unit volume, perhaps the commonest measure is that of milligrams per liter of air.

Table 18–1 shows some thresholds that have been published, all based on milligrams of odorant per liter of air, and are mostly from the work of Allison and Katz (1919) and Wenger, Jones, and Jones (1956). That such

TABLE 18–1

Thresholds in Milligrams of Odorant per Liter of Air for Several Typical Odorants

Substance	Odor	Concentration
Ethyl ether		5.83
Carbon tetrachloride	Sweet	4.533
Chloroform		3.30
Ethyl acetate		0.69
Amyl alcohol		0.225
Methyl salicylate	Wintergreen	0.100
Amyl acetate	Banana oil	0.039
N-butyric acid	Perspiration	0.009
Benzene	Kerosene	0.0088
Safrol	Sassafras	0.005
Ethyl acetate	Fruity	0.0036
Pyridine	Burned	0.00074
Hydrogen sulfide	Rotten eggs	0.00018
N-butile sulfide	Foul, sulfurous	0.00009
Citral	Lemony	0.000003
Ethyl mercaptan	Decayed cabbage	0.00000066
Trinitro-tertiary butylxylene	Musk	0.000000075

Most of these data are from M. A. Wenger, F. N. Jones, and M. H. Jones, *Physiological Psychology*, New York: Holt, Rinehart and Winston, 1956.

figures can be accepted only as relative and perhaps only suggestive of true thresholds was suggested by Moncrief. He pointed out that the threshold for ethyl mercaptan using laboratory olfactory methods was found to be 0.046 mg/liter of air and 0.00000066 mg/liter when distributed in a room with the subject able to sniff as desired. This is a difference of almost 1 million to 1. The most striking and useful feature of Table 18–1, however, is the extreme differences in sensitivity among the various substances, being about 100 million to 1 for musk as contrasted with carbon tetrachloride. It may also be significant that those odors of apparent importance for the survival of the primitive animal are still at the high-sensitivity end of the table.

The problem is even more difficult than merely choosing from among several methodological approaches. In all methods, odors are sensed in a background of air. But how often, even with extreme controls, is air perfectly odorless? It is almost like trying to determine visual brightness thresholds against a background of starlight. In the blast-injection technique it might be possible to fill the bottle with pure, odorless air, but once the odorant reaches the nasal cavity it is mixed with the residual air that must occupy this oddly shaped space. Except perhaps for highly artificial laboratory preparations, we may never be able to determine true absolute thresholds for olfaction.

Difference Thresholds. The determination of differences in strengths of odorants necessary for recognition of a difference presents an even more formidable methodological problem. We are probably safe in concluding that relatively large changes in concentration are needed in order for quantitative differences to be detected. Gamble in 1898 calculated Weber fractions from about $\frac{1}{6}$ to $\frac{1}{2}$—rather large values, compared with those for most other senses. Zigler and Holway (1935) calculated DL's more recently; they too found that rather large differences are required in order for two odors to differ in strength. They found values of $\Delta I/I$ on the order of $\frac{1}{3}$ to $\frac{4}{5}$ for different concentrations of India rubber, a relatively strong odorant material frequently used in laboratory research. More recently, Engen (1970) stated that the concentration of an odorant had to change by more than 25 percent in order for an intensity change to be detected. We can conclude that intensity discrimination is quite poor in spite of (or because of?) the extreme sensitivity of the modality.

An interesting, modern approach, resulting in much better apparent discriminations, has been described by Cain (1977). Recognizing that the olfactory sense involves the detection and discrimination of signals in "noise," Cain applied signal detection techniques to the study of olfactory intensity differences. Cain discovered, by chromatographic analysis, that there was often extreme variability in the actual odorant concentrations. With careful control and the use of receiver operating characteristic (ROC) curves derived from chromatographic analysis, he found differences in concentrations as low as 5 percent to be detectable in some instances. According to Cain, many difference thresholds rivaled those of high-quality chromatographs. This work would lead one to believe that the traditional poor difference thresholds for olfactory intensity discrimination were the result of less precise methodology, rather than any limitation inherent in the physiological mechanism involved.

ADAPTATION

Another serious problem besetting the researcher in olfaction is that of adaptation. The speed and extent (even completeness) of olfactory adaptation is very great. Recollect how quickly one can adapt to odors in a room, or, over time, to the odors of his own home or place of business. Other persons may notice the odors, but not the person regularly inhabiting the area. But note too that adaptation is one of the most important problems in psychophysics. Much can be learned of the functioning of the organism by means of adaptation studies. For example, as we suggested in vision, we can utilize selective adaptation to determine what the primary stimuli are. The course of olfactory adaptation is so certain and predictable that it has been used as a model for adaptation in other, more complex senses. We try to explain visual adaptation, for example, in light of our knowledge of olfactory and gustatory adaptation. Yet our knowledge of olfactory adaptation is seriously limited by methodological problems such as those we have mentioned.

Figure 18–4 is an example of results from a laboratory experiment on adaptation to two substances, benzoin and rubber. The abscissa of this curve shows the adaptation time, in seconds, to two different concentrations of each of the two substances. The ordinate shows the threshold for the substances, in olfacties. Note how rapidly the adaptation takes place.

More recent work by Cain and Engen (1969) has verified and elaborated on the older adaptation curves of Zwaardemaker (1925). These investigators demonstrated the interrelation of adapting time and concentration of the adapting odorant on the course of adaptation. They also showed the influence of adaptation on the power function for detection. For additional, more detailed information on the psychophysics of olfaction, including the application of power function techniques, the interested reader should consult the reference by Engen (1971).

Figure 18–4 is an example of *self-adaptation*, in which the adapting and test odorants are the same. But olfactory adaptation is not limited to self-adaptation. To be sure, *cross-adaptation* also takes place, wherein adaptation to one odorant substance results in higher thresholds for a second substance. Although the time for adaptation to any substance may be proportional to the molecular concentration of the odorant in the air (Woodrow and Karpman, 1917), the matter of cross-adaptation is much more complex. Adaptation to one substance may or may not affect the sensitivity to another stimulus. For example, exposure to camphor elevates thresholds for eucalyptal and eugenol. Indeed, there is a mutual effect among all three. On the other hand, benzaldehyde has little effect among all three.

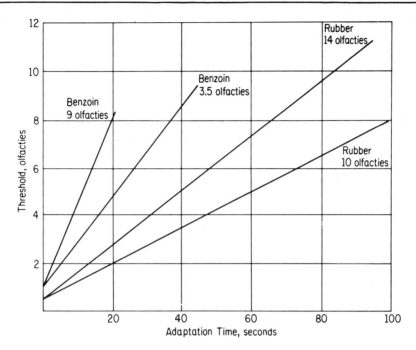

Figure 18–4

Olfactory adaptation curves. (From C. Pfaflman, "Taste and Smell," in S. S. Stevens, *Handbook of Experimental Psychology*, New York: John Wiley & Sons, Inc., 1951.)

It should be apparent to the reader that cross-adaptation studies provide a basis for attempting to classify odors. It was hypothesized that if two odors resulted in mutual adaptation effects, they were of a similar "class" and were probably mediated by the same type of receptor. Hence classes of odorants could be developed, thereby reducing the number of specific odors, each with its own tuned receptor, necessary to describe the sense of olfaction. Indeed, Pfaffman (1951) proposed that such findings suggest a receptor mosaic made up of groups of sensitive units, each of which is sensitive to a different family of chemical stimuli.

Although Moncrief (1956) experienced difficulty in finding enough cross-adaptation effects to classify odors with any degree of confidence, other workers are continuing the search. Cain and Engen have been somewhat more successful, but the problem is far from being resolved, being complicated, for example, by subjective preferences and psychological factors difficult to control.

ODORANT MIXTURES

Most of the research we have mentioned deals with pure odors. In fact, getting pure, uncontaminated odorants in known concentrations has been traditionally the most difficult problem confronting olfactory researchers.

But what happens when different odors are mixed intentionally? Several different things may happen: (1) both odors may be identified in the mixture; (2) one odor may mask the other, as is true for many so-called commercial deodorants; (3) compensation may result, such that there is a mutual alteration between odorants. Schiffman (1976), for example, suggests that the odor of paraffin or cedarwood cancels out the odor of India rubber. (Does chlorophyll actually cancel out bad odors, as certain manufacturers claim?)

An interesting approach to odorant mixture might involve dichorhinic stimulation, in which two different odors are presented separately to the two nostrils, thereby reducing the likelihood of chemical interaction. The writer has been unable to find any generalizable results utilizing this technique that shed light on the enigmatic functioning of the olfactory system. We can conclude very simply that the entire matter of odorant mixtures is still unresolved.

INDIVIDUAL DIFFERENCES IN SENSITIVITY

Yet another complication in the study of human olfaction is the existence of rather extreme differences among individuals. Individual differences in olfactory sensitivity are very great. Amoore (1971) suggests that the variability between most-sensitive and least-sensitive persons may be as much as a thousandfold.

Some individuals are *anosmic* to some or all odors. They simply cannot smell some smells. Complete anosmia can result only from a loss of both olfactory and trigeminal nerve functioning, but specific anosmias and *hyposmias* (lowered sensitivity) have a much more poorly understood etiology.

Several specific anosmias have been studied with genetic determination in mind. Although not conclusive, they are highly suggestive, seeming to indicate that dominant genes are responsible for the ability to detect some odors and that recessive genes are responsible for anosmias. The study of specific anosmias should be of great value in determining classes of odorants. Amoore discusses this matter and is actively working toward an odor classification scheme based largely on groups of odors exhibiting common anosmias or hyposmias.

Hyposmias can, of course, be acquired. We have already mentioned adaptation effects that can result in temporary threshold elevations. Perhaps long-term adaptation can result in permanent hyposmias. In addition, everyone has experienced hyposmias caused by head colds and similar infections, although such symptoms may be due primarily to blockage of the nasal passages rather than to any true loss of olfactory sensitivity. Hyposmias are also a common symptom in some psychiatric disorders, perhaps involving other hysterical symptoms.

Hyperosmias are increased sensitivities to olfactory stimuli. Some are probably the result of genetic influences, some are acquired, and some are the result of disease. Amoore suggests that cystic fibrosis can result in increasing the sensitivity to some odorants by a factor of 10,000.

It has been disclosed that the absolute threshold for one musklike odorant used in perfumes varies for the human female in accordance with the menstrual cycle (Elsberg, Brewer, and Levy, 1935; Vierling and Rock, 1967). It was found that peak sensitivity to this odorant occurred 17 and 8 days prior to the menses, at the time when estrogen secretion levels reach their maximum. About half of a sample of males were completely anosmic to this odorant, but the other half showed thresholds 1,000 times higher than those for the females at peak sensitivity. Additional research indicated that women who had ovariectomies had higher thresholds than other women. The significance of hormonal influences in olfaction cannot be denied.

A final source of variability in olfactory psychophysics is that of *parosmia*. In some mysterious way (like color blindness?) the same odorant may result in different experiences for different people. The quality of the experience is not determined by the odorant alone, but by an interaction with the person. Indeed, the odor is in the nose of the beholder! Very little is known concerning the basis or nature of parosmia, but it is a nice little word to add to your vocabulary.

Odor Classification

Olfactory theory has progressed over the centuries from the early attempts at classifying and defining odors, all the way to current theory involving the "how" of olfactory sensitivity. But even with our modern "how" theories, a truly parsimonious classification system is still elusive.

LINNAEUS'S ODOR CLASSIFICATION

Probably the first attempt at classifying odors that remains of importance today was that of Carl Linné (latinized as Carolus Linnaeus), the eminent botanist and father of taxonomy. In his cataloguing of plants he attempted to establish a meaningful system for the description of their odors. In 1752 he presented a system made up of seven classes of odors:

1. Aromatic
2. Fragrant
3. Ambrosia
4. Alliaceous
5. Hircine
6. Foul
7. Nauseous

In addition to Linnaeus's classification, the eighteenth century saw several additional classifications. Albrecht von Haller, the physiologist, described a three-component theory, consisting of (1) sweet-smelling or ambrosiac odors; (2) intermediate odors; and (3) stenches. There were also two theories developed in the nineteenth century by D. Lorry, in 1784, and A. F. de Fourcroy, in 1798, both based on chemical characteristics of odorants. After five or six additional, less popularized attempts at classification in the nineteenth century, Hendrik Zwaardemaker, the Dutch physiologist, came onto the scene.

ZWAARDEMAKER'S CLASSIFICATION

In 1895 Zwaardemaker presented his nine-class system of olfactory taxonomy that was to have such a profound effect on olfactory thinking. Even today this system is sometimes used, because the nine odors described by Zwaardemaker do indeed appear to be unique, and because most complex odors can be fitted into one or more of his categories without undue straining of the imagination. On the basis of more recent research with such techniques as cross-adaptation, it is clear that Zwaardemaker's nine classes are not mutually exclusive and that some changes in the system are called for. Nevertheless, it was and still is a useful classification and worth noting for practical as well as historic interest.

Zwaardemaker's classification utilized the seven odors of Linnaeus, with the addition of one from each of Haller's and Lorry's systems. His classification, with examples to help define the basic odor names, follows:

1. Aromatic—camphor, cloves, citron, almonds, anise
2. Fragrant—flowers, vanilla, balsam, violet
3. Ambrosiac—amber, musk
4. Alliaceous—onion, acetylene, iodine, chlorine
5. Hircine (also called caprylic)—goaty, cheese, rancid fat, sweaty
6. Foul—narcotics, some bugs, nightshade
7. Nauseous—carrion, feces
8. Ethereal (from Lorry)—ether, beeswax, fruits
9. Empyreumatic (from Haller)—roasted coffee, tobacco smoke, benzene

With numerous subclasses within the nine major classes, Zwaardemaker's classification met with universal acceptance, at least until the advent in 1915 of Henning's smell prism.

HENNING'S PRISM

The result of an elaborate investigation of qualitative similarities in odors, Hans Henning (1924) constructed a prism with six primary groups of odors and many intermediate odors lying on the edges and surfaces of the prism. In Henning's system all odors lie on one of the five surfaces or edges of the prism; no odors are found inside the prism. The six primary classes of odors as shown in Fig. 18–5 were related to Zwaardemaker's nine classes and were identified thus:

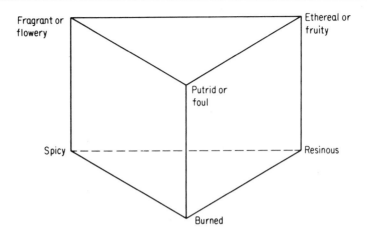

Figure 18–5
Henning's smell prism.

1. Ethereal (E)—Corresponds to Zwaardemaker's ethereal
2. Fragrant (F)—Corresponds to Zwaardemaker's fragrant
3. Spicy (S)—Corresponds to part of Zwaardemaker's aromatic
4. Resinous (R)—Corresponds to the remainder of Zwaardemaker's aromatic
5. Burned (B)—Corresponds to Zwaardemaker's empyreumatic
6. Putrid (P)—Corresponds to Zwaardemaker's foul and nauseous

Henning considered some odors to be duplex—that is, lying on a line between two primary classes. Geranium, for instance, lies on the line between fragrant and ethereal, whereas cinnamon occupies a point on the line between spicy and putrid. Other odors were quadruplex—that is, lying on the surface of the prism, hence defined by four primary classes. Cedar is located on the FESR plane, whereas garlic occupies a point on the FPSB plane (see Figure 18–6).

The alliaceous odors of Zwaardemaker fall in the middle of the FPSB surface, but the hircine (caprylic) odors really do not have a specific locus. Myrtle, for example, would be hircine in Zwaardemaker's system but falls on the line between spicy and resinous for Henning; balsam is resinous for Henning, fragrant for Zwaardemaker.

Most recent investigations have shown that, at least by gross approximation, the classification of Henning seems to work, but in details of the system, there are pronounced difficulties. As in all systems up to this time, Henning's classification was based purely on phenomenology, the way the substances "smell" to human subjects. Any classification based on more fundamental chemical or physical parameters of the stimulus was to wait until relatively recent times.

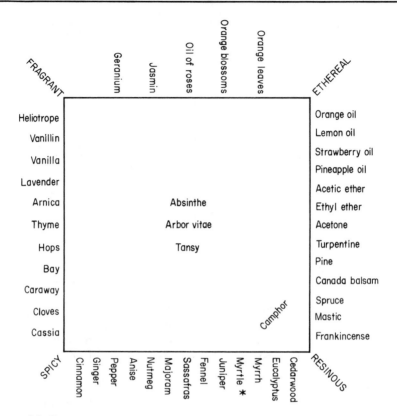

Figure 18-6
A face of Henning's prism. The odors lying along any edge resemble the odors located at the two corners, and resemble most the nearer corner. Notice, for example, the location of myrtle, between spicy and resinous, but closer, and therefore more similar, to the resinous substances.

CROCKER AND HENDERSON (1927)

A more pragmatic system, utilized "because it works," was developed by Ernest P. Crocker and Lloyd F. Henderson of the Arthur D. Little Laboratories. Although it may indeed be an oversimplification to try to describe all odors in terms of just four basic types, for practical applications the system seems to work, and a trained observer can, according to the authors, recognize the degree to which a substance contains the four basic odors. The primary odors proposed by Crocker and Henderson are as follows:

1. Fragrant or sweet
2. Acid or sour
3. Burnt or empyreumatic
4. Caprylic or goaty

Trained observers, evaluating foodstuffs, perfumes, and deodorants, are able to assign numbers from 1 to 8 to each of the four components making up any complex odor. For example, ethyl alcohol has an odor defined as 5414, vanillin as 7122 (considerable fragrant or sweet), and a rose as 6423. The Crocker Henderson system is not based on any elegant analytical chemical or physical basis. It is purely pragmatic, the result of years of research in the applied-flavor field. For describing commercial foodstuffs and the like, the system appears quite adequate.

AMOORE (1964)

The modern system of classification, proposed by Amoore, a researcher at the Oxford University, should also be mentioned at this time. Amoore proposed the existence of seven basic odors as shown in Table 18–2. The rationale for their selection is discussed in the next section when we present information on olfactory theory.

Olfactory Theory

Theories to explain the sense of smell have been with us for many years, perhaps millennia would be more precise. Yet even today the matter is far from settled. We cannot even identify with certainty the adequate stimulus necessary for the olfactory experience. Let us, however, look into the situation as it existed in history and as it exists today.

HISTORICAL

Two thousand years ago the Roman poet Lucretius (1951) suggested that the "palate" contained minute pores of various shapes and sizes. Every odorous substance, he speculated, gave off tiny "molecules" of a particular shape that fitted into these pores. The identification of the odor depended, then, on which pores were occupied by appropriate molecules. Although we may have once laughed at his naiveté, modern olfactory theory has made a wide circle and has now come back to an explanation that would surely have warmed the heart of Lucretius.

In the interim between Lucretius and such modern theorists as Mon-

TABLE 18–2
Primary Odor Classes of Amoore

Odor Class	Substance
Camphoraceous	Camphor, moth repellent
Musky	Angelica root, musk
Floral	Roses, lavender
Pepperminty	Mint candy
Ethereal	Dry-cleaning fluid
Pungent	Vinegar, roasted coffee
Putrid	Rotten eggs

crief, Amoore, Davies, and Wright numerous attempts at explaining olfactory phenomena have been described. Faraday noted, for example, that many odorous substances strongly absorb radiation in the infrared region of the spectrum. Thus a theory of olfaction based on possible infrared sensitivity was engendered. Even today, numerous investigators emphasize the importance of infrared radiation (Beck, 1950; Beck and Miles, 1947). However, even though infrared absorption can be shown to be correlated with odorant strength, it is obvious to the scientific mind that it cannot therefore of necessity be used as an explanation. The explanation for odorant efficacy may be simply the same as that for the existence of the marked infrared absorption, some characteristic of the atomic or molecular nature of the odorous substance.

MODERN THEORY

Moncrief's Theory. In 1949 R. W. Moncrief proposed a hypothesis not entirely unlike that offered some 2,000 years earlier by Lucretius. He suggested that there are a limited number of types of receptor cells, each representing a different "primary" odor, and that molecules of odorant material produce their effects by fitting into the correct "slots." Actually, Moncrief's explanation is similar to the "lock and key" concept currently employed in explaining the action of enzymes with their substrates, antibodies with antigens, and a host of similar relationships so popular with modern theorists working in fields other than sensory physiology and psychology.

Amoore's Theory. Recently a classification based largely on the shape of complex molecules, and hence the nature of the olfactory receptor sites, has resulted in a very promising theory of odors. Probably influenced by the earlier work of Moncrief, John E. Amoore (1964) at Oxford University succeeded in identifying seven primary odor classes and their characteristic molecular natures, five being identified by their shape (and hence the shape of the receptor "slot") and two by their electrical charges. The seven primary odor classes of Amoore and their identifying substances are shown in Table 18–2.

Of more significance than the remarkable agreement with both Linnaeus's and Zwaardemaker's odor classifications is the relation between Amoore's primary odors and the molecular shape of the odorant substances. It was found that substances with the camphoraceous odor had molecules of a generally spherical nature and were all of about the same size, on the order of seven angstrom units (0.7 mμ) in diameter. Thus it was hypothesized that the "slot" for the camphoraceous odor must be shaped like a hollowed-out bowl and must have a diameter on the order of seven angstrom units.

When the characteristic molecules of the other odorants were examined, it was found that they fell into four additional shape groups and that their odors could be largely predicted on the basis of the shape of their

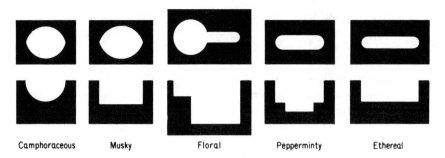

| Camphoraceous | Musky | Floral | Pepperminty | Ethereal |

Figure 18-7
Approximate shapes of several hypothetical "slots" into which odorant molecules fit. The top row shows the approximate shapes of the hypothesized sites, and the bottom row shows the same "slots" in cross section.

molecules. Musk, floral, pepperminty, and ethereal seemed to result from additional molecular shapes for which appropriate receptor "slots" could be hypothesized. Figure 18-7 is a schematic drawing of the approximate shapes hypothesized for the first five primary odorant classes in both vertical and cross-sectional view. Can you see why this theory has been called the "lock-and-key" theory?

For pungent and putrid odors no characteristic shapes were evident. Fortunately, it was discovered that a characteristic electrical charge identified these two remaining odor classes—that pungent substances carried a positive electrical charge and that putrid substances could be identified by a negative charge.

More recently, Amoore (1967, 1969) has improved our understanding of the apparent relationship between molecular shape and olfactory quality by a series of studies involving specific anosmias. These studies led Amoore to accept the suggestion of Guillot (1948) that each specific anosmia is the result of a defect in some primary odor detector. On the basis of this later research, Amoore has proposed that there may be as many as 20 or 30 primaries.

Another interesting contribution to the theory is exemplified by Schiffman (1974). She applied the mathematical techniques of multidimensional scaling to the identification and prediction of olfactory quality. Her methods give promise of a much more analytic approach to the isolation and identification of specific chemical substances and the qualitative experiences that result from them.

Although they have not received the attention of Amoore's stereochemical theory, several additional theories should be mentioned.

Molecular Vibration Theory. The molecular vibration theory was advanced by Wright (1966). He pointed out that molecules vibrate whenever they collide, that is, whenever any energy is applied to them. As a refinement of Amoore's theory, he suggests adding to the shape-coded lock-and-key approach, qualitative experiences due to frequency of vibration of colliding molecules. Differences in odors that would not be predicted by Amoore's model could be accounted for by differences in vibratory frequency.

Penetration or Puncturing Theory. Davies (1962, 1971) suggests that olfactory stimulation occurs when a puncture hole is made in the receptor membrane by one or more odorous molecules. Through this hole potassium and sodium ions may interchange, resulting in a neural impulse. The hole presumably closes in short order and the membrane is again ready to be penetrated by additional molecules. There is little direct evidence for this theory, but Davies does present some indirect evidence to support it. The interested reader should read the Davies chapter in Beidler (1971).

Pigment Theory. First advanced by Rosenberg, Misra, and Switzer (1968), the pigment theory contends that the pigments in the cell membrane of the olfactory receptors are the true receptor sites. Odorous molecules form weak bonds with the pigment molecule, eventually depolarizing the cell; this depolarization manifests itself as a neural impulse. Olfactory quality is a function of the bonding and the type of pigment involved. No data adequate to prove or disprove the pigment theory are as yet available. The interested reader might do well to read both the Rosenberg et al. article and the Moulton (1971) chapter on olfactory pigments.

That is about where we are today in the circuitous history of olfactory theory. We certainly do not understand olfaction with the perceptive insights we hold for vision and audition. But there are many unanswered questions with respect to these senses, and experts differ widely in their explanations for many visual and auditory phenomena. The stereochemical theory of odor answers many questions, but it also leaves many questions unanswered. The necessity of appending the two odor classes resulting from molecular charges raises more than a grain of doubt. However, until a better, more complete theory is advanced, we will have to admit to the likelihood that this one is most nearly correct.

Summary

In this chapter we tried to examine what is known about the human olfactory sense, the sense of smell. After considering the anatomy of the olfactory organ, we looked into the problem of sensitivity, including the determination of absolute and difference thresholds, adaptation, individual differences in sensitivity, and the result of odorant mixtures. Emphasizing throughout the monumental difficulties encountered in conducting adequately controlled research in the olfactory area, we stressed the imprecision of psychophysical techniques when applied to olfaction. Finally, we examined olfactory classification and concluded with a brief examination of olfactory theory.

Suggested Readings

Several of the following suggested readings are appropriate for both the preceding chapter, on olfaction, and the following chapter, on gustation.

1. From Lloyd M. Beidler (ed.). *Handbook of Sensory Physiology,* vol. IV, *Chemical Senses, part 1, Olfaction.* Berlin: Springer-Verlag, 1947. This is a very fine, relatively complete book on the physiology of olfaction. It is a quite advanced collection of specialized articles by persons eminent in the field. Although the book is quite expensive and not readily available in most libraries, it is important reading for the advanced student with sufficient background and interest in the area. The average undergraduate student might not profit greatly from its contents, but if you can find a copy, take a look at it; you might be surprised at what is known about olfaction. For example, chap. 1, "Anatomy of Nasal Structures from a Comparative Viewpoint" by Parsons; chap. 2, "The Olfactory Mucosa of Vertebrates," by Graziadei, and chap. 3, "The Olfactory Pigment," by Moulton, are all highly informative and related to our superficial treatment of the anatomy of the olfactory mechanism. Chapter 10, "Olfactory Psychophysics," by Engen should be of value to the advanced student interested in details of thresholds and adaptation. His stressing of detection theory in olfactory psychophysics is especially intriguing. Other chapters of this excellent reference are of equal value and have been referred to in the text, both in the preceding chapter and in this chapter.

2. Hessel De Vries and Minze Stuiver. "The Absolute Sensitivity of the Human Sense of Smell," in Walter A. Rosenblith (ed.), *Sensory Communication.* New York: Wiley, 1962. This is a short article, limited to the matter of absolute thresholds. It is a good, short (eight pages) summary of the subject.

3. H. R. Schiffman. *Sensation and Perception: An Integrated Approach.* New York: Wiley, 1976. Chapter 10 of this fine book is directed toward the olfactory sense. It is a highly recommended reading because of its complete coverage and comfortable level of presentation.

4. E. C. Crocker. *Flavor.* New York: McGraw-Hill, 1945. R. W. Moncrief. *The Chemical Senses* 3rd ed. (London: Hill, 1967. These two references are recommended reading for this and the following chapter. They are somewhat old, but still worth reading.

5. From C. G. Mueller. *Sensory Psychology.* Englewood Cliffs, N.J.: Prentice-Hall, 1965. Chapter 6 is devoted entirely to olfaction. Its 19 pages are well written and recommended as highly pertinent to the material covered in this chapter. It is interesting and fairly easy reading.

6. D. Wolsk. "Chemical Sensitivity," in M. Alpern, M. Lawrence and D. Wolsk, *Sensory Processes.* Belmont, Calif.: Brooks/Cole, 1967. This should prove of value for both chapters on the human chemical senses. This is a good reading, somewhat more technical than the Mueller reference, but less difficult than some of the other readings recommended for this chapter.

7. Thomas S. Brown. "Olfaction and Taste," in Bertram Scharf (ed.), *Experimental Sensory Psychology.* Glenview, Ill.: Scott, Foresman, 1975. This is a relatively short, interesting presentation of both olfaction and taste. It is about 28 pages long and has a very fine bibliography. The student who can find

time for only one reading might concentrate on this one. It is, of course, applicable to both this and the following chapter.

8. C. Pfaffman. "Taste and Smell," in S. S. Stevens (ed.), *Handbook of Experimental Psychology*. New York: Wiley, 1951. This is a relatively old reference, but it is still very useful. It is excellently organized and touches on just about everything discussed in this and the next chapter. As a source of additional references it is dated, but for general background reading it is unsurpassed. It should be available in your library.

9. A. J. Haagen-Smit. "Smell and Taste," *Scientific American*, March 1952. A short article of six pages which presents the available knowledge on the chemical senses in a highly readable manner. A brief history is included and an introduction to chemical theory is presented. This is a good starting point for someone interested in the chemical senses. The article is perhaps more directly applicable to the sense of olfaction than taste, hence its inclusion here rather than in the preceding chapter.

10. J. E. Amoore, J. W. Johnston, Jr., and M. Rubin. "The Stereochemical Theory of Odor," *Scientific American*, February 1964. One of the more recent and better descriptions of modern thinking on olfactory theory. It is somewhat technical, presenting the theory involving shapes and charges of molecules and their fitting into "slots" on the olfactory endings. This is good reading for the student interested in modern olfactory theory.

11. From Carl Pfaffman (ed.). *Olfaction and Taste: Proceedings of the Third International Symposium*. New York: The Rockefeller University Press, 1969. The first half of this book, recommended for the preceding chapter, is also pertinent to the material we have just been considering. This is a good source of supplemental reading.

19/the gustatory sense

The second major chemical sense of importance to man is gustation, the sense of taste. Like olfaction, it is a very primitive sense, perhaps only slightly better understood than olfaction, and of similar limited utility to man. To be sure, the sense of taste helps many lower animals identify nutritious substances and avoid spoiled or noxious materials that might otherwise be ingested. However, although it is still of some survival value to man, the sense of taste is probably more important as a source of pleasure, because it can no longer be relied on to guarantee a proper diet or ensure the avoidance of noxious or poisonous substances. Nonnutritious foods can be made to taste so good that we can literally starve to death while gorging ourselves on sweets and other good-tasting foods that have little, if any, nutritive value.

In this chapter we examine the gustatory sense in a manner similar to that employed for the olfactory sense in the preceding chapter. We look first into the anatomy and physiology of the taste system. We consider gustatory psychophysics: absolute and difference thresholds, the scaling of gustatory experience, adaptation, and taste quality—that is, the primary tastes. We touch on several features related to taste, such as the common chemical sense, flavor, and appetite. Although several of these topics may sound familiar, they are discussed in the context of taste rather than olfaction, where they were first mentioned. We also consider theories of taste before leaving the chemical senses.

Morphology and Physiology of Gustation

GUSTATION IN SUBHUMAN SPECIES

All animals are sensitive to the chemical nature of their environment. Kare (1971) points out that the amoeba withdraws from acid and that the sea anemone has separate sense areas for tactile and chemical stimuli. Many insects have sense organs, called sense hairs, on their *hypopharynx* (a tonguelike mouthpart) that seem to provide taste discrimination for sweet, salt, and water. Indeed, research has shown that there are one sugar, one water, and two salt receptors within the same taste hair (Hansen, 1969). Additional chemoreceptors, which seem to function as taste receptors, are also found on the legs, the antennae, and even the body of some insects. These cells are described as projecting hairs arising from bipolar cells anchored in the substrate, with direct axonal connections quite reminiscent of the olfactory sense cells we encountered earlier. Perhaps we are back to the earlier question: taste or smell?

With few exceptions, the gustatory sense of vertebrates is restricted to receptors located in the oral cavity. Two noteworthy exceptions are fish and amphibians. The chemoreceptors of some fish, although structurally similar to higher animals' taste buds, are located on the surface of their bodies. Amphibians, in addition to having taste buds in their mouths, also respond to chemical stimuli applied to their skins and can sense the pH and salinity of the water they are in.

ANATOMY OF THE VERTEBRATE GUSTATORY ORGAN

Complicated end organs for taste are found on the tongue and other oral structures of man, the adult *Homo sapiens* having about 9,000 of these *taste buds*, although younger members of the species frequently have more. First appearing in the human fetus at the age of about three months, taste buds in the young child are found over the entire upper surface of the tongue and much of the inside of the mouth. Ontogenetic development results in a pronounced decrease in the total number of taste buds and concentrates them in limited loci in the oral cavity.

Table 19–1 shows that the number of taste buds varies widely from species to species, being as high as 100,000 for catfish and apparently nonexistent for snakes. Incidentally, gustatory sensitivity does not appear to be determined by the number of taste buds; animals with limited num-

TABLE 19–1
Number of Taste Buds for Several Animals

Animal		Source
Snake	0	Payne, 1945
Chicken	24	Lindenmaier and Kare, 1959
Pigeon	37	Moore and Elliot, 1946
Duck	200	Bath, 1906
Bat	800	Moncrief, 1951
Man	9,000	Cole, 1941
Rabbit	17,000	Moncrief, 1951
Catfish	100,000	Hyman, 1942

bers of taste buds often show greater sensitivity than those with more taste buds. Taste buds in the human adult are largely limited to the areas of the tongue shown in Fig. 19–1. However, the sense of taste is not completely restricted to the tongue. There are also some taste buds, in limited numbers, on the palate, pharynx, and other areas of the oral cavity. Indeed, persons who have recently been fitted with dentures that cover the roof of the mouth often complain of an impaired sense of taste. Perhaps some taste buds located on surfaces other than the tongue have persisted beyond infancy and youth. Interestingly, different areas of the tongue are said to be sensitive to different tastes. The rear portion of the dorsal surface tends to have taste buds sensitive to bitterness. Near the lateral edges of the dorsal surface, areas sensitive to sourness are found, with experiences of saltiness and sweetness being localized nearer the tip of the tongue. The area near the central midline of the dorsal surface has no taste buds and is insensitive to any taste.

Taste buds are generally located on *papillae*, small elevations such as those illustrated in the middle drawing of Figure 19–1. Several different types of papillae have been identified: *foliate, fungiform, vallate,* and *filiform*. Identified by shape and location, as well as by their neural terminations, all these papillae, except the filiform, contain taste buds. Each taste bud has from 40 to 60 cells, known as *microvilli,* that appear to increase the functional surface area of the cell. Chemical materials in solution reach the microvilli by way of tiny pores in the papillae and, in some manner not yet fully understood, produce a neural response in the sensitive taste receptors. (See the bottom two drawings from Figure 19–1 and Figure 19-2.)

A remarkable bit of information regarding taste cells concerns their life span. Taste cells in the cat and rabbit have a life span of about three to five days (Beidler, 1963). Graziadei (1969) has put the life span of human taste cells at eleven days. Investigators who once thought they had identified different types of sensory cells (corresponding to different taste sensitivities) were probably observing the same cells in different stages of development. Recent investigators have shown that the same cell, in different stages of development within the several days' life cycle, responds differentially in accordance with its developmental status. Thus discriminability appears to be a function not of *which* cells are stimulated, but rather of what stage of development they are in when activated.

The problem of differential areas of the tongue still remains something of an enigma. It is not reasonable to believe that the base of the tongue should always have receptor cells in a state of development unlike those, for example, on the tip of the tongue. Recent work on the importance of enzymatic reactions in the mediation of taste may help clarify the issue.

What happens to the impulse generated by a taste receptor? There is no such thing as a "taste nerve," analogous to the optic, auditory, or olfactory nerves. Instead, gustatory experiences are mediated by the *chorda tympani* branch of the facial nerve (for the front part of the tongue), the

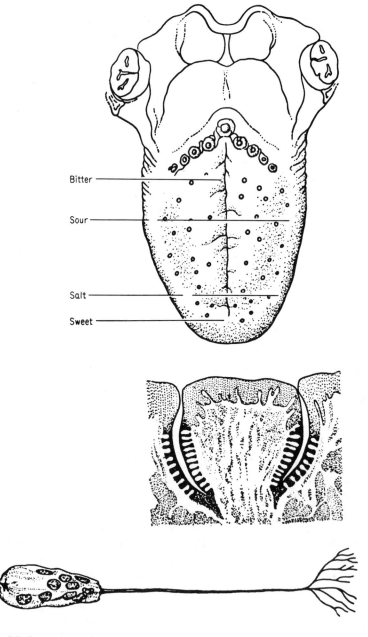

Bitter

Sour

Salt

Sweet

Figure 19–1

The gustatory sense. Taste receptors are located at the surface of tongue, as shown in the top drawing. The middle drawing illustrates one papilla containing many individual taste buds. The many taste buds are shown on the figure as the white fingerlike processes. The bottom drawing shows an individual taste bud with its nerve fiber.

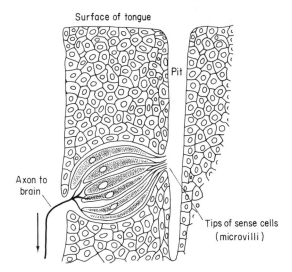

Surface of tongue

Pit

Axon to brain

Tips of sense cells (microvilli)

Figure 19–2
Schematic cross section of a taste bud. Clusters of such structures form papillae.
(From R. S. Woodworth, *Psychology*, 4th ed., New York: Holt, 1940.)

glossopharyngeal nerve (for the back of the tongue), and the vagus nerve (for the deeper portions of the throat, larynx, and pharynx).

Primary Tastes

In color vision, we found primary hues or qualities that, in combination, can account for all possible nuances of hue. The existence of analogous primary taste qualities has long been suggested. Aristotle said there were two primary tastes: sweet and bitter. All other tastes were said to fall between these two extremes. In later years the number of primary tastes was thought by some to be as high as nine or ten. The current view is that there are four taste qualities: salt, sweet, sour, and bitter being advanced by Fick in 1864. There is, to be sure, still some question whether these four should be considered qualities of a single modality or the result of four separate sensory modalities. We will see this problem again when we examine the so-called skin senses, where we are probably dealing with separate modalities rather than qualities of a single modality. For the purposes of this chapter, however, let us consider different tastes as qualities rather than modalities.

There may, indeed, be more than four primary taste qualities. Schiffman and Erickson (1971), for example, identify five primary tastes, adding *alkaline* to the conventional four. Still more recently, Schiffman and Dackis (1975) have reported evidence for two additional tastes: *sulfurous* and *fatty*. For the time being, however, the smaller number appears adequate to account for most taste experiences. There have also been some successful experiments in combining these four basic tastes to match other more complex compounds for taste equivalency.

According to Moncrief (1951), salt and sour are the more primitive evolutionary tastes, because of their survival value for water-inhabiting creatures. Probably the salt taste is more primitive, followed by the acid (sour) taste, with its warning function. Later in evolution the sweet taste, associated with edible substances, evolved, along with the bitter taste which identifies noxious or poisonous substances.

The stimuli necessary to produce these four primary tastes are not perfectly clear, but considerable progress is being made through current laboratory research.

SOUR

The stimulus necessary to produce the experience of sour has probably been best defined. It almost surely results from the presence of a weak acid in solution interacting with the oral saliva. The existence of an H^+ ion in solution is apparently necessary for the normal experience of sour. The experience of sour, however, is not simply related to the acid concentration. A weak solution of acetic acid tastes just as sour as a hydrocloric acid solution of four or five times the strength of the acetic acid. In general, organic acids taste more sour than inorganic ones. But not all acids taste sour; amino acids and sulfonic acids taste sweet, and some substances other than acids may taste sour. The relationship, whatever it is, is not a simple monotonic function of acidity.

SALTY

The most characteristic stimulus for the experience of salty is common table salt, sodium chloride. It is the only substance that elicits a pure salty taste, independent of other conflicting tastes. Other salts, such as potassium chloride or sodium bromide, produce additional tastes of bitter or sweet. It is apparent that the negative ion plays an important role in the experience of salty. Although the process is not fully understood, there is a high degree of relationship between cations (H^+) and the experience of sour and anions (e.g., Cl—) and the experience of salty. Note that a bit of salt on a sour grapefruit reduces the sourness quite effectively. (The anions of the salt presumably react with the cations of the fruit's acid, changing the overall result to a more nearly neutral [less sour] taste.)

SWEET AND BITTER

The situation with respect to the experience of sweet and bitter is even less clear. As a matter of fact, some organic substances may be changed from sweet to bitter, or from bitter to sweet by changing only a small portion of their complex molecules. Some persons even feel that a single receptor mechanism may be involved in sweet-bitter sensitivity. Others feel there should be two taste classifications: sour-salty, mediated by ionic activity, and sweet-bitter, mediated perhaps by enzymatic reactions. Only a few generalizations might be made: Most, but not all, compounds of sugars, saccharins, and the like, produce a sweet taste, but the alkaloids, such as quinine, strichnine, and other toxic agents, frequently have a bitter taste. Whereas the inorganic salts provide the salty taste, heavier salts based on organic compounds, frequently taste bitter. To be sure, the sweet taste is commonly associated with nutrients, but such substances as saccharin and beryllium salts also taste sweet. Cagen (1973) points out that two proteins found in some tropical fruits taste sweet, even though the fruits contain no carbohydrates.

The matter of primary tastes and their adequate stimuli is not at all resolved. Consider some additional complications: When saccharin is injected directly into the blood, a taste of sweetness results; when vitamin B_4 is injected directly into the bloodstream a peanutlike taste results; when camphor is injected into the bloodstream, both taste and olfactory experiences are produced (Geldard, 1972). Moreover, taste experiences can be produced by electrical stimulation, with direct current producing tastes different from those produced by alternating currents (Pfaffman, 1959). Our ignorance of the chemical senses is indeed profound. A proper understanding of how the primary tastes (assuming there are any) are mediated will have to await the results of current and future efforts by chemists and by those studying primitive chemotaxes.

Gustatory Psychophysics

Measurements of sensitivity aimed at determining thresholds for various sapid substances vary tremendously. Techniques for introducing the agents vary widely, and there are numerous variables, such as locus and area of application of the substance, its concentration, its temperature, and the adaptation level and overall condition of the organism. With respect to the latter, pregnant women show a marked threshold elevation for both sodium chloride and acid (Hansen and Langer, 1935). Anyone who has tasted an orange immediately after eating a piece of candy knows how sour the normally sweet fruit may taste, and everyone is aware of how long many tastes remain in the mouth, long after the food has been swallowed. The level of sugar in the blood has a noticeable effect on the taste threshold for sweet. In addition, there are inherited characteristics, such as the sensitivity or lack thereof to phenylthiocarbamide, the PTC so often used in genetic studies.

Nevertheless, we may attempt some broad generalizations, keeping in mind the dictum "other things being equal." With maximum attention to methodology, extreme control of stimuli, and careful selection of experi-

TABLE 19-2
Absolute Thresholds for Several
Gustatory Stimuli
(Molar Concentrations)

Substance	Threshold
Glucose	0.08
Sodium iodide	0.028
Sucrose	0.01
Sodium chloride	0.01
Citric acid	0.0023
Acetic acid	0.0018
Hydrochloric acid	0.0009
Caffeine	0.0007
Sadium saccharin	0.000023
Nicotine	0.000019
Quinine sulfate	0.000008

From C. Pfaffman, "The Sense of Taste,"
in J. Field, H. W. Magoun, and V. E. Hall
(eds.), *Handbook of Physiology*, vol 1,
Washington, D.C.: American Physiological
Society, 1959.

mental subjects, relatively precise measurements of psychophysical functions have been obtained.

INTENSITY CONSIDERATIONS

One study has shown threshold molar concentrations* of sucrose, sodium chloride, hydrochloride acid, saccharin, and quinine sulfate to be, respectively, 0.02, 0.035, 0.002, 0.00002, and 0.0000004 (Pfaffman, 1951). At least it would appear that the bitter taste for quinine can be experienced at a much lower level of concentration than can the other tastes. Note also that, as we indicated previously, acetic acid is more effective in eliciting the experience of sour than is hydrochloric acid. The results of later studies are shown in Table 19–2, again expressed in molar concentrations.

The function of the experience as a result of the concentration of the stimulus has also been studied. Utilizing the method of magnitude estimation, Stevens (1969) examined several tastes. Subjective intensity of the experience was scaled. (The results are shown in Figure 19–3.) Taste intensity was found to increase as a power function of the concentration. Representative exponents for the power function were 1.3 for sucrose and sodium chloride and 1.0 for quinine sulfate.

Different substances that may result in similar qualitative taste experiences may differ widely in their potency for eliciting a similar psychophysical response. Figure 19–4, for example, shows differences in perceived

* Molar concentration is the number of grams of the substance divided by its molecular weight per liter of total solution.

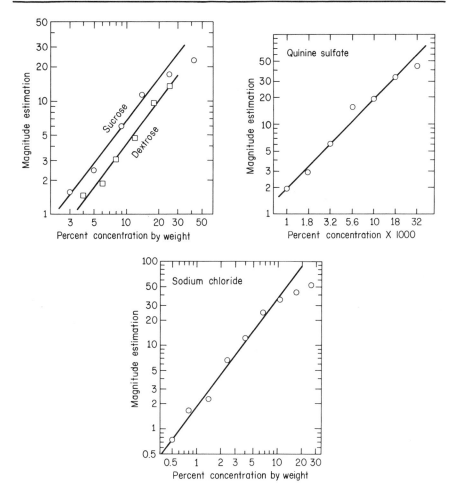

Figure 19-3

Psychophysical functions for sweetness, saltiness, and bitterness. The slope of the lines for sweet and salt indicates an exponent of about 1.3, with an exponent of 1.0 for bitter. [From S. S. Stevens, *Perception and Psychophysics* 6 (1969).]

sweetness as a result of several specific sugars. This figure shows the relative concentration of fructose, glucose, and glycerol needed to produce subjective equality with the sweetness experience of sucrose. It can be seen that in order for frustose to taste as sweet as a 0.050 g-mol percent solution of sucrose, it must have a concentration of about 0.080 g-mol percent.

For purposes of neurological examination, an interesting graded series of stimuli has been found to be of practical use (Börnstein, 1940). To the normal subject the concentrations in Table 19–3 were found to produce

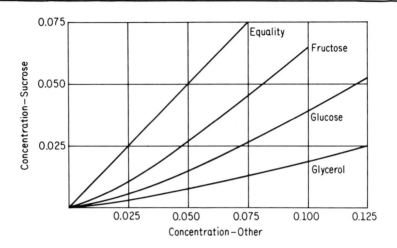

Figure 19–4
Comparative sweetness of various substances. Values of the abscissa are the concentrations of the listed agents necessary to produce subjective equality of sweetness with concentrations of sucrose shown on the ordinate. All concentrations are in gram-mol percent, i.e., 1/10 the value of the molar concentration. (Adapted from C. Pfaffman, "Taste and Smell," in S. S. Stevens, *Handbook of Experimental Psychology*, New York: John Wiley & Sons, Inc., 1951.)

the indicated experiences when drops of the solution were applied to different parts of the tongue.

The utilization of such a technique makes it possible to detect or at least suggest the presence of lesions or other damage in the gustatory portions of the central nervous system. To be sure, such thresholds are crude, and perhaps only radical departures from normal taste sensitivity can be detected.

Let us look in slightly more detail at a few of the factors already referred to that make precise determination of taste thresholds so difficult.

TABLE 19–3
Concentrations of Stimuli*

	Easily Recognizable	Moderately Strong	Very Strong
Sucrose	4.0	10.0	40.0
Sodium chloride	2.5	7.5	15.0
Citric acid	1.0	5.0	10.0
Quinine monohydrochloride	0.075	0.5	1.0

* In grams per 100 cm³ of water.

Area and Duration. In general, there is an inverse relation between the area stimulated and the concentration of a substance necessary to elicit a taste response. A weaker solution spread over a wider area will apparently encounter more taste receptors and, as a general rule, produce an experience more quickly than if a more limited area is stimulated. Presumably the apparent specificity of individual papillae results in less likelihood of a response if the area stimulated is sufficiently restricted. The factor of duration also influences thresholds, but apparently not in such a simple, straightforward manner as in the retinal elements discussed in a previous chapter.

Temperature. The temperature of the solution influences taste thresholds, but this relation is not at all simple. Even substances that evoke the same experience do not behave in the same way. Some sweet-eliciting substances increase in their evocation potential with an increase in temperature; others remain relatively constant. Although most chemical reactions are enhanced by a rise in temperature, only the tasting of some sweet-producing substances seems to follow this principle. At the other extreme, the experience of salt seems to follow a reverse curve, with higher temperatures resulting in higher thresholds, whereas the bitter taste produced by quinine seems to show an exponential function in the same direction.

Adaptation. It has long been known that adaptation plays an important part in taste sensitivity. In some ways it resembles the adaptation effects of vision, but in other ways it is much more complex, and certainly less well understood. Taste does decrease as the sapid material is held in the mouth; in some cases adaptation may be complete, with the taste actually disappearing. Here again, despite some confusion, adaptation and recovery curves *have* been plotted for many substances. Figure 19–5 is an example of the results of one such study. These curves show the threshold concentrations of sodium chloride required for various adaptation times, up to 30 seconds, and for recovery times up to the same limit. Note the rapid recovery when the adapting substance is removed. Somewhat similar curves have also been demonstrated for cane sugar and glycol (sweet) (Hahn, Kuckulies, and Taeger, 1938).

With the exception of such short durations for adapting to and recovering from the same substance, surprisingly few generalizations about gustatory adaptation can be made.* For example, adaptation to sour substances generally lowers sensitivity to all sour-producing agents, but adaptation to salty materials appears quite specific. It has been shown, for example, that with 24 different salts, adaptation to any one does not affect the threshold for the others (Pfaffman, 1951). There is some evidence that adaptation to sucrose (sweet) or to sodium chloride tends to enhance sensitivities for

---

* The long-lasting "taste in your mouth" and apparently long-lasting changes mentioned earlier are probably due not so much to changes in the sensitivity of individual receptors as to the presence in the saliva of the adapting agent. Researchers are very careful to remove all traces of the material being tested before continuing with precise laboratory studies.

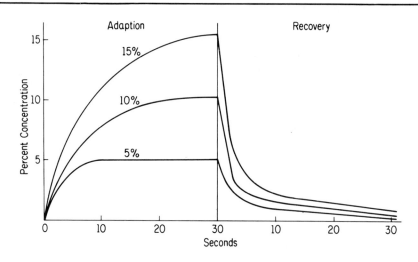

Figure 19–5
Adaptation and recovery for NaCl. Ordinate shows threshold for adaptation with indicated concentrations, for times shown on abscissa. [Adapted from H. Hahn, *Z. Sinnesphysiol.* 65 (1934).]

other qualities, whereas quinine increases the sensitivity to salt and sour, but not to sweet.

It has been suggested that gustatory adaptation is due to changes in the permeability of the taste-cell membrane for a specific agent. Thus the cell is still able to respond to other, noninhibited substances. Cross-adaptation and cross-enhancement among various substances still remain something of a puzzle to the student of taste. About all that can be said is that adaptation phenomena occur, but general principles to predict taste experience cannot be established with any degree of reliability.

Internal Factors. There is no question that the internal condition of the organism influences its gustatory sense, as was mentioned earlier with respect to olfaction. Similar shifts in gustatory sensitivity could be mentioned. For example, the chemical state of the mouth must be considered, for saliva has a complex chemical composition that interacts with the gustatory stimulus. Such physiological conditions as the menstrual period, with its hormonal changes, must also influence at least some gustatory sensitivities. The interested reader should consult Henkin, Kare, Gentile, Denton et al., and Fregly, all from Part VI of Pfaffman (1969), as well as Beidler (1971), chap. 15.

GUSTATORY INTERACTIONS

We have already mentioned interactions between taste quality and intensity, but what about qualitative interactions? Food manufacturers spend millions of dollars trying to produce appealing flavors (which also include

TABLE 19-4
Gustatory Interactions

Affect on	Sweetness	Saltiness	Sourness	Bitter
Sweet		no effect	reduces	reduces
Salty	reduces		*	no effect
Sour	enhances	enhances		enhances
Bitter	no effect	no effect	enhances	

* Enhances at high and low concentrations.

olfactory and other sensory considerations), but scientific research on combinations of taste qualities is less than abundant. Some tentative conclusions, based on what results are available, are shown in Table 19-4.

Several substances have been found that profoundly influence the sense of taste in unknown ways. Monosodium glutamate (MSG) has long been used as a so-called flavor enhancer. By itself it is said to elicit all four primary tastes; when used with foods it seems to accentuate normal taste qualities for all four primary tastes. In theory MSG serves as a taste stimulant, in some way modifying the taste receptors, perhaps to lower their thresholds and thus accentuate the character of food. You can, of course, obtain MSG from your neighborhood grocery, packaged and sold under various eye and ear appealing names.

Still other substances, such as the leaves of an Indian plant, *Gymnema sylvestre*, seem to alter taste quality, often in a highly selective fashion. These leaves reduce the experience of sweetness by some means not yet understood. That the effect is genuine has been demonstrated by reductions in neural impulses from the chorda tympani nerve after tongue stimulation with the juice from the leaves. Miraculin, a chemical derived from a fruit plant found in West Africa, works somewhat differently. Although tasteless itself, when it is placed on the tongue for several minutes, it causes sour substances to taste sweet. In addition, the much-maligned artichoke seems to have magical qualities, for exposing the tongue to an artichoke for a short time can make water taste sweet! For a more thorough discussion of taste modifiers see Kurihara (1971) or Bartoshuk et al., Henning et al., and Kurihara et al., all from Pfaffman (1959).

Gustatory Theory

The science of taste does not have such an abundance of theory as has developed for some of the other senses. The existence of four taste qualities is generally accepted, although even here there is some difference of opinion. The existence of taste buds that seem to exhibit sensitivities, at least partially determined by their maturational stage, complicates any theory requiring specificity of receptors, such as we found for color vision. In addition, microelectrode recordings show that a single taste cell may respond to several different primary stimuli. Recordings from afferent fibers of the chorda tympani show no specificity of the stimulating substance.

Pfaffman (1959) proposes an "afferent code" for taste. He contends that taste is determined by the relative activity across a population of fibers. Thus taste quality is determined not by a single element "tuned" to sweet, for example, but by the pattern of discharges. Erickson (1963) conducted some interesting research that seems to support Pfaffman's views.

Békésy (1964, 1966) has proposed a "duplexity" theory of taste. Based largely on taste interaction studies, Békésy suggests that two different types of receptors, along with cutaneous experiences of warm and cold, can account for all taste experiences. In his theory bitter and sweet are paired, as are salt and sour. The interested reader should consult the preceding references.

Summary

In this chapter we discussed the sense of taste or gustation. We examined briefly the anatomy of the taste organ and the receptors, known as taste buds. We considered primary tastes and gustatory sensitivity. With respect to the latter, we indicated the amazing complexity of taste sensitivity relationships. We considered as important factors the area of application of sapid substance, its temperature, and the nature of adaptation and internal factors as determinants of taste experience. We also approached the subject of taste interaction and taste modifiers. We concluded the chapter with a brief look at taste theory.

Suggested Readings

1. Lloyd M. Beidler (ed.). *Handbook of Sensory Physiology*, vol. IV, *Chemical Senses*, part 2, *Taste*. Berlin: Springer-Verlag, 1971. This book is the second volume in the series referred to in a preceding chapter. It too is a fine reference. My comments in the Suggested Readings for Chapters 17 and 18 also apply here: a difficult, expensive, and hard-to-obtain reference, but one quite useful for the advanced student with sufficient interest and background. For example, you will be intrigued by the remarkable drawings and photomicrographs of the tongue found in chap. 1. Other articles from this reference have been specifically cited in the text.

The following three references were recommended for either Chapter 17 or 18. They are also pertinent to the taste sense and are, therefore, repeated. Each has separate sections or chapters devoted to olfaction and gustation.

2. From Carl Pfaffman (ed.). *Olfaction and Taste: Proceedings of the Third International Symposium*. New York: The Rockefeller University Press, 1969.

The second half of this excellent collection of readings is devoted to taste and is highly recommended for the serious student. Several specific chapters are cited in your text.

3. From H. R. Schiffman. *Sensation and Perception: An Integrated Approach.* New York: Wiley, 1976. Chapter 9 is devoted to taste. It is very good reading, not too difficult, yet complete enough to satisfy all but the most advanced student.

4. Thomas S. Brown. "Olfaction and Taste," in Bertram Scharf (ed.), *Experimental Sensory Psychology.* Glenview, Ill.: Scott, Foresman, 1975. The part of the chapter dealing with taste is excellent and highly recommended. It is fairly easy reading and has a wealth of information.

5. E. C. Crocker. *Flavor.* New York: McGraw-Hill, 1945.

6. R. W. Moncrief. *The Chemical Senses,* 3rd ed. London: Hill, 1967. This and the preceding book have been listed together because they represent the standard references in the area of taste and smell. They are relatively old books, and recent chemical research has tended to clarify some of the problems and controversies they originally presented. The interested student need not read these two volumes in their entirety. They are, however, useful reference books and do much to set the stage historically for more recent research. The interested student should at least be familiar with these two important volumes.

7. From C. G. Mueller. *Sensory Psychology.* Englewood Cliffs, N.J.: Prentice-Hall, 1965. Chapter 5, consisting of ten easy-to-read pages, is devoted entirely to taste. It examines taste qualities, adaptation and contrast, taste thresholds, and possible physiological mechanisms. One cannot present a complete description of taste in ten pages, but these come about as close to presenting the full story as any short reference available.

8. D. Wolsk. "Chemical Sensitivity," in M. Alpern, M. Lawrence and D. Wolsk, *Sensory Processes.* Belmont, Calif.: Brooks/Cole, 1967. Another fairly elementary treatment of the subject, in keeping with the coverage of this book. The 21 pages of this selection are perhaps a little more advanced than the Mueller reference, but less technical than the following reference by Pfaffman. The last ten pages of this reference are devoted to taste, and the first eleven pages are concerned primarily with olfaction.

9. C. Pfaffman. "Taste and Smell," in S. S. Stevens (ed.), *Handbook of Experimental Psychology.* New York: Wiley, 1951. These 26 pages are particularly recommended. The first 16 pages are devoted to taste, the last ten to olfaction. A must for the serious student.

20 / the skin senses

The remaining two sensory areas are, first, those related to physical events acting directly on the living tissue of the organism from the outside and, second, those resulting from forces inside the organism. For the sake of simplicity we treat these experiences in separate chapters, divided in a somewhat arbitrary manner. In this chapter we deal primarily with events originating from the outside that stimulate the organism through its skin, or outer integumental covering. The matter of internally generated stimulation is considered in the final chapter.

The mammalian integument is indeed a complex organ. In addition to keeping the animal from falling apart and flowing about like a mass of jelly, the skin serves many organic purposes. It aids in temperature regulation, it is an excretory organ, it serves a respiratory function, and it has numerous important protective functions. Of particular significance to us in this book is the functioning of the skin as a sensory organ, the specialization of protoplasm's irritability function. Perhaps more accurately, we should recognize that the skin serves as a locus for many different sensory organs and, presumably, several different modalities.

The Skin

That the skin is a very complex organ can be seen from Figure 20–1. Indeed, it is a much more complicated organ than this figure would appear to indicate. This figure shows nerve endings in the form of tactile corpuscles as well as dendritic fibers entwined about a hair follicle. There are perhaps dozens of additional primary forms and secondary modifications of nerve endings in the skin. Sensory nerve endings are found in the walls of the blood vessels and there are free nerve endings in the skin, as well as several additional specialized receptors to which various sensory experiences, such as cold or warm, have been attributed.

As can be observed from Figure 20–1, the skin can be divided into two primary layers, the outer *epidermis* and the inner *dermis*. The former can in turn be divided into an outer, dead layer, containing neither nerves nor blood vessels, and an inner, living layer (*Malpighian layer*), containing free nerve endings but no vascular supply. The dermis, on the other hand, is richly endowed with numerous nerve endings, specialized receptors, blood vessels, cutaneous glands, and so on. The dermis tends to merge, without clear lines of demarcation, into the subcutaneous tissue.

Cutaneous Receptors

Traditionally, the student of cutaneous sensitivity has spent considerable time identifying receptors in the skin and attempting to determine their roles in the experience of cutaneous sensations. Since the latter part of the nineteenth century it has been recognized that the skin is not uniformly sensitive throughout its area. If a small area is mapped by means of different types of stimuli, such as those producing warmth, cold, touch, and pain, particular loci for sensitivity to the various stimuli may be found. Most companies supplying equipment for use in psychological laboratories still include in their inventories rubber stamps to be used for transferring an inked grid to a portion of skin, thus enabling an experimenter to "map" the skin for areas sensitive to the various cutaneous stimuli. When stimuli such as a warm object, a cool or cold object, a needle (for pain), and a hair (for touch) are applied within the inked grid, punctiform loci sensitive to the various stimuli can be plotted with relative precision. Many of these spots will remain stable over long periods of testing (Gilmer, 1942).

A commonsense assumption, and one that served as a primary motivating force for such pioneers as Max von Frey, would be that there must be some sort of specialized organs in the skin with differential sensitivities to the various stimuli. With this in mind, several exceptionally well-motivated gung-ho researchers have been known to strip off pieces of their previously mapped skin, stain them appropriately, and subject them to microscopic analysis. As a result of some of this early work, there were many accounts of what end organs were sensitive to what stimuli. Unfortunately, the data were highly contradictory and did not serve to prove that *any* end organs served *any* cutaneous modalities exclusively. For example, according to some experimenters a healthy cornea is sensitive to most if not all of the cutaneous modalities, such as cold, warm, touch, and pain; yet there are no specialized end organs to be found there, only free nerve endings.

As a reaction to the specific receptor theories, which certainly do not appear to be entirely adequate, John Paul Nafe presented his pattern theory (1927; Kenshalo and Nafe, 1962). He contends that there are no receptors

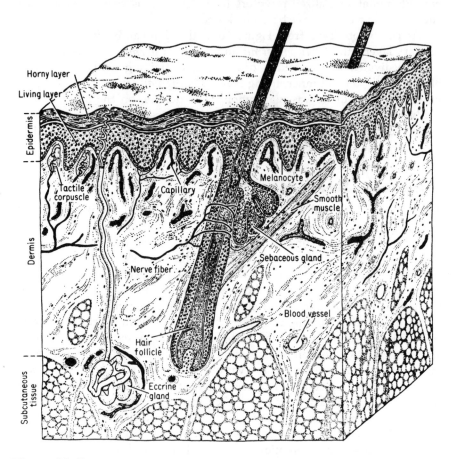

Figure 20-1
Schematic cross section of skin. (From "The Skin," W. Montagna. Copyright © 1965 by Scientific American, Inc. All rights reserved.)

or nerve fibers that carry information specific to a given stimulus and hence producing a corresponding experience. Rather, the result of cutaneous stimulation is a complex temporal and spatial pattern of impulses that, in effect, is interpreted by the brain. Thus a single fiber could mediate touch at one instance in time and pain, cold, or warmth at another. Unfortunately, the pattern theory of Nafe, although highly provocative, is not complete, for it fails to explain what happens at the receptor site.

A reconciliation of the specific receptor theory and the pattern theory of Nafe was attempted by Melzack and Wall (1962). They reject the idea of specific receptors in the manner of von Frey yet retain the idea that all endings are not alike, differing in the pattern of impulses they transmit. They contend that presynaptic terminations of the peripheral fibers selectively block or pass various aspects of the neural pattern. Finally, at the level of central nerve cells, the patterning of impulses is sensed as the appropriate *somesthetic* experience. The theory is not simple and has not yet been adequately subjected to test.

Although the assigning of a specific function to a particular structure, as suggested by von Frey, does not appear completely satisfactory, neither do the more modern pattern theories. Because there are a number of relations between structure and experience that appear to be relatively consistent, we might do well to look at them before proceeding to the psychophysical data, such as absolute thresholds, difference thresholds, and adaptation phenomena.

CUTANEOUS PAIN

Probably the most widely distributed neural receptors in the skin—indeed in the entire body—are the free nerve endings. It would be reasonable to assume that they represent more primitive stages of development than do the more specialized receptors and that they would be most useful in the preservation of the species.

It is generally agreed that free nerve endings mediate cutaneous pain. W. L. Jenkins (1951) suggests that throughout the body only free nerve endings exist in sufficient abundance to account for the almost universal presence of pain spots. Furthermore, the cornea, particularly susceptible to pain, has only free nerve endings. Some pain, as Nafe has suggested, may also rise from spastic activity of the blood vessels, but even then it is probably the free nerve endings associated with the blood vessels that, in the final analysis, actually mediate the sensation of pain.

An alternative suggestion is that pain is a unique experience resulting from specialized receptors (i.e., receptors that respond to a wide variety of harmful or injurious stimuli. Indeed, there are parts of the skin where pain appears to be the only possible sensation. In addition, pain spots seem to be more numerous than loci for touch and temperature. Table 20–1 shows the distribution of pain sensitivity for various areas of the body. Pain can often be eliminated by the application of morphine or codeine without seriously disturbing other cutaneous senses.

In light of the preceding observations, a universally accepted explanation for pain is not possible at this time. Some research, for example, has pointed to the existence of specific pain spots, so that the prick of a pin may miss a spot and thereby avoid causing pain. At the other extreme, under some conditions of *hyperalgesia,* even a light touch may result in excruciating pain. Although pain is often associated with tissue damage, it is obvious that not all tissue damage results in pain, and some pain can be produced in the absence of tissue damage. On the other hand, it is clear that increasing the intensity of an otherwise nonpainful stimulus may very well result in the experience of pain. Perhaps it is the number of sensory fibers evoked, or the rate of their discharge, that is significant for pain.

TABLE 20–1
Distribution of Pain Sensitivity
(Stimulation With a Spine-Tipped Hair)

Skin Region	"Points per cm²
Back of knee	232
Bend of elbow	224
Shoulder blade	212
Back of hand	188
Forehead	184
Buttocks	180
Eyelid	172
Scalp	144
Middle finger (radial surface)	95
Ball of thumb	60
Sole of foot	48
Tip of nose	44

From F. A. Geldard, *The Human Senses*, Copyright
© 1972. Reprinted by permission of John Wiley &
Sons, Inc.

Many experts believe there is more than one "pain," that they arise from different classes of stimuli and behave differently. According to Lewis (1942), there are two types of pain mediated by two types of fibers, one myelinated and rapid in conduction, the other unmyelinated and relatively slow. There is a commonly made distinction between "sharp" or "bright" pain and the so-called dull pain. The former tend to be well localized and are responded to promptly, unlike the latter, which are often poorly localized and may, in addition, produce more general reactions, such as sweating, vomiting, and so on. The physiological distinction between such pains is not at all clear, but may be related to fiber type.

There is also *referred* pain. Pain originating from internal organ malfunction may appear to be localized in more external regions of the body, such as the skin. As an example, the pain resulting from *angina pectoris* (a heart problem) may be experienced on the outer surface of the chest or the inner surface of the arm.

Theories of Pain. It might be well to summarize now some of the current thinking on pain. The specific receptor theory and the simple pattern theory have, in general, failed to explain the experience of pain. Of considerably more promise is the *Gate Control Theory* of Melzack and Wall (1965) and Melzack (1973). This theory, a duplex theory, posits two different kinds of nerve fibers that provide for a competitive interaction between themselves. The theory assumes that some sort of gate control system exists at the top of the spinal cord. This control system modulates or gates the nerve impulse from peripheral fibers, with pain resulting when the impulses reach some critical level. Two different types of fibers are involved: Large-diameter, myelinated fibers convey sharp pain as well as other cutaneous events, whereas small-diameter, unmyelinated, slower-conducting fibers mediate burning pain. Experience of pain is determined by the interaction of the large and small fibers. When large-fiber activity dominates, small-fiber activity is inhibited and nonpainful sensations result; when small-fiber activity dominates, pain is the result. Of course, central control mechanisms can influence the activity of the separate systems.

It has been demonstrated that bombarding the cutaneous afferent systems with nonpainful stimuli that activate the large afferent neurons can reduce severe pain. It would appear that large-fiber activity dominates small-fiber activity, thereby "closing the gate" to painful impulses. The use of electrical implants to alleviate pain is, presumably, an extreme example of artificially induced inhibition. The application of acupuncture to reduce or eliminate pain may be a further example of experimentally induced inhibitory effects, blocking the effective functioning of the small fibers.

There is also a theory that contends that injured tissue releases a substance called *neurokinin* that is the real physiological stimulus for pain. Although fluids extracted from particularly sore areas of the body have revealed the existence of chemical substances of this sort, very few investigators consider neurokinin to be a necessary accompaniment of pain. Pain can occur with or without tissue damage. Although tissue damage may once have been the only stimulus to produce pain, the process of evolution has brought us far beyond such an uncomplicated, simple state.

Pain is also a psychological experience. We can experience pain when we expect it; under conditions of extreme stress we can endure what would normally be excruciating pain; and some people can even ignore pain. It is certainly not a simple experience whose cause can be identified and measured in the same way we measure the intensity of sound. A student of the author's once expressed it this way: "Pain, we now believe, refers to a category of complex experiences, not to a single sensation produced by a specified stimulus. We are aware that in the lower part of the brain, at least, the patterns of impulses produced by painful stimuli travel over multiple pathways going to widespread regions of the brain and not along a single path going to a 'pain center.' The psychological evidence strongly supports the view of pain as a perceptual experience whose quality and intensity is influenced by the unique past history of the individual, by the meaning he gives to the pain-producing situation and by his 'state of mind' at the moment. We believe that all these factors play a role in determining the actual pattern of nerve impulses ascending to the brain and traveling within the brain itself. In this way, pain becomes a function of the whole individual, including his present thoughts and fears as well as his hopes for the future." (Colangelo, 1973)

For an interesting, highly readable discussion of how the body inhibits pain, the interested reader should see Marx (1977).

TOUCH OR PRESSURE

With touch and the perception of pressure the case for specific receptors seems to be much more defensible than was true for pain. Although the simplistic approach may not be entirely correct, it does seem to have value. Some forms of tactile sensitivity are almost certainly due to action of well-defined and well-identified structures. Let us look at several of these.

Deep Pressure. There are two types of sensitivity to touch or pressure. The basis for one of these, the relatively deep-lying sense of pressure or movement, is almost certainly attributable to deformations in the *Pacinian corpuscle*. This organ is a multilayered spherical body, about 0.02 to 0.06 in. in length, much like an onion, with alternate cellular and liquid layers and containing an unmyelinated nerve ending in its core (see Figure 21–1). It lies generally beneath the dermis in subcutaneous tissue and is found throughout the body, around muscles, in mesenteries, and so on. It is a very sensitive organ, research having shown that a movement of about 0.0001 in. is all that is necessary to evoke a response from it. (Were it not for the fact that they do appear to mediate deep pressure, as when one presses firmly against the skin, we would not have mentioned Pacinian corpuscles until the next chapter, where they really seem to be more applicable.)

In the second broad category of touch sensitivity, those experiences apparently mediated by nerve endings nearer the surface of the skin (generally in the Malpighian layer), at least three types of endings appear to be of importance.

Encapsulated Nerve Endings. There are a number of corpusclelike bodies found in the skin that have been credited with mediating tactual sensitivity; two in particular are *Meissner* corpuscles and *Merkel's* cells (see Figure 20–2). Although each of these organs, as well as such other specialized endings as *Ruffini* cylinders, *Krause* end bulbs, and *Glomus* bodies, was once thought to be structurally distinct and truly unique, some modern workers contend that they are simply different stages of development. A group at Oxford University denies there are separate capsules for different stimulus modalities (Wolsk, 1967). Jenkins (1951) further points out that there are so many intermediate forms of encapsulated endings that "any strict division into types is of dubious merit." On the other hand, it has been found that Meissner corpuscles are abundant in those parts of the body that are relatively hairless, such as the palms of the hands and soles of the feet. Conversely, on parts of the body that are richly endowed with hair, the next type of nerve endings to be discussed, *basket endings*, are found, and Meissner corpuscles are nonexistent. Circumstantial evidence points to the importance of Meissner corpuscles as mediators of tactual sensitivity.

Basket Endings. The existence of basketlike entwining of nerve endings around the hair bulbs (see Figure 20–1) help lend additional credence to the idea that Meissner corpuscles are responsible for tactual sensitivity. There can be little doubt that these fibers, entwined about the roots of the hair, signal any slight movement of the hair itself. Where hairs do not exist,

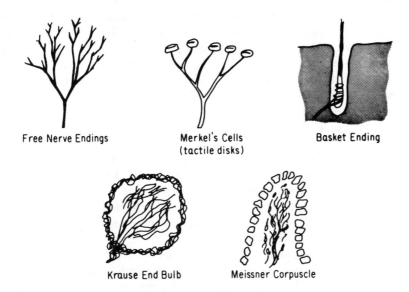

Free Nerve Endings   Merkel's Cells (tactile disks)   Basket Ending

Krause End Bulb   Meissner Corpuscle

Figure 20–2
Some representative cutaneous nerve endings.

tactual sensitivity is often still quite acute, and there and only there does one find Meissner corpuscles. Where hair exists, tactual sensitivity can be aroused by simply moving the hair, without actually touching the skin. But destroying hair root endings does not completely remove such sensitivity; moving the hair apparently also results in distorting the skin, so that other touch receptors are activated.

Free Nerve Endings. Sensitivity to touch is apparently the result, also, of a deformation gradient in the skin, particularly where hair follicles do not exist. If a finger is immersed in mercury, there is contact all over the finger, but the touch experience is only elicited at the surface of the liquid, where the pressure gradient must exist. Or if a small object is glued to the skin and alternately depressed and pulled gently, most persons cannot distinguish between the two activities. Deformation of the skin surface is clearly a necessary concomitant of touch sensitivity where hair does not exist. Probably both free nerve endings and Meissner corpuscles are involved in the sense of touch. In the cornea, for example, as indicated earlier, free nerve endings must be responsible; in other parts of the body, who can say for sure?

TEMPERATURE

Separate Receptors. Jenkins suggests that our ignorance about receptors for warm and cold is profound. The early suggestion of von Frey that Ruffini cylinders are the receptors for warmth and that Krause end bulbs serve the same function for cold has never been verified. The case for assigning cold sensitivity to Krause end bulbs has some plausibility. Often a topological relationship is found between sensory cold spots and the existence of Krause end bulbs in the skin. Areas of the body that are particularly sensitive to cold, such as the nipple, are found to be richly supplied with Krause end bulbs. Negative evidence, on the other hand, is equally abundant. Many areas of the body with excellent sensitivity to cold do not evidence Krause end bulbs. Perhaps the best that can be said is that the endings may be cold receptors in some parts of the body, but in other portions of the body some other mediational unit must be responsible for the sensation of cold.

There has never been any evidence in support of the Ruffini cylinders as receptors for warmth. To his credit, von Frey did not assign the sensation of warmth to these organs. He simply said the they *might* be responsible. Some weak evidence for the importance of Ruffini cylinders as mediators of warmth evolved about comparative depths of the various receptors and consequent time delays in sensing the nature of the stimuli. Early research had placed receptors for warmth at a greater depth than cold receptors. Hence the deeper Ruffini cylinders were indicated as receptors for warmth. But the evidence for shallow and deep temperature sensitivity is not good, both warm and cold can be sensed with a wide range of temporal delays and presumably with receptors at varying depths.

Evidence for the existence of some sort of specific receptors for warm and cold is also found as a result of stimulation with nonadequate stimuli. The jab of a fine needle or an electric shock can produce either an experience of warmth or one of cold, depending apparently on what receptor is stimulated. As early as 1883 one experimenter succeeded in producing either cold or warm experiences by means of electric shock. Various chemicals can produce the experience of either cold or warmth, further leading one to accept the existence of separate receptors for the two temperature conditions.

The existence of *paradoxical cold*, and perhaps *paradoxical warmth*, has long been recognized and often employed as evidence for separate receptors for warm and cold. Paradoxical cold can be produced by stimulating an area (or point) on the skin with a temperature on the order of 45°C (113°F), and on occasion paradoxical warmth has been achieved as a result of stimulation with temperatures lower than the normal skin temperature. The assumption might be made that there must be separate receptors for the two temperature extremes.

"Warm' 'and "Cold" Fibers. Another important approach considers the thickness of the afferent fibers to be significant. Although there does seem to be some relation between the primary modality (including pain, touch, and temperature) and the size of nerve fibers, the relationship is not at all clear, and there is considerable overlapping in size of fibers serving the different modalities. Evidence from higher levels, such as the spinal cord, does point to different fibers for pain or touch, as contrasted with temperature. But for distinguishing between warm and cold, such evidence is far from convincing.

Some fibers have been found that increase their rate of firing when temperature is increased; other fibers show an increase in firing rate with a decrease in temperature. Under conditions of high temperature, both types of fibers increase their rate of firing, producing an experience of heat. An interesting demonstration can be made that tends to support the conclusion that a sensation of heat results when both warm and cold receptors fire simultaneously. If one stimulates the forearm with an arrangement of parallel thin strips, alternately warm and cool, the experience is that of heat. Presumably some fibers increase their rate of firing as a result of the warm stimuli, whereas others increase their rate because of the cool stimuli. The result is the same as if all the fibers were stimulated by a hot stimulus.

Perhaps some of the difficulty in identifying temperature receptors may be due to the fact that warm and cold are not unitary experiences. Some writers hold that there are two forms of temperature stimulation, and hence appropriate receptor mechanisms: radiant and contact application (Hardy and Oppel, 1937). There are puzzling differences between the effects of radiant and contact stimulation, and the attempt to lump the temperature sense into only two so-called modalities may be impossible.

Vascular Theory. An interesting theory, which lacks sufficient evidence either to support or to disprove it, is the vascular theory advanced by John Paul Nafe (1938). According to this theory free nerve ending in the walls of the fine blood vessels indicate changes in the diameter of the vessels as they either dilate or constrict as a function of impinging temperature changes. This theory capitalizes on one particular fact: that the temperature sense is basically a sense of *change* in temperature. As we shall see in a later section, adaptation to temperature is quite profound and, by and large, only changes in temperature are sensed. It is an interesting theory, but not entirely defensible. If the cornea is indeed sensitive to cold, there must be some basis other than changes in capillary size in this admittedly nonvascular tissue. In addition, such phenomena as nonadequate stimulation seem to point to the existence of specific receptors (Jenkins, 1939).

Cutaneous Experience—Sensitivity

Some of the various phenomena associated with cutaneous experience are discussed in the following pages, the experience being related to the physical event wherever possible and viewed in the context of the various explanations for cutaneous sensitivity we have considered. Most of the psychophysical methods referred to earlier have been employed in studying the skin senses, and we consider, for example, absolute thresholds, difference thresholds, adaptation, and subjective scaling.

In spite of the universal problems inherent in determining absolute and differences thresholds for the cutaneous senses, including adaptation, bodily location, and even identification of the adequate stimulus, many researchers have attacked the problem, and the results have been surprisingly consistent and worth noting.

Before examining the data in more detail, we might point out that in general the cutaneous senses are much less sensitive than vision or audition. The almost infinitesimal amounts of energy required for these senses are inadequate to evoke most of the cutaneous receptors. It has been suggested that some of the skin receptors are more than a billion times less sensitive than the auditory or visual receptors.*

TOUCH

Several different experimental approaches to the study of the touch or pressure sense suggest themselves. These include the determination of absolute thresholds, the two-point threshold, and thresholds for vibration.

Absolute Threshold. Thresholds for touch are generally obtained by gently pressing against the skin with an object of known weight, and hence pressure or force. Frequently a fine bristle or hair is used to minimize areal effects and assure punctiform stimulation. By pressing with a hair of known stiffness just to the point where it begins to bend, a known force may be applied. One set of hairs, graded in stiffness and thereby permitting differing forces, in known as von Frey hairs, named after the early cutaneous experimenter already cited. A similar set may still be obtained from manufacturers of psychological laboratory equipment. Modern techniques, of course, permit much better control of pressure and rate of application of the stimuli.

Sensitivity to tactile stimuli varies with the region of the body stimulated. Table 20–2, based on the early work of von Frey, shows some typical absolute thresholds for different areas of the body. Although these values were obtained many years ago and might not agree in absolute value with data obtained by more recent, better-controlled methods, the relative differences for the various regions of the body would probably hold.

The area of surface being stimulated is an important factor. As the areal size of the stimulus is increased, the force exerted must be increased to maintain threshold. It would appear that the critical measure is the force per unit area, rather than the total force exerted. Above some maximum area, the relationship no longer holds, causing some theorists to suggest that the important factor in determining thresholds is not the vertical force applied, but the lateral tension in the cutaneous membranes that result from the vertical distortion.

Two-Point Threshold. A well-known measure of tactile acuity is the two-point threshold, which is analogous to resolving power in the visual

---

* If the reported experiments by the Russians in which persons are able to "read" with their fingertips are verified, then some change in thinking about the cutaneous receptors might be called for.

TABLE 20–2
Absolute Thresholds for Touch

Skin Region	AL, grams/mm²
Tip of tongue	2
Tip of finger	3
Back of finger	5
Front of forearm	8
Back of hand	12
Calf of leg	16
Back of forearm	33
Loin	48
Sole of foot	250

system. The two-point threshold is defined as the minimum distance between two tactile stimuli that can be reliably detected as two. A device known as an *esthesiometer* is used to measure the two-point threshold. This instrument is similar to a pair of draftsman's dividers, except that it has somewhat blunted points. The experimenter touches the two points to the subject's skin simultaneously and the subject reports whether he feels one point or two. The experimenter repeats the procedure many times, with many different separation of the points, such that, at one extreme, consistent reports of "two points," and at the opposite extreme, consistent reports of "one point" are obtained. By psychophysical methods similar to those we described for calculating difference thresholds, the experimenter can determine two-point thresholds for various regions of the body.

One might expect that sensitive areas of the body, such as the fingertips, would show small two-point thresholds as contrasted with relatively unsensitive areas such as the back or the feet. Generally speaking, this is precisely what is found. Typical two-point thresholds are given in Table 20–3.

One might suppose that the two-point threshold is determined solely by the richness of nerve endings in the skin or the number of pressure receptors available, as did von Frey. The matter does not appear to be quite that simple. Many years ago A. W. Volkman showed that changes in the two-point threshold could be obtained with practice and that improvements obtained on one forearm might be transferred to the bilateral arm. Learning apparently plays an important role, and the two-point threshold is not simply an indication of the richness of the neural supply. Perhaps touch receptors are no more plentiful in the fingertips than in the back; greater sensitivity in the fingertips may simply result from their more frequent use in touching.

Like visual acuity, the two-point tactile threshold is much more significant than as simply a sterile psychophysical measure. The Braille alphabet shown in Figure 20–3 uses the ability of the skin to discriminate and local-

TABLE 20-3
Two-Point Tactile Thresholds

Region of Skin	Threshold, mm
Middle finger	2.5
Index finger	3.0
Thumb	3.5
Upper lip	5.5
Nose	8.0
Palm	11.5
Forehead	15.0
Sole of foot	22.5
Forearm	38.5
Back	44.0
Calf	47.0

From S. Weinstein, "Intensive and Extensive Aspects of Tactile Sensitivity as a Function of Body Part, Sex, and Laterality," in D. R. Kenshalo (ed.), *The Skin Senses*, Springfield, Ill.: Charles C Thomas.

ize multiple points or raised dots on a piece of paper. An experienced reader can read as many as 50 words per minute by moving the tip of the finger over the raised surface.

A device called the Opticon has recently been developed to convert printed material into tactile form. According to Bliss (1971), users can read these tactile printouts at rates of up to 60 words per minute.

Vibration. If not a separate cutaneous sense, sensitivity to tactile vibration is certainly a highly specialized capability of the skin. Vibratory sensitivity is similar in many ways to auditory pitch sensitivity, a fact recognized by many contemporary researchers. The curve for vibratory thresholds (frequency on the abscissa and amplitude on the ordinate) looks surprisingly like the curve for auditory sensitivity (Figure 14–1), but there are several differences. First, considerably more power is required to obtain vibratory thresholds—perhaps a difference of 100,000 to 1. Second, the frequency spectrum for the vibratory sense is quite different from that for the auditory sense, being displaced in a downward direction by a factor of about 10. The 50- to 20,000-Hz auditory range corresponds roughly to a 10- to 2,000-Hz cutaneous vibration-sensitivity range, although it is said that this range can be considerably expanded if sufficiently intense signals are employed. Furthermore, the point of maximum sensitivity for the auditory sense, of about 2,000 Hz, corresponds to a point of maximum sensitivity for the vibratory sense of about 200 Hz. At this point of maximum sensitivity a movement of the skin on the order of 0.001 mm can be sensed. Contrast this with minimum detectable movements of the ear drum of

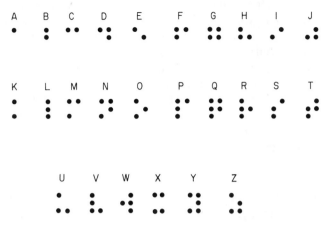

Figure 20–3
The Braille alphabet.

0.00000001 mm, and movements of one hundredth of this value at the basilar membrane!

There appear to be other parallels between the skin's sensitivity to vibration and the basilar membrane's response to acoustic stimuli. The matter of sharpening or funneling, which we referred to in a previous chapter, seems to play a role in the cutaneous vibratory sense too. Might not the skin be used as an auditory organ? Actually, attempts have been made to do just that. By reducing frequencies by a factor of 10 and activating a tactual vibrator against the skin of the forearm, some experimenters have succeeded in "teaching" subjects to recognize quite a few of the many vocal sounds or phonemes.

In a somewhat different approach, aimed at providing the deaf with a communication code of their own, Geldard (1960, 1966) attached vibrators to the skin, employing a code made up of three intensity levels and three durations (0.1, 0.3, and 0.5 seconds). Utilizing five separate locations on the chest, a total of 45 different signals was possible. Geldard reported that his *Vibratese* alphabet could be mastered in a few hours. One skilled subject was able to receive signals at the rate of about 36 words per minute. A still more recent technique utilizes the *Optohapt* system, which scans printed material and converts it into tactile stimuli that in effect write on the skin (Geldard, 1968).

A still more imaginative system to enable the blind to "see" pictorial material via the skin has been developed. White et al. (1970) developed a system employing a bank of 400 vibrators in a 29 × 20 matrix 25 cm square mounted on the back of a chair. A video camera views a scene and activates appropriate groups of vibrators, which in effect draw the visual scene on the subject's back by tactile vibratory stimulation. The system seems successful. With minimum training subjects have been able to "see" simple geometric figures, and with sufficient experience, such articles as a coffee cup, telephone, and so on, have been identified. It appears that even some three-dimensionality can be sensed by the more experienced subjects.

Craig (1977) reports on two extraordinary observers who could read up to 90 words per minute using an *Opticon*. This device, designed as a reading aid for the blind and currently in use by about 2,000 blind people, employs a "reading camera" to activate a 24 × 6 array of tactile pins (Bliss et al., 1974). An observer senses patterned vibrations with a fingertip. Usually a reading rate of 30 to 60 words per minute is achieved.

PAIN

As suggested earlier, pain is a very difficult experience to examine by conventional psychophysical methods. There are different kinds of pain; for example, both "sharp" and "dull" pain may be experienced as a result of the same stimulus. There is referred pain, and perhaps itching is a form of pain; it certainly has a warning function. As described earlier, pain can be inhibited, or, at the other extreme, it can exist with little or no observable cause.

Nevertheless, attempts have been made to examine the psychophysics of pain. Thresholds for pain can be determined in much the same manner as was done for the determination of touch or pressure thresholds, except that in this case a pain-producing stimulus must be used, and if we are to believe the earlier workers in the field, specific pain "spots" must be located.

Absolute Thresholds. To produce the data found in Table 20–4, von Frey used a very sharp needle to locate and measure sensitivity to point "spots." Note the extreme variability in sensitivity to pain, a range of 1,500 to 1, as contrasted with a range of 125 to 1 in pressure or touch thresholds, determined by the same man and described in Table 20–2.

One might note the marked differences between this table and that presented earlier for touch sensitivity. Notice in particular the difference in

TABLE 20–4
Threshold for Pain

Skin Region	AL for pain, grams/mm^2
Cornea	0.2
Conjunctiva	2.
Abdomen	15.
Front of forearm	20.
Back of forearm	30.
Back of hand	100.
Sole of foot	200.
Fingertip	300.

sensitivity for touch and pain in the fingertips. The fingertips seems to be quite sensitive to touch but relatively insensitive to pain. The soles of the feet, on the other hand, are relatively insensitive to both types of stimuli.

Difference Thresholds. In spite of the difficulty in even specifying the stimulus, numerous attempts have been made to determine difference thresholds for pain. Possibly the most successful of these attempts was first reported by Hardy, Wolff, and Goodell (1948), who used radiant heat as the pain-producing stimulus. They were able to employ nine values of heat intensity, ranging from one that barely evoked threshold pain to the most intense stimulus, just below a level that would blister the skin. These investigators proposed a scale of pain, based on the *dol*,* where 1 dol is a unit of painfulness equal in size to 2 jnd's in pain intensity. By subjecting 73 subjects to a stimulus of 8 dols (16 jnd's above threshold) and utilizing a fractionation method of scaling, the authors felt that they had developed a truly subjective scale of pain intensity, linearly related to sensed painfulness.

TEMPERATURE

An absolute threshold for sensing temperature is probably a meaningless concept, because changes in temperature are sensed, not absolute values. All temperatures experiences are experiences of differences, rather than absolute values. As contrasted with absolute judgments of pitch, sweetness, or weight, absolute judgments of temperature are virtually impossible. Because of the efficiency of visual adaptation, one cannot make absolute judgments of light intensity; possibly for similar reasons, one cannot make absolute judgments of temperature. For light, however, there is a true zero; with temperature, the concept of no temperature is completely alien to our experience. All temperatures exist only to the extent that they differ from our basic, underlying, physiological reference point. Hence temperature experience is essentially a function of difference, rather than absolute thresholds.

The ability to detect changes in temperature is apparently the result of several factors and varies widely according to the method used to investigate it. Wolsk, for example, suggests that we are able to detect changes in temperature as slight as 0.01° per second. This speed, incidentally, is one piece of evidence militating against Nafe's vascular theory. It is unlikely that the smooth muscle-mediated changes in capillary size could be rapid enough to account for such prompt recognition of temperature changes.

At the opposite extreme, adaptation effects, over broad areas of skin, are such that changes at a relatively rapid rate often cannot be detected. Gertz found that changes of about 0.2°C per minute were threshold, quite a difference from the previously cited 0.01° per second. With changes at the rate of roughly 10° over a period of thirty-five to forty-five minutes, no change in experienced temperature could be detected by Gertz's subjects. The

---

* The word *dol* is derived from the Latin word *dolar*, meaning "pain" or "grief."

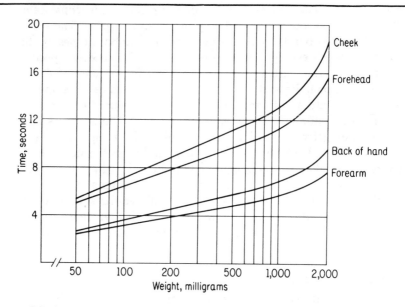

Figure 20–4
Tactile adaptation times for different body areas. [Data from M. J. Zigler, *Amer J. Psychol.* 44 (1932).]

matter is quite complex, and we still have much to learn about temperature sensitivity.

Cutaneous Experience–Adaptation

In light of our frequent references to difficulties in determining psychophysical measures because of adaptation effects, it might be well to consider adaptation for the cutaneous senses in more detail.

TOUCH

In touch, adaptation is very pronounced, even complete, over a relatively short period of time. Note how quickly you become oblivious to your clothing in contact with your skin. The time required for such complete adaptation is a function of the particular individual, as well as the pressure of the stimulus, the area of skin involved, and the particular location on the body. Figure 20–4 shows mean times for eight subjects required for complete adaptation to different pressures on several body locations. In this experiment a weight, shown on the abscissa, was lowered gently to the skin and allowed to rest there until the subject reported that it could no longer be felt. This then is the time for total adaptation (Zigler, 1932).

Another approach to tactile adaptation involves a matching procedure,

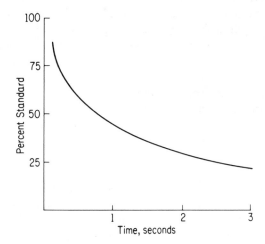

Figure 20-5
Course of pressure adaptation. [After M. von Frey and A. Goldman, *Z. Biol.* 65 (1915).]

and, in a sense, evaluates the pressure sensation. In one experiment, a stimulus of known weight was applied for four seconds to a point on the forearm. A nearby area was simultaneously stimulated periodically with weights of varying size to determine subjective equality. As can be seen from Figure 20–5, after three seconds a weight of only 20 percent as great was judged equal to the standard. In other words, the pressure experience had declined to only 20 percent of its original sensory magnitude in a mere three seconds.

It is unlikely that any explanation for tactile adaptation in the manner of that suggested for the chemical senses and for vision is either warranted or needed. The sense of touch is a sense of movement or change; it is produced by externally induced movements—compression, bending, shearing, in sensitive receptor endings. When the movement ceases, the stimulation ceases. The short adaptation times that do exist may reflect mechanical adaptation of the skin and underlying tissues as they readjust to the original deformation. Such a description accounts for the advantage of "active" touch over "passive" touch. If you wish to feel the texture of something you slide your fingers over it, producing a series of changes, of tactual experience. Sandpaper feels like sandpaper only if the fingers "scan" it. Note too that the reader of Braille must move his fingertips over the raised characters if he is to perceive them properly.

PAIN

The reader might question whether there is true adaptation to pain. Evidence indicates that adaptation to pain does indeed exist, and can be, like adaptation to touch, complete. But it seems to take longer. In one study, involving pain produced by inserting needles in the forearm, as long as five minutes were required for complete disappearance of the pain. For shallower insertions of the needle (2.5- to 25-g pressure) adaptation times on the order of one and one-half minutes or less were found.

The longer adaptation times commonly reported in the case of pain provide additional evidence for the theory that pain is in some way associated with damage-producing stimuli and is possibly mediated by receptors other than those mediating pressure or touch. Pain appears to be more than just rapid, intense firing of conventional tactile fibers.

TEMPERATURE

No one need be apprised of the existence of temperature adaptation. Stepping into a tub of water can result in a rude awakening if one has been adapted to a noticabley different air temperature. At the other extreme, with gradual adaptation, one can actually hold his hand in water so hot as to damage the tissue. Probably some cases of severe sunburn may be due to an unawareness of the temperature adaptation taking place.

A very great number of studies on temperature adaptation have been published in the scientific literature. Some of these bear on the extent to which complete adaptation can take place—that is, the extent to which a cold or hot stimulus may, with time, achieve a neutral apparent temperature. The human cannot adapt completely to as wide a range of temperatures as can the frog in the hot water we referred to earlier (if the whole matter is not simply an old wive's tale). At extreme temperatures, adaptation to a point of neutrality simply does not occur. If you place your hand in boiling water it will not reach an experience of neutral temperature, at least not before it is severely damaged. Yet for a rather wide but restricted range of temperatures on either side of the normal skin temperature, complete adaptation can occur.

The time required to adapt completely to various temperatures depends on how far away the adapting temperature is from the normal skin temperature. Figure 20–6, based on studies of Hensel (1950), show times required for adaptation to various temperatures indicated on the abscissa. These data are based on a single resting skin temperature, represent only one form and size of stimulating device, and are for only one body location. They are, however, fairly representative and serve to show the general trend. Note that an increase of 5° requires about ten minutes for complete adaptation, whereas a decrease of the same amount adapts in only five minutes.

Another approach to temperature adaptation is to study the course of the adaptation and involves the stimulation of different skin areas. We might adapt both hands to the same level by immersing them in water of a known temperature—for example, 38°C (100°F). At the end of the pre-adaptation we immerse the left hand in water of a different temperature,

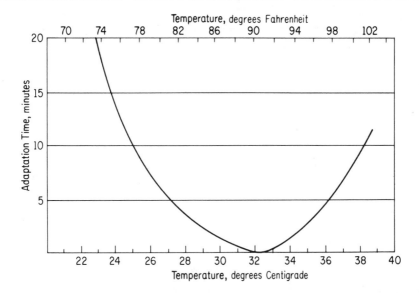

Figure 20-6

Adaptation to different temperatures. See text for explanation. (Smoothed curve
based on data from H. Henset, "Physiologie der Thermoreception," Ergebmisse der
Physiologie, Biologischen Chemie und Experimentellen Pharmakologie, 1952, 47,
166–368.)

such as 26°C (79°F). At regular intervals following this new adaptation of
the left hand, we present test stimuli to the right hand and ask the subject
to report whether the test temperatures are warmer, colder, or equal to the
temperature of the left hand, still being adapted to the new level. As can
be seen from Figure 20–7, at time 0, the right hand requires a 26° stimulus
to achieve equality with the left hand's 26° adaptation stimulus. (Both had
been adapted to the same temperature immediately before.) After about
one minute a temperature of 34°C (93°F) applied to the right hand feels
equal to the 26° of stimulation of the left hand. By four minutes, adaptation is complete, and a 38° stimulus feels the same temperature to both
hands. What has apparently happened is that both hands have, in four
minutes, achieved a physiological zero, such that the 26° stimulus to one
hand feels the same as a 38° stimulus to the other.

Experiments like these show the possible range of temperature adaptation, and time for adaptation, and disclose many critical variables, such as
the size of the stimulated area and its location. What apparently is happen-
ing in all these instances of temperature adaptation is a distortion, either
moderate or profound, of the underlying sensory scale. The manner in
which such distortions take place is a problem we cannot answer at this
time.

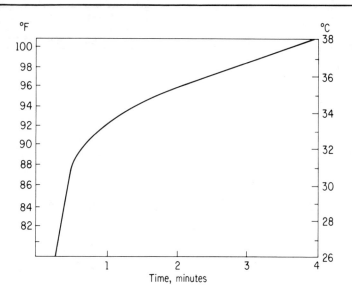

Figure 20–7
Course of temperature adaptation. [Smoothed curve based on data from H. Hahn,
Z. Sinnesphysiol. 60 (1930).]

Summary

In this chapter we tried to cast light on a subject of which surprisingly
little is known with certainty. We first examined the nature of the cutaneous receptors, describing several possible receptors for pain, touch, and
temperature experiences. We referred to such possible receptors as free
nerve endings, basket endings, and the encapsulated endings, such as
Krause end bulbs, Ruffini cylinders, Meissner corpuscles, Pacinian corpuscles, and Merkel's cells. Evidence available to attribute particular cutaneous experience was considered and evaluated. We examined the available
knowledge on the psychophysics of cutaneous experience, absolute and
difference thresholds, including the important two-point threshold for tactile experience. We touched on the application of vibratory stimulation for
communication purposes. We examined in some detail the phenomenon of
cutaneous adaptation, describing adaptation for touch, pain, and temperature. We closed the chapter with the some note of uncertainty with which
we began it, recognizing that our ignorance of the skin senses is indeed
profound.

Suggested Readings

1. W. Montagna. "The Skin," *Scientific American* 212 (1965), 56–66. These ten
   pages are relatively easy reading, covering such topics as a little anatomy, the
   nature and function of hair, finger prints, and sweat glands. The article is not

particularly germane to the subject of sensory processes of the skin, but does provide considerable background on the skin from a general point of view. Not must reading, but certainly an interesting addition to the information provided in this chapter.

2. H. H. Donaldson. "On the Temperature-Sense," in W. Dennis (ed.), *Readings in the History of Psychology*. New York: Appleton, 1948. This selection is not must reading either. It does, however, present an interesting historical perspective. The nine pages are not especially difficult to read, considering the publication date of 1885, and the serious student may find the endeavor rewarding.

3. W. L. Jenkins. "Somesthesis," in S. S. Stevens (ed.), *Handbook of Experimental Psychology*. New York: Wiley, 1951. Pages 1172 to 1185 are of particular value to the student interested in cutaneous sensitivity. This reference should be familiar to the serious student.

4. From R. S. Woodworth and H. Schlosberg. *Experimental Psychology*, rev. ed. New York: Holt, 1954. Chapter 10, "The Cutaneous Senses," provides in 30 pages one of the best short accounts of the cutaneous senses. It is very well referenced and covers in greater detail just about all the topics referred to in the preceding chapter. Its bibliography is excellent, though somewhat old. A very important reference for the interested student.

5. From C. G. Mueller. *Sensory Psychology*. Englewood Cliffs, N.J.: Prentice-Hall, 1965. Chapter 7 of this previously suggested book is a good, short (16-page) summary of current information on touch and temperature sensitivity. It is recommended as rather easy reading, interesting, and informative.

6. From S. H. Bartley. *Principles of Perception*, 2d ed. New York: Harper & Row, 1969. Chapter 12, "The Senses of the Skin," provides a detailed description of much of the material covered in this chapter. Its 35 pages are well worth reading, and provide a wealth of detailed information beyond that which we have just covered. This reference is highly recommended for the interested student.

7. E. R. Kenshalo (ed.). *The Skin Senses*. Springfield, Ill.: Thomas, 1968. This is a relatively complete collection of works on the cutaneous senses and should be consulted by any student who is serious about learning more about this difficult area.

8. From H. R. Schiffman. *Sensation and Perception: An Integrated Approach*. New York: Wiley, 1976. Chapter 7, "Somesthesis I: Kinesthesis and Cutaneous Sense," and chap. 8, "Somesthesis II: Temperature and Pain," are both quite applicable to the material covered in this chapter. These two chapters should be consulted to elaborate on our relatively restricted presentation.

9. Ronald T. Verrillo. "Cutaneous Sensation," in Bertram Scharf (ed.). *Experimental Sensory Psychology*. Glenview, Ill.: Scott, Foresman, 1975. This is also a fine reading that is highly recommended. It is fairly easy to read but is loaded with valuable information.

10. From Edward C. Carterette and Morton P. Friedman (eds.). *Handbook of Perception*, vol. III, *Biology of Perceptual Systems*. New York: Academic Press, 1973. Chapter 11, "Cutaneous Mechanoreceptors," by Burgess; chap. 12, "Tactual Perception of Texture," by Taylor et al.; and chap. 15, "Temperature Reception," by Hensel all provide valuable reading for the interested

student. These are not introductory presentations, but they should prove of value to the advanced student.

11. From Walter A. Rosenblith (ed.). *Sensory Communication.* New York: Wiley, 1962. Chapters in this book by Geldard, Wall, and Rosner are particularly appropriate to our chapter on the cutaneous senses. Again, not the easiest reading in the world, but worth the effort.

12. Solomon H. Snyder. "Opiate Receptors and Internal Opiates," *Scientific American*, March 1977. This is a fine, detailed article on the effects of opiates on pain reduction. It is a rather technical and advanced article, perhaps too advanced for the average undergraduate, but worth looking into. It is equally appropriate for the following chapter.

21 / organic and internal senses

For this, the last chapter of our description of the senses, we have reserved discussion of more actual sensory receptors than were considered in all the previous chapters combined. There are probably more individual receptors and sensory nerve endings under the heading of this chapter than the entire total of receptors involved in all the preceding chapters.

Sensory nerve endings and/or specialized receptors are to be found in virtually every organ of the body—from tiny blood vessels to the heart, from large muscles to deep centers of the brain. Indeed, many sense organs have other sense organs in them. The muscles inside the eye have sensory nerve endings that presumably indicate the state of the muscles for accommodation and pupillary adjustment. Many of the responses from such sensory entities do not reach a level of consciousness, but they are still part and parcel of our vast sensory system.

But we are not devoting a corresponding amount of space to the receptors for such a vast range of stimuli and of such importance. There are several reasons for this; for one thing, many of them are "silent" systems—they do not provide an output that involves our conscious experience, except in some cases where the absence of some "normal" experience is observable. For the most part they are probably conspicuous only by their absence. We walk about, sit, stand, and perform countless skeletal muscular actions without ever realizing the importance of the steady flow of impulses from sensory cells in our joints or muscles, and from our *vestibular* (inner-ear) apparatus. Outputs from delicate sensory endings in the brain maintain a continuous equilibrium in animate processes. The level of oxygen in the blood, sugar level, respiration, and pulse rate are all conditions that are self-adjusting, and by virtue of internal receptors cooperate to maintain the condition known as *homeostasis*. Only when the departure from normal is extreme do we even become aware of such things as low blood sugar or oxygen deficiency. Then it is probably secondary results of such imbalances that produce the awareness, rather than activity of the primary, organic sense organs.

A second reason for not devoting more space to the internal senses is that we actually know much too little about them. Much of what we do "know" is based on supposition and secondary or circumstantial evidence. Direct experimentation with such inaccessible and difficult to identify organs is indeed difficult.

To simplify our discussion and to bring a little order to a confusing situation, it might be well to divide the internal senses into perhaps four rather arbitrary categories. We will discuss in order first the deep pressure or subcutaneous sense referred to in the previous chapter; second, the *proprioceptive* sense, involving movement and positioning of the body and limbs; third, the visceral-organic senses; and last, the highly specialized vestibular sense, located in the inner ear.

Subcutaneous Senses

The two principal experiences provided by receptors lying in tissue beneath the skin would appear to be those of pressure and pain. The latter is probably mediated by free nerve endings, but as was the case with cutaneous pain, our lack of specific knowledge is indeed vast.

Large end organs known as Pacinian corpuscles are believed to mediate deep pressure (see Figure 21–1). This receptor organ has been studied quite thoroughly. As mentioned in the preceding chapter, its rather large, laminated, onionlike body has been excised and shown to respond to pressure, movements as small as 0.0001 in. being sufficient to produce a discharge in its axial nerve fiber (Lowenstein, 1960). Located in mesenteries and in tissue around muscles, as well as in subcutaneous tissue, this organ is most surely involved in pressure sensitivity. It is one of the few receptors concerning whose function we can be reasonably certain.

Proprioception

Two of the three examples of subcutaneous nerve endings shown in Figure 21–1 are most certainly involved in proprioception, the sense of movement and bodily position. Although much of our awareness of bodily position is mediated by the semicircular canals of the *vestibular body*, which are often included in the proprioceptor domain, we reserve consideration of that organ until a later section. In the meantime, we will survey the other possible receptors or nerve endings that help us to remain aware of the position of our body and limbs.

ROLE OF VISION

In addition to the proprioceptive senses and their associated neural structures to be considered in this section, vision plays a very important

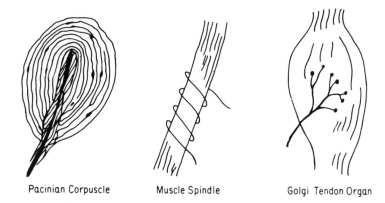

| Pacinian Corpuscle | Muscle Spindle | Golgi Tendon Organ |

Figure 21-1
Some subcutaneous nerve endings involved in proprioception.

role in maintaining bodily position. The association, at a neurological level, between vision and the vestibular mechanism must be quite intimate, as evidenced by nystagmic movements of the eyes, possible nausea, and other symptoms that may be produced when conflict exists between the visual experience and those of the vestibular and proprioceptive systems.

TACTILE RECEPTORS

Although they are not too often emphasized, the tactile and stretch receptors of our skin play an important role in proprioception. Bending an arm results in tightening the skin on one side and relaxation or compression on the other side. Surely such sensations arising from the skin must aid us in knowing which joints are being flexed and which are being extended.

KINESTHESIS

Notice that most proprioceptive experiences are also *kinesthetic* experiences. They are the result of movement, of change. Without continuous movement of some sort we would be unable to know for long just how our bodies are oriented. It is actually possible, as when flying an airplane or a trainer, to be upside-down for some time and not know it. Even the sensed internal strains and altered blood-pressure relationships may be adapted to, and unless there are suprathreshold changes in position one may in effect not know which end is up.

Several different receptors for kinesthesis, or the sense of movement, have been identified. Endings associated with muscles are most certainly of significance. As can be seen from Figure 20-1, free nerve endings (*muscle spindles*) are found wrapped around small bundles of muscle fibers. These sensory endings appear to be stretch fibers, ostensibly firing when the muscle is extended, not when it contracts. Thus the response from a given muscle arises only when the antagonistic muscle contracts, thereby stretching the former.

The *Golgi tendon ending,* on the other hand, appears to respond when the muscle contracts. In the form of spirals around the end of a tendon where it attaches to a muscle, the Golgi endings seem to complement the muscle spindles. Thus afferent impulses from a single muscle can disclose whether the muscle is contracting, stretching, or, in the absence of any clear signal, remaining at rest.

Although the existence of receptors at the joints is still a matter of conjecture, a mounting consensus holds that spray-type endings in the capsules of the joints play an important role. According to Boyd and Roberts (1953), each spray-type receptor covers a 15° to 30° range of movement and provides a beautifully simple coding of body posture. Although it is not entirely clear how they do it, there is evidence that *spray-type* endings in the joint are able to indicate static position of the joints, rather than simply movement, as appears to hold for the muscle and tendon receptors.

Pacinian corpuscles, previously referred to as receptors for deep pressure, probably play a role in kinesthesis. Located often in the *fascia* (sheaths) of muscles, these receptors must be activated as a result of pressure variations set up by movements of limbs and other muscular activity.

LOCOMOTOR ATAXIA

A classic example of what may happen when proprioceptive functioning is impaired can be seen in the disorder *locomotor ataxia.* As described in Chapter 1, this disease was so named because it appears that the shuffling or foot-slapping gait of the victim is the result of problems in the motor or musculature system. The patient does not appear to have adequate control of his legs and feet. In truth, the trouble is sensory rather than motor. Usually it is the result of a syphilitic infection of the *dorsal horn* of the spinal cord, that part of the cord containing afferent fibers leading from the sense organs of the limbs to the central nervous system. When the ascending tracts are destroyed (*tabes dorsalis*), impulses from proprioceptors in the joints and muscles of the extremities can no longer reach the brain. Hence the victim must look at his feet to see exactly where they are, and with the uncertainty he has, he either shuffles carefully or slaps his feet firmly against the ground to maximize any feedback cues that may be produced.

PROPRIOCEPTIVE EXPERIENCE

The bellwether of the senses for psychophysical study was that of proprioception. Some of the earliest studies were done, for example, with lifted weights; experiments wherein judgments of weight were made on the basis of conscious experiences arising from proprioceptive sensitivities. Even today, practically all psychological supply houses list sets of calibrated weights so that any student can replicate the psychophysical studies of

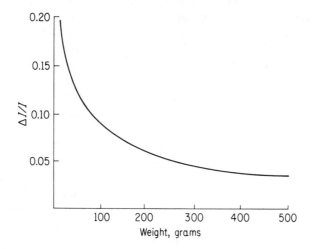

Figure 21–2
Hypothetical difference threshold function for lifted weights.

Weber and his followers and come up with difference threshold curves such as those shown in Figure 21–2.

Current interest in the proprioceptive and kinesthetic senses often concerns the ability of people to make specific movements with known time durations and levels of accuracy. For example, "blind positioning" movements, so necessary for the operation of many complex equipments, may be studied. The science of human engineering studies the variables that determine how well a person can set a control or track a moving target, all as a function of his proprioceptive feedback. Repetitive movements, also based on adequacy of proprioceptive feedback, are a further subject of study.

Visceral Senses

Because of difficulties in experimentation, not too much is known concerning the sensitivity of the internal parts of the body. Conventional touch sensitivity, as one might guess, appears to be lacking throughout most of the internal organs. It is also unlikely that many internal organs contain receptors for temperature, at least very few that effect conscious experience. Both the esophagus and stomach, however, are said to have temperature sensitivity, but no sensitivity to light touch (Boring 1915a and b). On the other hand, both must have something like deep pressure or strain sensitivity, since moderate distention produces an experience different from simple touch or conventional pain. With extreme distention, of course, an unquestionable experience of pain may result.

The general existence, or lack thereof, of visceral pain presents additional problems. Most solid organs such as the kidneys and liver are insensitive to painful stimuli. They can be cut, burned, and crushed without producing pain. The brain itself is presumably devoid of pain receptors, as is the heart muscle. Pain receptors are plentiful, however, in the mesenteries, connective tissues, and body walls. The peritoneum is quite sensitive to pain from stretching. "Gas on the stomach" produces pain, but undoubtedly not so much from the intestines themselves as from the mesenteries and abdominal walls which take the brunt of the spasmodic stretching and "thrashing about." It is these structures, not the visceral organs themselves, which appear to contain the free nerve ending which mediate pain.

An interesting aspect of visceral pain is the matter of referred pain, mentioned in the preceding chapter. Pain arising from specific internal disturbances is often referred (localized) to other, more external and hence accessible portions of the body. Attacks of *angina pectoris* often leave a tenderness in the skin on the left side of the chest (Lewis, 1942). Frequently following the segmented arrangement of the spinal nerves, such localizations can often be used to pinpoint an internal problem and facilitate diagnosis.

There are numerous additional complex experiences arising from within our bodies that might be called senses. Is hunger a sense? Is nausea a sense? What about such difficult to describe experiences as those associated with suffocation, sexual arousal, fear, and the like? The best that can be said is that such experiences are simply recognition, at a conscious level, of patterns of basic underlying sensory responses of the type we have been describing. Perhaps they are more than this; no one knows for sure.

Most of our internal receptors never produce a response that evokes a conscious experience. Receptors that maintain our internal homeostasis and regulate such variables as body temperature, calcium metabolism, water intake, or excretion rarely fall within the domain of sensory psychology.

Most of these internal receptors are either mechanoreceptors (stretch, pressure) or chemoreceptors and are deeply involved with low-level organismic processes of the central nervous system. For example, cells have been found in the hypothalamus highly sensitive to temperature change (Nakayama et al., 1961), and most certainly the presence or absence in the blood of such substances as calcium, oxygen, and carbon dioxide must excite to action specific receptors. Many internal receptors must be considered as part of the endocrine system, contributing to the constant give-and-take that is life, and whose absence would mean the ultimate in homeostasis, death.

Such sensory processes as these are certainly critical for our survival. But they are not a part of our sensory experience, hence not a suitable subject for inclusion in this book. With that one statement we can write off as inappropriate a sensory system, far more extensive than the total of all those previously considered.

Vestibular Sense

The "sense of balance" is mediated largely by a remarkable organ, located deep in the bone of the skull, and identified as a part of the inner ear. The entire inner ear, as indicated in Chapter 13, is known as the *labyrinth* and consists of two major divisions, the *cochlear* apparatus, responsible for audition, and the *vestibular* apparatus of importance for balance and equilibrium (see Figure 21–3). We will briefly examine the anatomy of this vestibular apparatus before considering some of the ramifications of its functioning.

ANATOMY OF VESTIBULAR APPARATUS

The vestibular apparatus consists of three *semicircular canals* and the so-called *otolith organs*, the *utricle* or *utriculus*, and the *saccule* or *sacculus*, along with assorted blood vessels and a generous nerve supply. The three semicircular canals lie roughly one in each of the three possible physical planes. As a result, turning the head in any direction will, by centrifugal force, set the fluid in motion in at least one of the three canals. Thus an awareness of which canal is involved in the movement, and in which direction the fluid is moving, will serve to indicate changes in the position of the head.

The semicircular canals are continuous at their bases with the utricle (sometimes called the *vestibular organ*), from which they arise, and the saccule, which is joined to the utricle by a short duct. All three canals and the two chambers are filled with endolymph, the same primitive and nutritive fluid referred to earlier as occupying the cochlear or endotic duct of the cochlear canal.

Receptors for the semicircular canals are found in the three *ampullae*, thickened bulges at the base of each canal. Each ampulla contains many ciliated receptor cells (hair cells) that respond in a manner, as yet not clear, to movement of the fluid therein. It is generally presumed that a gelatinous mass, the *cupula*, has enough inertia to act like a swinging door in the ampulla, thereby stimulating the sensitive hair cells.

The utricle and saccule seem to have a function somewhat different from that of the semicircular canals. They appear to be more responsive to movement and vibration than do the positional-directional sensitive ampullae of the semicircular canals. The utricle appears to be sensitive to linear rather than rotational movement, and also to gravity. The function of the saccule is not entirely clear, and in fish it is believed by some to still be a vibratory (sound?) receptor.

The vestibular organs contain an *otolithic membrane* lying over the hair cells that is free to move about somewhat as a function of gravity. Such movement stimulates the hair cells, especially as a result of linear movement of the head. Both the utricle and saccule also contain tiny calcareous crystals, up to 14 μ in diameter in mammals, called *otoliths*. As-

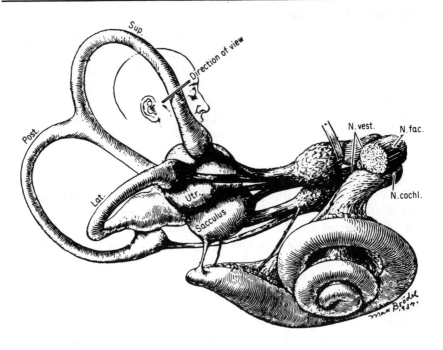

Figure 21–3
Vestibular and cochlear organs. [From M. Hardy, *Anat. Rec.* 59 (1934).]

sociated with the otolithic membrane, these little stones are perhaps able to move about in the viscous endolymph and presumably elicit responses from delicate hair cells attached to the walls of the chambers. Thus the semicircular canals provide a primary response to rotation, and the utricle and saccule indicate linear movement.

Nerve fibers from the delicate hair cells combine and leave the labyrinth by way of the vestibular portion of the VIIIth cranial nerve. One major branch arises from each of the three ampullae, one branch comes from the utricle, two from the saccule, and a seventh (Oort's nerve) from the cochlea. The vestibular fibers number about 19,000 and make up roughly half of the VIIIth nerve, the other half being auditory fibers from the basilar membrane of the cochlea.

BALANCE AND EQUILIBRIUM

The vestibular apparatus is of extreme importance in maintaining balance and equilibrium. The ability of a cat to right itself in midair upon being dropped is a function of the reflexive vestibular reaction alone. Even in complete darkness a cat will succeed in righting itself unless the vestibular organs have been destroyed, in which case it will land in a heap, with no attention to top or bottom.

Over 130 years ago Flourens showed that a bird with damage to just one of the three canals will not fly voluntarily; if forced to fly, its behavior is crude and uncoordinated and it quickly descends. The removal of all three canals on one side leaves an animal unable even to maintain a standing position.

In the normal adult human, much of the balance-equilibrium function is also a result of vision and the numerous proprioceptive and kinesthetic impulses constantly bombarding the brain. With a poorly performing vestibular apparatus, one can survive, but closing the eyes can result in loss of balance and general disorientation. For immediate, automatic, reflexive awareness of bodily position, the inner-ear-mechanism is essential. In addition, damage to the inner ear, or disorders resulting from serious infections, can produce nausea, extreme dizziness, and even changes in heartbeat and blood pressure.

EYE MOVEMENTS

Reflexive relationships between the vestibular apparatus and the positioning of the eyes have been well established, although not worked out in complete detail. As a result of feedback from the vestibular apparatus, as well as proprioceptive and visual stimuli, eye movements to maintain fixation tend to be quite automatic and comparatively effortless. Such involuntary movements often result in a phenomenon called *nystagmus*, reflexive eye movements, generally in the horizontal plane.

One method of studying nystagmus is to rotate a blindfolded subject in a chair at a constant speed. When the rotation is stopped, horizontal eye movements may be observed. A primary nystagmus may be observed, followed by a long-lasting secondary nystagmus in the opposite direction. There are usually slow sweeping movements followed by rapid, saccadic-like movements, the cycle repeating itself perhaps many times, depending on the original angular velocity and duration. Nystagmus apparently results from the involuntary, reflexive adjustments arising from the interaction of the various "senses" of motion and position. The eyes make an adjustment; having overadjusted, they return but then overadjust in the opposite direction until finally a point of neutral or balanced enervation is reached.

The association between nystagmus and such organismic symptoms as dizziness and nausea is certainly recognized, although the cause-and-effect relations are not always evident. It is said that performers who must spin rapidly on their vertical axes, such as ice skaters and dancers, thus causing the visual scene to rotate rapidly about them, have a unique way of preventing the ill effects of nystagmus. They allegedly fixate, for an instant, a stationary object as they spin past it, allowing one fixation per revolution, thus avoiding the rotary pursuit movements of the eye which, if not eliminated, apparently contribute to nystagmus and, in many cases subsequent dizziness.

Many persons have studied nystagmus in considerable detail and the matter is much too complex and controversial to be treated in depth here. The interested reader is encouraged to read the Wendt reference and the pertinent bibliographical entries at the end of it.

MOTION SICKNESS

Motion sickness is an interesting, albeit unpleasant phenomenon arising largely from activity of the vestibular apparatus. Producing nausea, headache, sweating, and feelings of muscular weakness, the disorder may persist after termination of the motion and last in some cases for several days. In general, slow, vertical movements and movements in several planes at once are most effective in producing motion sickness. There also is a psychological factor, both of expectation, which may enhance the effect, and habituation, which may ultimately result in its nonexistence. Visual activity also plays a role in motion sickness, as might be expected, because the relation between the vestibular apparatus and reflexive eye movements is so intimate. That motion sickness is largely a result of vestibular activity is evidenced by the fact that some deaf individuals who lack vestibular sensitivity do not become motion sick.

RESULTS OF VESTIBULAR DAMAGE

Surgical removal of the entire labyrinth or cutting of the VIIIth nerve may or may not produce profound effects. In lower animals the effects seem to be much more serious than in man. Bilateral destruction in the case of the pigeon results in violent movements and an inability to maintain an upright posture. After several days some recovery occurs, probably through use of proprioceptors and visual senses. Although it can still stand and walk, albeit unsteadily, the animal does not fly or even feed itself.

The effects in mammals are much less striking. Unsteadiness in standing, head tremors, and impaired movements may result, but nothing as severe as what is found in the case of the lower animals.

Deaf people are often lacking in their vestibular response. According to Wendt, about 20 percent of deaf people lack all vestibular response. Such people have somewhat impaired equilibrium, but not severe enough to handicap them noticeably. In Ménière's disease, the vestibular nerve is sometimes sectioned, thus eliminating the vestibular function entirely. Patients, especially if the disease was severe, appear to get along much better with no vestibular function than with a diseased one.

Summary

In this final chapter we examined the remaining sense organs, those of an organic, reflexive nature, frequently lying deep within the body. We considered them under four general, arbitrary classes: the subcutaneous senses, such as the deep pressure sense mediated by the Pacinian corpuscle; the visceral senses, evoked by mechanical and chemical means; proprioception and its dependency on movement and pressure; and the vestibular sense, mediated by the semicircular canals and the otolith organs of the inner ear. With respect to these various organs we considered briefly their structure, functioning, and significance for human behavior.

Suggested Readings

1. G. R. Wendt. "Vestibular Functions," in S. C. Stevens (ed.), *Handbook of Experimental Psychology*. New York: Wiley, 1951. This chapter from the Stevens handbook is probably the best moderate length description of vestibular functions. Its 33 pages include a particularly excellent bibliography of over 200 entries. It is relatively difficult reading, including a considerable amount of detail. For the serious student it should prove to be a valuable source of information.
2. From C. G. Mueller. *Sensory Psychology*. Englewood Cliffs, N.J.: Prentice-Hall, 1965. Chapter 8 of this previously cited reference covers the vestibular and kinesthetic senses. The 12 pages are quite easy to read and provide a treatment somewhat different from what we have presented. It is recommended for the general reader as a source of additional information.
3. From W. L. Jenkins. "Somesthesis," in S. S. Stevens (ed.), *Handbook of Experimental Psychology*. New York: Wiley, 1951. There are four pages in this reference that do justice to the topic of this chapter. Pages 1184–1188 include excellent, short descriptions of deep sensitivity, kinesthesis, and internal or organic sensitivities. A reference as short as this, and at the same time so well presented, is a must reading for the serious student.
4. W. D. Neff. "Studying Proprioception," in T. G. Andrews (ed.), *Methods of Psychology*. New York: Wiley, 1948. This 30-page chapter is more than just methodology. Although methodology is indeed covered adequately, the reference includes valuable information on structure, physiology, and general functioning of the proprioceptive senses that are defined so as to include kinesthesis and the vestibular function. This is very worthwhile reading. Its age should not detract seriously from its value for the interested student.
5. From S. H. Bartley. *Principles of Perception*, 2d ed. New York: Harper & Row, 1969. Chapter 13 includes 24 well-written pages that elaborate on the material we have just covered. For additional general material, of a somewhat more technical nature, this reference is highly recommended.
6. I. P. Howard. "The Spatial Senses" and "Orientation and Motion in Space," in Edward C. Carterette and Morton P. Friedman (eds.), *Handbook of Perception*, vol. III, *Biology of Perceptual Systems*. New York: Academic Press, 1973. These two chapters (13 and 14) include worthwhile discussions of joint receptors, muscle spindles and tendon organs, and the vestibular system, as well as information on kinesthesis, orientation, and sensorimotor coordination. The chapters recommended here are worth reading by the serious student.

bibliography

Adler, J. "Chemoreceptors in Bacteria," *Science* 166 (1969): 1588–1597.

Adrian, E. D. *The Physical Background of Perception*. London: Oxford University Press, 1947.

Allen, W. F. "Effects on Respiration, Blood Pressure, and Carotid Pulse of Various Inhaled and Insufflated Vapors," *Amer. J. Physiol.* 88 (1929): 117–129.

Allison, V. C., and S. H. Katz. "An Investigation of Stenches and Odors for Industrial Purposes," *J. Indust. Eng. Chem.* 11 (1919): 336–338.

Alpern, M., M. Lawrence, and D. Wolsk. *Sensory Processes*. Belmont, Calif.: Brooks/Cole, 1967.

Amoore, J. E., J. W. Johnston, Jr., and M. Rubin. "The Stereo-Chemical Theory of Odor," *Scientific American*, February, 1964.

———. "Specific Anosmia: A Clue to the Olfactory Code," *Nature* 214 (1967): 1058–1098.

———. "A Plan to Identify Most of the Primary Odors," in C. Pfaffman (ed.), *Olfaction and Taste*, vol. III. New York: The Rockefeller University Press, Press, 1969.

———. "Olfactory Genetics and Anosmia," in L. M. Beidler (ed.), *Handbook of Sensory Physiology*, vol. IV, *Chemical Senses*, part 1, *Olfaction*. Berlin: Springer-Verlag, 1971.

Andreas, B. G. *Experimental Psychology*. New York: Wiley, 1960.

Andrews, T. G. (ed.). *Methods of Psychology*. New York: Wiley, 1948.

Annis, R. C., and B. Frost. "Human Visual Ecology and Orientation Anisotropies in Acuity," *Science* 182 (1973): 729–731.

Arbib, M. *Brains, Machines and Mathematics*. New York: McGraw-Hill, 1964.

Arey, L. B. *Developmental Anatomy*, 7th ed. Philadelphia: Saunders, 1965.

Atema, J., J. H. Todd, and J. E. Bardach. "Olfaction and Behavioral Sophistication in Fish," in C. Pfaffman (ed.), *Olfaction and Taste*, vol. III. New York: The Rockefeller University Press, 1969.

Attneave, F. *Applications of Information Theory to Psychology.* New York: Holt, Rinehart and Winston, 1959.

Bardach, J. E., and J. E. Todd. "Chemical Communication in Fish," in J. W. Johnston, Jr., D. G. Moulton, and A. Turk (eds.), *Advances in Chemoreception*, vol. I, *Communications by Chemical Signals.* Englewood Cliffs, N.J.: Prentice-Hall, 1970.

Barlow, H. B., and J. M. B. Sparrock. "The Role of After-images in Dark Adaptation," *Science* 144 (1964): 1309–1314.

Bartley, S. H. *Vision.* New York: Van Nostrand Reinhold, 1941.

———. "The Psychophysiology of Vision," in S. S. Stevens (ed.), *Handbook of Experimental Psychology.* New York: Wiley, 1951.

———. *Principles of Perception*, 2d ed. New York: Harper & Row, 1969.

Bath, W. "Die Geschmacksorgane der Vögel und Crocodile," *Arch. Biontol.* (Berlin) 1 (1906): 1–47.

Beck, L. H. "Osmics: Theory and Problems Related to the Initial Effects in Olfaction," in O. Glasser (ed.), *Medical Physics. Chicago:* Year Book Medical Publishers, 1950.

———, and W. R. Miles. "Some Theoretical and Experimental Relationships between Infra-red Absorption and Olfaction," *Science* 106 (1947): 511.

Begbie, G. H. *Seeing and the Eye.* Garden City, N.Y.: Doubleday, 1973.

Beidler, L. M. "Dynamics of Taste Cells," in Y. Zotterman (ed.), *Olfaction and Taste.* New York: Macmillan, 1963.

——— (ed.). *Handbook of Sensory Physiology*, vol. IV, *Chemical Senses*, part 1, *Olfaction.* Berlin: Springer-Verlag, 1971.

——— (ed.). *Handbook of Sensory Physiology*, vol. IV, *Chemical Senses*, part 2, *Taste.* Berlin: Springer-Verlag, 1971.

Békésy, G. von. "Current Status of Theories of Hearing," *Science* 123 (1956): 779–783.

———. "The Ear," *Scientific American*, August 1957.

———. "Similarities Between Hearing and Skin Sensations," *Psychol. Rev.* 66 (1959): 1–22.

———. *Experiments in Hearing.* Trans. and edited by E. G. Wever. New York: McGraw-Hill, 1960.

———. "Duplexity Theory of Taste," *Science* 145 (1964): 834–835.

———. "Taste Theories and the Chemical Stimulation of Single Papillae," *J. Appl. Physiol.* 21 (1966): 1–9.

———, and W. A. Rosenblith. "The Early History of Hearing—Observations and Theories," *J. Acoust. Soc. Amer.* 20 (1948): 727–748.

———. "The Mechanical Properties of the Ear," in S. S. Stevens (ed.), *Handbook of Experimental Psychology.* New York: Wiley, 1951.

Bell, D. W., and G. Fairbanks. "TTS Produced by Low-Level Tones and the Effects of Testing on Recovery," *J. Acoust. Soc. Amer.* 35 (1963): 1725–1731.

Beranek, L. L. "The Design of Speech Communication Systems," *Proc Inst. Radio Engrs.* 35 (1947): 880–890.

———. *Acoustic Measurements.* New York: Wiley, 1949.

———. *Acoustics.* New York: McGraw-Hill, 1954.

———, W. E. Blazier, and J. J. Figwer. "Preferred Noise Criterion (PNC) Curves and Their Application to Rooms," *J. Acoust. Soc. Amer.* 50 (1971): 1223–1228.

Bird, C. "Maturation and Practice: Their Effects upon the Feeding Reaction of Chicks," *J. Comp. Psychol.* 16 (1933): 212–234.

Blackwell, H. B., and O. M. Blackwell. "Rod and Cone Mechanisms in Typical and Atypical Congenital Achromatopsia," *Vision Res.* 1 (1961): 62–107.

Blakemore, C., and P. Sutton. "Size Adaptation: A New Aftereffect," *Science* 166 (1069): 245–247.

Bliss, J. "A Reading Machine with Tactile Display," in T. D. Sterling, E. A. Bering, S. V. Pollack, and H. G. Vaughan (eds.), *Visual Prosthesis*. New York: Academic Press, 1971.

Bloemendal, Hans. "The Vertebrate Eye Lens," *Science* 197 (1977): 127–137.

Bock, R. D., and L. V. Jones. *The Measurement and Prediction of Judgment and Choice*. San Francisco: Holden-Day, 1968.

Bolt, R. H., S. J. Lukasik, A. W. Nolle, and A. D. Frost. *Handbook of Acoustic Noise Control*, vol. I, *Physical Acoustics*. WADC-TR-42-40, Wright Air Development Center, Ohio, 1952.

Boring, E. G. "The Sensations of the Alimentary Canal," *Amer. J. Psychol.* 26 (1915): 1–57.

———. "The Thermal Sensitivity of the Stomach," *Amer. J. Psychol.* 26 (1915): 484–494.

———. *Sensation and Perception in the History of Experimental Psychology*. New York: Appleton, 1942.

———. *A History of Experimental Psychology*. 2d ed. New York: Appleton, 1950.

Börnstein, W. S. "Cortical Representation of Taste in Man and Monkey," vol. II. *Yale J. Biol. Med.* 13 (1940): 133–156.

Bouman, M. A. "History and Present Status of Quantum Theory in Vision," in W. A. Rosenblith (ed.), *Sensory Communication*. New York: Wiley, 1962.

Boyd, I. A., and T. D. M. Roberts. "Proprioceptive Discharges from the Stretch Receptors in the Knee Joint of the Cat," *J. Physiol.* 122 (1953): 38–58.

Brindley, G. S. *The Physiology of the Retina and Visual Pathway*. London: Edward Arnold, Publishers Ltd., 1960.

———. "Afterimages," *Scientific American*, October 1963.

Brink, F., Jr. "Excitation and Conduction in the Neuron," in S. S. Stevens (ed.), *Handbook of Experimental Psychology*. New York: Wiley, 1951.

Brown, C. W., and E. E. Guiselli, *Scientific Method in Psychology*. New York: McGraw-Hill, 1965.

Brown, T. S. "Olfaction and Taste," in B. Scharf (ed.), *Experimental Sensory Psychology*. Glenview, Ill.: Scott, Foresman, 1975.

Brownell, P. H. "Compressional and Surface Waves in Sand: Used by Desert Scorpions to Locate Prey," *Science* 197 (1977): 479–481.

Buddenbrock, M. von, *The Senses*. Ann Arbor: University of Michigan Press, 1958.

Burnham, R. W., R. M. Hanes, and C. J. Bartleson. *Color: A Guide to Basic Facts and Concepts*. New York: Wiley, 1963.

Burtt, H. E. *The Psychology of Birds*. New York: Macmillan, 1967.

Cabanac, M. "Physiological Role of Pleasure," *Science* 173 (1971): 1103–1107.

Cagan, R. H. "Chemostimulatory Protein: A New Type of Taste Stimulus," *Science* 181 (1973): 32–35.

Cain, W. S. "Differential Sensitivity for Smell: 'Noise' at the Nose," *Science* 195 (1977): 796–798.

———, and T. Engen. "Olfactory Adaptation and the Direct Scaling of Odor Intensity," in C. Pfaffman (ed.), *Olfaction and Taste,* vol. III. New York: The Rockefeller University Press, 1969.

Cameron, A. T. "The Taste Sense and the Relative Sweetness of Sugars and Other Sweet Substances," Scientific Report Series No. 9, Sugar Research Foundation, 1947.

Carterette, E. C., and M. P. Friedman (eds.). *Handbook of Perception,* vol. I, *Historical and Philosophical Roots of Perception.* New York: Academic Press, 1973.

———. *Handbook of Perception,* vol. II, *Psychophysical Judgment and Measurement.* New York: Academic Press, 1974.

———. *Handbook of Perception,* vol. III, *Biology of Perceptual Systems.* New York: Academic Press, 1973.

Chapanis, A. "The Dark Adaptation of the Color Anomalous Measured with Lights of Different Hues," *J. Gen. Physiol.* 30 (1947): 423–437.

Cherry, C. *On Human Communications,* New York: Wiley, 1957.

Christman, R. J. "Figural After-effects Utilizing Apparent Movement as Inspection-Figure," *Amer. J. Psychol.* 66 (1953): 66–72.

———. "Shifts in Pitch as a Function of Prolonged Stimulation with Pure Tones," *Amer. J. Psychol.* 67 (1954): 484–491.

———. "The Perception of Direction as a Function of Binaural Temporal and Amplitude Disparity," in G. Finch and F. Cameron (eds.), *Air Force Human Engineering, Personnel, and Training Research.* Baltimore: Air Research and Development Command, 1956.

———. "Noise Reduction in Air Force Control Towers," *Noise Control* 5 (1959): 24–29.

———. "Person-to-Person Communication in an Atmosphere-Free Environment," in D. P. LeGalley (ed.), *Bioastronautics and Electronics, and Invited Addresses.* Proceedings of the Fifth Symposium on Ballistic Missiles and Space Technology. New York: Academic Press, 1960.

———, and W. E. Williams. "Influence of the Time Interval on Experimentally Induced Shifts in Pitch," *J. Acoust. Soc. Amer.* 35 (1963): 1030–1033.

Cohen, J., and D. A. Gordon. "The Prevost-Fechner-Benham Subjective Colors," *Psychol. Bull.* 46 (1949): 97–136.

Cohn, R. "Differential Cerebral Processing of Noise and Verbal Stimuli," *Science* 172 (1971): 559–601.

Colangelo, Donald, "Pain," Term paper submitted for college course (1972).

Cole, E. C. *Comparative Histology.* Philadelphia: Blakiston, 1941.

Committee on Colorimetry of the Optical Society of America. *The Science of Color.* New York: Crowell, 1953.

Corning, W. C., and M. Balaban (eds.). *The Mind: Biological Approaches to Its Functions.* New York: Wiley, 1968.

Cornsweet, Tom N. *Visual Perception.* New York: Academic Press, 1970.

Corso, J. F. *The Experimental Psychology of Sensory Behavior.* New York: Holt, Rinehart and Winston, 1967.

———, and D. A. Norman. "Neural Controversy in Sensory Psychology," *Science* 181 (1973): 467–469.

Crafts, L. W., T. C. Schneirla, and R. W. Gilbert. *Recent Experiments in Psychology*, 2d ed. New York: McGraw-Hill, 1950.

Craig, J. C. "Vibrotactile Pattern Perception: Extraordinary Observers," *Science* 196 (1977): 450–452.

Crocker, E. C. *Flavor*. New York: McGraw-Hill, 1945.

———, and L. F. Henderson. "Analysis and Classification of Odors," *Amer. Perfum.* 22 (1927): 325–356.

Crombie, A. C. "Early Concepts of the Senses and the Mind," *Scientific American*, May 1964.

Crozier, W. J. "Regarding the Existence of the Common Chemical Sense in Vertebrates," *J. Comp. Neurol.* 26 (1916): 1–8.

Cruze, W. W. "Maturation and Learning in Chicks," *J. Comp. Psychol.* 19 (1935): 371–409.

Dallenbach, K. M. "A Bibliography of the Attempts to Identify the Functional End-Organs of Cold and Warmth," *Amer. J. Psychol.* 41 (1929): 344–378.

Dartnall, H. J. A. *Visual Pigments*. New York: Wiley, 1957.

Davenport, D. "Bee Language," *Science* 186 (1974): 975.

Davies, J. T. "The Mechanism of Olfaction," *Symposia of the Society for Experimental Biology*, 16 (1962): 170–179.

———. "Olfactory Theories," in L. M. Beidler (ed.). *Handbook of Sensory Physiology*, vol. IV, *Chemical Senses*, part 1, *Olfaction*. Berlin: Springer-Verlag, 1971.

Davis, H. "Psychophysiology of Hearing and Deafness," in S. S. Stevens (ed.), *Handbook of Experimental Psychology*. New York: Wiley, 1951.

———. "The Excitation of Nerve Impulses in the Cochlea," *Ann. Otol. Rhinol. Laryngol.* 61 (1954): 469–481.

———, and S. R. Silverman (eds.). *Hearing and Deafness*. New York: Holt, Rinehart and Winston, 1970.

———, et al. "Final Report on Physiological Effects of Exposure to Certain Sounds," OSRD Report 889, Harvard University, 1944.

Davson, H. (ed.). *The Eye*. New York: Academic Press, 1962.

De Beer, Sir G. *Embryos and Ancestors*, 3d ed. Oxford: Clarendon Press, 1958.

De Lange, H. "Research into the Dynamic Nature of the Human Fovea-Cortex System with Intermittent and Modulated Light," *J. Opt. Soc. Am.* 48 (1958): 777–784.

De Lorenzo, A. J. "Studies on the Ultrastructure and Histophysiology of Cell Membranes, Nerve Fibers, and Synaptic Junctions in Chemoreceptors," in Y. Zotterman (ed.), *Olfaction and Taste*. New York: Macmillan, 1963.

De Valois, R. L. "Analysis and Coding of Color Vision in the Primate Visual System," *Cold Spring Harbor Symposium on Quantitative Biology* 30 (1965): 567–579.

De Vries, H., and M. Stuiver. "The Absolute Sensitivity of the Human Sense of Smell," in W. A. Rosenblith (ed.), *Sensory Communications*. New York: Wiley, 1961.

Dennis, W. (ed.). *Readings in the History of Psychology*. New York: Appleton, 1948.

Dethier, V. G. *To Know a Fly*. San Francisco: Holden-Day, 1962.

———. *The Physiology of Insect Senses*. New York: Wiley, 1963.

Deutsch, J. A., and M. L. Wang. "The Stomach as a Site for Rapid Nutrient Reinforcement Sensors," *Science* 195 (1977): 89–90.

Diehn, Bodo. "Phototaxis and Sensory Transduction in Euglena," *Science* 181 (1973): 1009–1015.

Dobelle, W. H., M. G. Mladejovsky, and J. P. Girvin. "Artificial Vision for the Blind: Electrical Stimulation of Visual Cortex Offers Hope for a Functional Prosthesis," *Science* 183 (1974): 440–443.

Du Verney, J. G. "Traité de l'Organe de l'Ouie," Paris: 1683.

Eckert, R. "Biolectric Control of Ciliary Activity," *Science* 176 (1972): 473–481.

Egan, J. P. "Articulation Testing Methods II," OSRD Rpt. 3802, Contract OEMsr-658, Psycho-Acoustic Lab., Harvard University, 1944.

————. "Articulation Testing Methods," PNR-36, Contract N5ori-76, ONR, Psycho-Acoustic Lab., Harvard University, 1947.

————. "Articulation Testing Methods," *Laryngoscope* 58 (1948): 955–991.

————, A. I. Schulman, and G. Z. Greenberg. "Operating Characteristics Determined by Binary Decisions and by Ratings," *J. Acoust. Soc. Amer.* 31 (1959): 768–773.

————, and F. M. Wiener. "On the Articulation Efficiency of Bands of Speech in Noise," *J. Acoust. Soc. Amer.* 18 (1946): 435–441.

Eisner, T., R. E. Silberglied, D. Aneshansley, J. E. Carrel, and H. C. Howland. "Ultraviolet Video-Viewing: The Television Camera as an Insect Eye," *Science* 166 (1969): 1172–1174.

Elsberg, C. A., E. D. Brewer, and I. Levy. "Concerning Conditions Which May Temporarily Alter Normal Olfactory Acuity," *Bull. Neurol. Inst. N.Y.* 4 (1935): 31–34.

————, and I. Levy. "A New and Simple Method of Quantitative Olfactometry," *Bull. Neurol. Inst. N.Y.* 4 (1935): 5–19.

Engen, T. "Man's Ability to Perceive Odors," in J. W. Johnson, D. G. Moulton, and A. Turk (eds.), *Advances in Chemoreception*, vol. I, *Communication by Chemical Signals*. Englewood Cliffs, N.J.: Prentice-Hall, 1970.

————. "Olfactory Psychophysics," in L. M. Beidler (ed.), *Handbook of Sensory Physiology*, vol. IV, *Chemical Senses*, part 1, *Olfaction*. Berlin: Springer-Verlag, 1971.

Enright, J. T. "Distortions of Apparent Velocity: A New Optical Illusion," *Science* 168 (1970): 464–467.

Erickson, R. P. "Sensory Neural Patterns and Gustation," in Y. Zotterman (ed.), *Olfaction and Taste*. New York: Macmillan, 1963.

Evans, R. M. *An Introduction to Color*. New York: Wiley, 1948.

Favreau, O. E., V. F. Emerson, and M. C. Corbalis. "Motion Perception: A Color-Contingent Aftereffect," *Science* 176 (1972): 78–79.

Favreau, O., and M. C. Corbalis. "Negative Aftereffects in Visual Perception," *Scientific American*, December 1976.

Fender, D. H. "Control Mechanisms of the Eye," *Scientific American*, July 1964.

Fitzhugh, R. "The Statistical Detection of Threshold Signals in the Retina," *J. Gen. Physiol.* 40 (1957): 925–948.

Fletcher, H. *Speech and Hearing*. New York: Van Nostrand Reinhold, 1929.

————. "Auditory Patterns," *Rev. Mod. Phys.* 12 (1940): 47–65.

————. *Speech and Hearing in Communications*. New York: Van Nostrand Reinhold, 1953.

————, and W. A. Munson, "Loudness, Its Definition, Measurement, and Calculation," *J. Acoust. Soc. Amer.* 5 (1933): 82–108.

Forgus, R. H. *Perception.* New York: McGraw-Hill, 1966.

Foster, D., E. H. Scofield, and K. M. Dallenbach, "An Olfactorium," *Amer. J. Psychol.* 63 (1950): 431–440.

Fox, R., S. W. Lehmkuhle, and D. H. Westendorf. "Falcon Visual Acuity," *Science* 192 (1976): 263–265.

————, S. W. Lehmkuhle, and R. C. Bush. "Stereopsis in the Falcon," *Science* 197 (1977): 79–81.

French, J. D. "The Reticular Formation," *Scientific American,* May 1957.

————. "The Reticular Formation," in J. Field (ed.), *Handbook of Physiology,* vol. II. Washington, D.C.: American Physiological Society, 1960.

French, N. R., and J. C. Steinberg. "Factors Governing the Intelligibility of Speech Sounds," *J. Acoust. Soc. Amer.* 19 (1947): 90–120.

Frey, M. von. "Beitrage zur Sinnesphysiologie des Haut," *Ber Sächs Ges Wiss Leipzig Math-Phys Cl.* 47 (1895): 166–184.

————, and A. Goldman. "Der zeitliche Verlauf der Einstellung bei den Druckempfindungen," *Z. Biol.* 65 (1915): 183–202.

Friend, A. W., Jr., and E. D. Finch. "Low Frequency Electric Field Induced Changes in the Shape and Motility of Amoebas," *Science* 198 (1975): 357–359.

Frisch, K. von. *The Dance Language and Orientation of Bees.* Cambridge, Mass.: Harvard University Press, 1967.

————. "Decoding the Language of the Bee," *Science* 185 (1974): 663–668.

Fulton, J. F. *Howell's Textbook of Physiology.* Philadelphia: Saunders, 1947.

Galambos, R. "Neural Mechanisms of Audition," *Physiol. Rev.* 34 (1954): 497–528.

Gamble, E. M. "The Applicability of Weber's Law to Smell," *Amer. J. Psychol.* 10 (1898): 82–142.

Gandelman, R., M. X. Zarrow, V. H. Denenberg, and M. Myers. "Olfactory Bulb Removal Eliminated Maternal Behavior in the Mouse," *Science* 171 (1971): 210–211.

Garner, W. R., and G. A. Miller. "The Masked Threshold of Pure Tones as a Function of Duration," *J. Exptl. Psychol.* 37 (1947): 293–303.

Geldard, F. A. "Adventures in Tactile Literacy," *Amer. Physiol.* 12 (1957): 115–124.

————. "Some Neglected Possibilities of Communication," *Science* 131 (1960): 1583–1588.

————. "Cutaneous Coding of Optical Signals: The Optohapt," *Perception and Psychophysics* 1 (1966): 377–381.

————. "Body English," *Psychology Today* 2 (1968): 42–47.

————. *The Human Senses,* 2d ed. New York: Wiley, 1972.

Gibson, E. J., and R. D. Wall. "The Visual Cliff," *Scientific American,* April 1960.

Gibson, J. J. *The Perception of the Visual World.* Boston: Houghton Mifflin, 1950.

————. "Observations of Active Touch," *Psychol. Rev.* 69 (1962): 477–491.

————. "The Useful Dimensions of Sensitivity," *Amer. Psychol.* (1963): 1–15.

————. *The Senses Considered as Perceptual Systems.* Boston: Houghton Mifflin, 1966.

Gibson, K. S. *Spectrophotometry.* Washington, D. C.: National Bureau of Standards, Circular 484, 1949.

Gilchrist, A. L. Perceived Lightness Depends on Perceived Spatial Arrangement," *Science* 195 (1977): 185–187.

Gilmer, B. von Haller. "The Glomus Body as a Receptor of Cutaneous Pressure and Vibration," *Psychol. Bull.* 39 (1942): 73–79.

————. "The Relation of Cold Sensitivity to Sweat Duct Distribution and the Neurovascular Mechanism of the Skin," *J. Psychol.* 13 (1942): 307–325.

Glickstein, M. "Organization of the Visual Pathways," *Science* 164 (1969): 917–925.

Gorman, A. L. F., and J. S. McReynolds. "Hyperpolarizing and Depolarizing Receptor Potentials in the Scallop Eye," *Science* 165 (1969): 309–310.

Gottlieb, F. J. *Developmental Genetics.* New York: Van Nostrand Reinhold, 1966.

Gouras, P. "Trichromatic Mechanisms in Single Cortical Neurons," *Science* 168 (1970): 489–492.

Graham, C. H. "Visual Perception," in S. S. Stevens (ed.), *Handbook of Experimental Psychology.* New York: Wiley, 1951.

————. "Color Theory," in S. Koch (ed.), *Psychology: A Study of a Science,* vol. I. New York: McGraw-Hill, 1959.

———— (ed.). *Vision and Visual Perception.* New York: Wiley, 1965.

Granit, R. *Receptors and Sensory Perception.* New Haven: Yale University Press, 1955.

Graziadei, P. P. C. "The Ultrastructure of Vertebrate Taste Buds," in C. Pfaffman (ed.), *Olfaction and Taste,* vol. III. New York: The Rockefeller University Press, 1969.

————. "The Olfactory Mucosa of Vertebrates," in L. M. Beidler (ed.), *Handbook of Sensory Physiology,* vol. IV, *Chemical Senses,* part 1, *Olfaction.* Berlin: Springer-Verlag, 1971.

Green, B. F. *Digital Computers in Research.* New York: McGraw-Hill, 1954.

Green, D. M. "Psychoacoustics and Detection Theory," *J. Acoust. Soc. Amer.* 32 (1960): 1189–1203.

————, and J. A. Swets. *Signal Detection and Psychophysics.* New York: Wiley, 1966.

Green, M., T. Corwin, and V. Zemon. "A Comparison of Fourier Analysis and Feature Analysis in Pattern-Specific Color Aftereffects," *Science* 192 (1976): 147–148.

Gregory, R. L. "Eye Movements and the Stability of the Visual World," *Nature* 182 (1958): 1214.

————. *Eye and Brain: The Psychology of Seeing.* New York: McGraw-Hill, 1966.

————, and O. L. Zangwill. "The Origin of the Autokinetic Effect," *Quart. J. Exptl. Psychol.* 15 (1963): 4.

Gross, C. G., and H. P. Zeigler (eds.). *Readings in Physiological Psychology: Neurophysiology/Sensory Processes.* New York: Harper & Row, 1969.

Grossman, S. P. *A Textbook of Physiological Psychology.* New York: Wiley, 1967.

Guilford, J. P. *Psychometric Methods.* New York: McGraw-Hill, 1936.

————. *Psychometric Methods,* 2d ed. New York: McGraw-Hill, 1954.

Guillot, J. P. "Anosmies Partielles et Odeurs Fondamentales," *Comptes Rendus Hebdomadaires des Séances de l'Académie des Sciences* (Paris) 226 (1948): 1307–1309.

Haagen-Smit, A. J. "Smell and Taste," *Scientific American,* March, 1952.

Haber, R. N. (ed.). *Contemporary Theory and Research in Visual Perception.* New York: Holt, Rinehart and Winston, 1968.

————. *Information-Processing Approaches to Visual Perception.* New York: Holt, Rinehart and Winston, 1969.

Hahn, H. "Die Psycho-physischen Konstanten und Variablen des Temperatursinnes," *Z. Sinnesphysiol.* 60 (1930): 198–232.

————. "Die Adaptation des Geschmacksinnes," *Z. Sinnesphysiol.* 65 (1934): 105–145.

————. G. Kuckulies, and H. Taeger, "Eine systematische Untersuchung der Geschmacksschwellen," *Z. Sinnesphysiol.* 67 (1938): 259–306.

Ham, A. W. *Histology.* Philadelphia: Lippincott, 1950.

Hansen, K. "The Mechanism of Insect Sugar Reception: A Biochemical Investigation," in C. Pfaffman (ed.), *Olfaction and Taste,* vol. III. New York: The Rockefeller University Press, 1969.

Hansen, R., and W. Langer. "Uber Geschmacksveränderungen in der Schwangerschaft," *Klin. Wschr.* 14 (1935): 1173–1176.

Hardy, J. D., and T. W. Oppel. "Studies in Temperature Sensation III: The Sensitivity of the Body to Heat and the Spatial Summation of the End Organ Responses," *J. Clin. Invest.* 16 (1937): 533–540.

————, H. G. Wolff, and H. Goodell, "Studies on Pain: An Investigation of Some Quantitative Aspects of the Dol Scale of Pain Intensity," *J. Clin. Invest.* 27 (1948): 380–386.

Hardy, M. "Observations on the Innervation of the Macula Saculi in Man," *Anat. Rec.* 59 (1934): 403–418.

Harris, C. S., and A. R. Gibson. "Is Orientation-Specific Color Adaptation in Human Vision Due to Edge Detectors, Afterimages, or 'Dipoles'?" *Science* 162 (1968): 1506–1507.

Harris, J. F., and R. I. Gamov. "Snake Infrared Receptors: Thermal or Photochemical Mechanisms," *Science* 172 (1971): 1252–1253.

Harth, M. S., and M. B. Heaton. "Nonvisual Photic Responses in Newly Hatched Pigeons (*Columbia livia*)," *Science* 180 (1973): 753–755.

Hartline, H. K. "Visual Receptor and Retinal Interaction," *Science* 164 (1969): 270–278.

————, and C. H. Graham. "Nerve Impulses from Single Receptors in the Eye," *J. Cell. Comp. Physiol.* 1 (1932): 277–295.

————, and R. Ratliff. "Inhibitory Interaction of Receptor Units in the Eye of Limulus," *J. Gen. Physiol.* 40 (1957): 357–376.

Hawkins, J. E., Jr., and S. S. Stevens. "The Masking of Pure Tones and of Speech by White Noise," *J. Acoust. Soc. Amer.* 22 (1950): 6–13.

Hecht, S. "Rods, Cones and the Chemical Basis of Vision," *Physiol. Rev.* 17 (1937): 239–290.

————, C. Haig, and A. M. Chase. "Influence of Light Adaptation on Subsequent Dark Adaptation of the Eye," *J. Gen. Physiol.* 20 (1937): 831–850.

———, and S. Shlaer. "Intermittent Stimulation by Light. V: The Relation Between Intensity and Critical Frequency for Different Parts of the Spectrum," *J. Gen. Physiol.* 19 (1936): 965–977.

———, and M. H. Pirenne. "Energy Quanta and Vision," *J. Gen. Physiol.* 25 (1942): 819–840.

Hartline, Peter H., Leonard Kass, and Michael S. Loop. "Merging of Modalities in the Optic Tectum: Infrared and Visual Integration in Rattlesnakes," *Science* 199 (1978): 1225–1229.

Held, R., and S. R. Shattuck. "Color- and Edge-sensitive Channels in the Human Visual System: Tuning for Orientation," *Science* 174 (1971): 314–316.

Helson, H. "Some Factors and Implications of Color Constancy," *J. Opt. Soc. Amer.* 33 (1943): 555–567.

———. *Adaptation Level Theory.* New York: Harper & Row, 1964.

Helmholtz, H. L. von. *Sensations of Tone.* A. J. Ellis (trans.). New York: Longman, 1930.

Henning, H. *Der Geruch,* 2d ed. Leipzig: Barth, 1924.

Hepler, N. "Color: A Motion-Contingent Aftereffect," *Science* 162 (1968): 376–377.

Hinde, R. A. *Animal Behavior.* New York: McGraw-Hill, 1966.

Hirsh, I. J. *The Measurement of Hearing.* New York: McGraw-Hill, 1952.

———, E. G. Reynolds, and M. Joseph. "Intelligibility of Different Speech Materials," *J. Acoust. Soc. Amer.* 26 (1954): 530–539.

Hölldobler, B., and C. P. Haskins. "Sexual Calling Behavior in Primitive Ants," *Science* 195 (1977): 793–794.

———, and E. O. Wilson. "Weaver Ants: Social Establishment and Maintenance of Territory," *Science* 195 (1977): 900–902.

Holst, E. von. "Relation between the Central Nervous System and the Peripheral Organs," *Brit. J. Anim Behav.* 2 (1954): 89.

Hornbostel, E. M. von, and M. Wertheimer. Über die Wahrnehmung der Schallrichtung," *Akad. Wiss.,* Berlin (1920): 288–296.

Horridge, G. A. "The Compound Eye of Insects," *Scientific American,* July 1977.

Howard, I. P., and W. B. Templeton. *Human Spatial Orientation.* New York: Wiley, 1966.

Hubel, D. H., and T. N. Wiesel. "Receptive Fields of Single Neurons in the Cat's Striate Cortex," *J. Physiol.* 148 (1959): 574–591.

———. "Receptive Fields and Functional Architecture of Monkey Striate Cortex," *J. Physiol.* 195 (1968): 215–243.

Huggins, W. H., and J. C. R. Licklider. "Place Mechanisms of Auditory Frequency Analysis," *J. Acoust. Soc. Amer.* 23 (1951): 290–299.

Hyman, L. H. *Comparative Vertebrate Anatomy.* Chicago: University of Chicago Press, 1942.

Jeffres, L. A. "A Place Theory of Sound Localization," *J. Comp. Physiol. Psychol.* 41 (1948): 35–39.

Jenkins, W. L. "Nafe's Vascular Theory and the Preponderance of Evidence," *Amer. J. Psychol.* 52 (1939): 462–465.

———. "Studies in Thermal Sensitivity: 17. The Topographical and Functional Relations of Warm and Cold," *J. Exptl. Psychol.* 29 (1941): 511–516.

———. "Somesthesis," in S. S. Stevens (ed.), *Handbook of Experimental Psychology.* New York: Wiley, 1951.

Johnson, J. W., D. G. Moulton, and A. Turk (eds.). *Advances in Chemoreception,* vol. I. *Communication by Chemical Signals.* Englewood Cliffs, N.J.: Prentice-Hall, 1970.

Journal of the Acoustical Society of America, "Békésy Commemorative Issue," *J. Acoust. Soc. Amer.* 34 (1962): 1319–1533.

Judd, D. B. "Chromaticity Sensibility to Stimulus Differences," *J. Opt. Soc. Amer.* 22 (1932): 72–108.

———. *Colorimetry.* Washington, D.C.: National Bureau of Standards Circular No. 478 (1950).

———. "Basic Correlates of the Visual Stimulus," in S. S. Stevens (ed.), *Handbook of Experimental Psychology.* New York: Wiley, 1951.

———, and G. Wyszecki. *Color in Business, Science and Industry,* 2d ed. New York: Wiley, 1963.

Kaissling, K. E. "Insect Olfaction," in L. M. Beidler (ed.), *Handbook of Sensory Physiology,* vol. IV, *Chemical Senses,* part 1, *Olfaction.* Berlin: Springer-Verlag, 1971.

Kare, M. "Comparative Study of Taste," in L. M. Beidler (ed.), *Handbook of Sensory Physiology,* vol. IV, *Chemical Senses,* part 2, *Taste.* Berlin: Springer-Verlag, 1971.

Kellicott, W. E. *Outlines of Chordate Development.* New York: Holt, 1934.

Kelly, K. L. "Color Designation for Lights," *J. Research* (National Bureau of Standards) 31 (1943): 271.

Kennedy, D. "Inhibition in Visual Systems," *Scientific American,* July 1963.

Kenshalo, D. R. *The Skin Senses.* Springfield, Ill.: Thomas, 1968.

———, and J. P. Nafe. "A Quantitative Theory of Feeling," *Psychol. Rev.* 69 (1962): 17–33.

Kistiakowsky, G. B. "On the Theory of Odors," *Science* 112 (1950): 154–155.

Klemm, O. "Untersuchungen über die Lokalisation von Schallreizen. Über den Einfluss des binauralen Zeitunterschiedes auf die Lokalisation," *Arch. Ges. Psychol.* 40 (1920): 117–146.

Koch, S. (ed.). *Psychology: a Study of a Science,* vol. I. New York: McGraw-Hill, 1959.

Köhler, W., and H. Wallach. "Figural After-Effects: An Investigation of Visual Processes," *Proc. Amer. Philos. Soc.* 88 (1944): 269–357.

Kolers, P. A., and M. von Grunau. "Visual Construction of Color Is Digital," *Science* 187 (1975): 757–759.

Koshland, D. E., Jr. "A Response Regulator Model in a Simple Sensory System," *Science* 196 (1977): 1055–1063.

Kruger, L., and B. E. Stein. "Primordial Sense Organs and the Evolution of Sensory Systems," in E. C. Carterette and M. P. Friedman (eds.), *Handbook of Perception,* vol. III, *Biology of Perceptual Systems.* New York: Academic Press, 1973.

Kryter, K. D. "Speech Communications in Noise," AFCRC-TR-54-52, Air Force Cambridge Research Center, USAF, Washington, D.C., 1955.

———. "On Predicting the Intelligibility of Speech from Acoustical Measurements," *J. Speech Hearing Disorders* 21 (1956): 208–217.

———. *The Effect of Noise on Man.* New York: Academic Press, 1970.

Kurihara, K. "Taste Modifiers," in L. M. Beidler (ed.), *Handbook of Sensory*

Physiology, vol. IV, *Chemical Senses,* part 2, *Taste.* Berlin: Springer-Verlag, 1971.

Land. E. H. "Experiments in Color Vision," *Scientific American* 200 (1959): 84–99.

———. "The Retinex," *American Scientist* 52 (1964): 247–264.

Larkin, R. P., and P. J. Sutherland. "Migrating Birds Respond to Project Seafarer's Electromagnetic Field," *Science* 195 (1977): 777–779.

Lashley, K. S., and J. T. Russell. "The Mechanism of Vision: A Preliminary Test of Innate Organization," *J. Genetic Psychol.* 45 (1934): 136–144.

Lawrence, M. "Hearing," in M. Alpern, M. Lawrence, and D. Wolsk, *Sensory Processes.* Belmont, Calif.: Brooks/Cole, 1967.

Le Grand, Y. *Light, Color and Vision.* Trans. by R. W. G. Hunt. New York: Wiley, 1957.

Lettvin, J. Y., H. R. Maturana, W. S. McCulloch, and W. H. Pitts. "What the Frog's Eye Tells the Frog's Brain," *Proc. Inst. of Radio Eng.* 47 (1959): 1940–1950.

Lewis, T. *Pain.* New York: Macmillan, 1942.

Lewison, L. *You and Your Eyes.* New York: Trinity, 1960.

Licklider, J. C. R. "Basic Correlates of the Auditory Stimulus," in S. S. Stevens (eds.), *Handbook of Experimental Psychology.* New York: Wiley, 1951.

———. "Auditory Frequency Analysis," in E. C. Cherry (ed.), *Information Theory.* London: Butterworth Scientific Publications, 1956.

———. "Three Auditory Theories," in S. Koch (ed.), *Psychology: A Study of a Science,* vol. I. New York: McGraw-Hill, 1959.

———, and N. Guttman. "Masking of Speech by Line-Spectrum Interference," *J. Acoust. Soc. Amer.* 29 (1957): 287–296.

Lindenmaier, P., and M. R. Kare. "The Taste Organs of the Chicken," *Poultry Sci.* 38 (1959): 545–550.

Lindsay, P. H., and D. A. Norman. *Human Information Processing, An Introduction to Psychology.* New York: Academic Press, 1972.

Loewenstein, W. R. "Biological Transducers," *Scientific American,* August 1960.

Lorenz, K. Z. "Analogy as a Source of Knowledge," *Science* 185 (1974): 229–234.

Lucretius. *The Nature of the Universe.* Trans. by R. E. Latham. Baltimore: Penguin Books, 1951.

Lukasik, S. J., and W. W. Nolle (eds.). *Handbook of Acoustic Noise Control,* Supplement 1 to vol. 1, *Physical Acoustics.* WADC-TR-52-204. Dayton, Ohio: Wright Air Development Center, 1955.

Lüscher, E., and J. Zwislocki. "The Decay of Sensation and the Remainder of Adaptation after Short Pure-Tone Impulses on the Ear," *Acta otolaryng* (Stockholm) 35 (1947): 428–445.

MacKay, D. M. "Interactive Processes in Visual Perception," in W. A. Rosenblith (ed.), *Sensory Communication.* New York: Wiley, 1962.

MacLean, P. D. "Studies on the Limbic System (Visceral Brain) and Their Bearing on Psychosomatic Problems," in E. D. Wittkover and R. A. Cleghorn (eds.), *Recent Developments in Psychosomatic Medicine.* Philadelphia: Lippincott, 1954.

MacNichol, E. F., Jr. "Three-Pigment Color Vision," *Scientific American,* December 1964.

Maffei, L., and F. W. Campbell. "Neurophysiological Localization of the Vertical and Horizontal Visual Coordinates in Man," *Science* 167 (1970): 386–387.

Maier, N. R. F., and T. C. Schneirla. *Principles of Animal Psychology.* New York: McGraw-Hill, 1935.

Manner, H. W. *Elements of Anatomy and Physiology.* Philadelphia: Saunders, 1963.

———. *Elements of Comparative Vertebrate Embryology.* New York: Macmillan, 1964.

Marks, W. B., W. H. Dobelle, and E. F. MacNichol, Jr. "Visual Pigments of Single Primate Cones," *Science* 143 (1964): 1181–1183.

Marsh, J. T., F. G. Worden, and J. C. Smith. "Auditory Frequency-Following Response: Neural or Artifact?" *Science* 169 (1970): 1222–1223.

Marx, J. L. "Analgesia: How the Body Inhibits Pain Perception," *Science* 195 (1977): 471–473.

Masland, R. H. "Visual Motion Perception: Experimental Modification," *Science* 165 (1969): 819–821.

Mason, E. *Internal Perception and Bodily Functioning.* New York: International Universities Press, 1961.

Maugh, T. H., II. "Diabetic Retinopathy: New Ways to Prevent Blindness," *Science* 192 (1976): 539–540.

Mavor, J. W., and H. W. Manner. *General Biology,* 6th ed. New York: Macmillan, 1966.

May, J. G., and H. H. Matteson. "Spatial Frequency-Contingent Color After-effects," *Science* 192 (1976): 145–147.

Mayer, C. L. *Sensation: The Origin of Life.* Yellow Springs, Ohio: Antioch Press, 1961.

Mayer-Gross, W., and J. W. Walker. "Taste and Taste Selection of Food in Hypoglycemia," *Brit. J. Exp. Path.* 27 (1946): 297–305.

Mazokhin-Porshnyakov, G. A. *Insect Vision.* New York: Plenum, 1969.

McClintock, M. K. "Menstrual Synchrony and Suppression," *Nature* 229 (1971): 244–245.

McCollough, C. "Color Adaptation of Edge-detectors in the Human Visual System," *Science* 149 (1965): 1115–1116.

Mellon, DeForest, Jr. *The Physiology of Sense Organs.* San Francisco: Freeman, 1968.

Melzack, R. *The Puzzle of Pain.* New York: Basic Books, 1973.

———, and P. D. Wall. "On the Nature of Cutaneous Sensory Mechanisms," *Brain* 85 (1962): 331–356.

———, and P. D. Wall. "Pain Mechanisms: A New Theory," *Science* 150 (1965): 971–979.

Michael, R. P., E. B. Keverne, and R. W. Bonsall. "Pheromones: Isolation of Male Sex Attractants from a Female Primate," *Science* 172 (1971): 964–966.

Miller, G. A. *Language and Communication.* New York: McGraw-Hill, 1951.

———. "The Magical Number Seven, Plus or Minus Two: Some Limits on Our Capacity for Processing Information," *Psychol. Rev.* 63 (1956): 81–97.

Miller, W. H., R. Ratliff, and H. K. Hartline. "How Cells Receive Stimuli," *Scientific American,* September 1961.

Mills, A. W. "On the Minimum Audible Angle," *J. Acoust. Soc. Amer.* 30 (1958): 237–246.

Milne, L., and M. Milne. *The Senses of Animals and Man.* New York: Atheneum, 1962.

422   Bibliography

Möglich, M., U. Maschwitz, and B. Hölldobler. "Tandem Calling: A New Kind of Signal in Ant Communication," *Science* 186 (1974): 1047–1049.

Moncrief, R. W. "Olfactory Adaptation and Odor Likeness," *J. Physiol.* 133 (1956): 301–316.

———. *The Chemical Senses*, 3d ed. London: Hill, 1967.

Montagna, W. *The Structure and Function of Skin*. New York: Academic Press, 1962.

———. "The Skin," *Scientific American*, February 1965.

Moore, C. A., and R. Elliot. "Numerical and Regional Distribution of Taste Buds on the Tongue of the Bird," *J. Comp. Neurol.* 84 (1946): 119–132.

Morgan, C. T. *Physiological Psychology*, 3d ed. New York: McGraw-Hill, 1964.

———, J. S. Cook, III, A. Chapanis, and M. W. Lund (eds.). *Human Engineering Guide to Equipment Design*. New York: McGraw-Hill, 1963.

Moser, J. C., R. C. Brownlee, and R. Silverstein. "Alarm Pheromones of the Ant *Atta Texana*," *J. Insect Physiol.* 14 (1968): 529–535.

Moulton, D. G. "The Olfactory Pigment," in L. M. Beidler (ed.), *Handbook of Sensory Physiology*, vol. IV, *Chemical Senses*, part 1, *Olfaction*. Berlin: Springer-Verlag, 1971.

Mueller, C. G. *Sensory Psychology*. Englewood Cliffs, N.J.: Prentice-Hall, 1965.

Munn, N. L. *Psychological Development*. Boston: Houghton Mifflin, 1938.

Murch, G. M. *Visual and Auditory Perception*. Indianapolis: Bobbs-Merrill, 1973.

Murphy, M. R., and G. E. Schneider. "Olfactory Bulb Removal Eliminates Mating Behavior in the Male Golden Hamster," *Science* 167 (1970): 302–303.

Nafe, J. P. "The Psychology of Felt Experience," *Amer. J. Psychol.* 39 (1927): 367–389.

———, and W. L. Jenkins. "On the Vascular Theory of Warmth and Cold," *Amer. J. Psychol.* 51 (1938): 763–769.

———, and D. R. Kenshalo. "Somesthetic Senses," *Annual Rev. Psychol.* 13 (1962): 201–224.

———, and K. S. Wagoner. "The Experiences of Warmth, Cold and Heat," *J. Psychol* 2 (1936): 421–431.

———, and K. S. Wagoner. "The Nature of Pressure Adaptation," *J. Gen. Psychol.* 25 (1941): 323–351.

Nakayama, J., J. S. Eisenmann, and J. D. Hardy. "Single-Unit Activity of Anterior Hypothalamus during Local Heating," *Science* 134 (1961): 560–561.

Neff, W. D. "Studying Proprioception," in T. G. Andrews (ed.), *Methods of Psychology*. New York: Wiley, 1948.

Nimeroff, I. *Colorimetry*. Washington, D.C.: National Bureau of Standards, Monograph 104, 1968.

Novomeiskii, A. S. "The Nature of the Dermo-optic Sense," *Int. J. Parapsychol.* 7 (4) (1965): 34–36.

Ochs, S. *Elements of Neurophysiology*. New York: Wiley, 1964.

Olds, J. "Self-stimulation of Hippocampus in Rats," *J. Comp. Physiol. Psychol.* 61 (1966): 353–359.

Optical Society of America, Committee on Colorimetry, *The Science of Color*. New York: Crowell, 1953.

Oster, G. "Auditory Beats in the Brain," *Scientific American*, October 1973.

Parducci, A., and L. F. Perrett. "Category Rating Scales: Effects of Relative Spacing and Frequency of Stimulus Values," *J. Exptl. Psychol. Monographs* 1971.

Parker, G. H., and E. M. Stabler. "On Certain Distinctions between Taste and Smell," *Amer. J. Physiol.* 32 (1913): 230–240.

Patten, B. M. *Human Embryology.* Philadelphia: Blakiston, 1946.

Payne, A. "The Sense of Smell in Snakes," *J. Bomb. Nat. Hist.* 45 (1945): 507.

Peele, T. L. *The Neuroanatomical Basis for Clinical Neurology,* 2d ed. New York: McGraw-Hill, 1961.

Peterson, A. P. G., and L. L. Beranek. *Handbook of Noise Measurement,* 3d ed. Concord, Mass.: GenRad, Inc., 1956.

———, and E. E. Gross, Jr. *Handbook of Noise Measurement,* 6th ed. West Concord, Mass.: GenRad, Inc., 1969.

Peterson, W. W., T. G. Birdsall, and W. C. Fox. "The Theory of Signal Detectability," *IRE Trans.* PGIT-4 (1954): 171–212.

Pettigrew, J. D. "The Neurophysiology of Binocular Vision," *Scientific American,* August 1972.

Pfaffman, C. "Taste and Smell," in S. S. Stevens (ed.), *Handbook of Experimental Psychology.* New York: Wiley, 1951.

———. "The Sense of Taste," in J. Field, H. W. Magoun, and V. E. Hall (eds.), *Handbook of Physiology,* vol. I. Washington, D.C.: American Physiological Society, 1969.

———. "The Pleasures of Sensation," *Psychol. Rev.* 67 (1960): 253–268.

——— (ed.). *Olfaction and Taste, Proceedings of the Third International Symposium.* New York: The Rockefeller University Press, 1969.

———, and J. K. Bare. "Gustatory thresholds in normal and adrenalectomized rats," *J. Comp. Physiol. Psychol.* 43 (1950): 320–324.

Pfeiffer, J., and the editors of *Life. The Cell.* New York: Time, Inc., 1964.

Pickett, J. M., and K. D. Kryter. "Prediction of Speech Intelligibility in Noise," AFCRC-TR-55-4. Washington, D.C.: Air Force Cambridge Research Center, USAF, 1955.

Pierce, R. R., and E. E. David, Jr. *Man's World of Sound.* Garden City, N.Y.: Doubleday, 1958.

Pirenne, M. H. *Vision and the Eye.* London: Chapman and Hall, Ltd., 1967.

———, and F. H. C. Marriott. "The Quantum Theory of Light and the Psycho-Physiology of Vision," in S. Koch (ed.), *Psychology: A Study of a Science,* vol. I. New York: McGraw-Hill, 1959.

Pollack, L. "Effects of High Pass and Low Pass Filtering upon Intelligibility of Bands of Speech in Noise," *J. Acoust. Soc. Amer.* 20 (1948): 259–266.

Polyak, S. L. *The Retina.* Chicago: University of Chicago Press, 1941.

Postman, L., and J. P. Egan. *Experimental Psychology: an Introduction.* New York: Harper, 1949.

Potter, R. K., G. A. Kopp, and H. C. Green. *Visible Speech.* New York: Van Nostrand Reinhold, 1947.

Rasmussen, A. T. *Outlines of Neuro-anatomy,* 3d ed. Dubuque, Iowa: Brown, 1943.

Raven, C. P. *An Outline of Developmental Physiology.* Trans. by L. D. Ruiter. New York: McGraw-Hill, 1954.

Regan, D., and K. I. Beverley. "Disparity Detectors in Human Depth Perception: Evidence for Directional Selectivity," *Science* 181 (1973): 877–879.

Restle, F. "Moon Illusion Explained on the Basis of Relative Size," *Science* 167 (1970): 1092–1096.

Richter, C. P. "Self-regulating Functions," *Harvey Lectures* 38 (1942): 63–103.

Riesen, A. H. "The Development of Visual Perception in Man and Chimpanzee," *Science* 106 (1947): 107–108.

———. "Arrested Vision," *Scientific American,* July 1950.

———. "Studying Perceptual Development Using the Technique of Sensory Deprivation," *J. Nerv. Ment. Dis.* 132 (1961): 21–25.

Riesz, R. R. "Differential Intensity Sensitivity of the Ear for Pure Tones," *Phys. Rev.* 31 (1928): 867–875.

Riggs, L. A. "Curvature as a Feature of Pattern Vision," *Science* 181 (1973): 1070–1072.

Rock, I. *An Introduction to Perception.* New York: Macmillan, 1975.

Rose, J. E., and V. B. Mountcastle. "Touch and Kinesthesis," in J. Fields (ed.), *Handbook of Physiology,* vol. I. Washington, D.C.: American Physiological Society, 1959.

Rosenberg, B., T. N. Misra, and R. Switzer. "Mechanism of Olfactory Transduction," *Nature* 217 (1968): 423–427.

Rosenblith, W. A. (ed.). *Sensory Communication.* New York: Wiley, 1962.

———, K. N. Stevens, and staff of Bolt, Beranek, and Newman. *Handbook of Acoustic Noise Control,* vol. II: *Noise and Man.* WADC-TR-52-204. Wright Air Development Center, Ohio, 1953.

Ruch, T. C. "Sensory Mechanisms," in S. S. Stevens (ed.), *Handbook of Experimental Psychology.* New York: Wiley, 1951.

Rushton, W. A. H. "The Difference Spectrum and Photosensitivity of Rhodopsin in the Living Human Eye," *J. Physiol.* 134 (1956): 11–29.

———. "Rhodopsin Measurement and Dark-Adaptation in a Subject Deficient in Cone Vision," *J. Physiol.* 156 (1961): 193–205.

———. *Visual Pigments in Man.* Liverpool: Liverpool University Press, 1962.

———. "Color Blindness and Cone Pigments," *Amer. J. Optom.* 41 (1964): 265–282.

Sauer, E. G. F. "Celestial Navigation by Birds," *Scientific American,* August 1958.

Schapiro, S., and M. Salas. "Behavioral Responses of Infant Rats to Maternal Odor," *Physiology & Behavior* 5 (1970): 815–818.

Scharf, B. "Critical Bands," in J. V. Tobias (ed.), *Foundations of Modern Auditory Theory,* vol. I. New York: Academic Press, 1970.

——— (ed.). *Experimental Sensory Psychology.* Glenview, Ill.: Scott, Foresman, 1975.

Schiffman, H. R. *Sensation and Perception: An Integrated Approach.* New York: Wiley, 1976.

Schiffman, S. S. "Physiochemical Correlates of Olfactory Quality," *Science* 185 (1974): 112–117.

———, and C. Dackis. "Taste of Nutrients: Amino Acids, Vitamins, and Fatty Acids," *Perception and Psychophysics* 17 (1975): 140–146.

———, and R. P. Erickson. "A Theoretical Review: A Psychophysical Model for Gustatory Quality," *Physiology and Behavior* 7 (1971): 617–633.

Schneider, D. "Electrophysiological Investigation of Insect Olfaction," in Y. Zotterman (ed.), *Olfaction and Taste.* New York: MacMillan, 1963.

———. "Insect Olfaction: Deciphering System for Chemical Messages," *Science* 163 (1969): 1031–1037.

Schouten, J. F. "The Perception of Pitch," *Philips Tech. Rev.* 5 (1940): 286–294.

Schwarz, R. "Über die Riechschärfe der Honigbiene," *Z. vergl. Physiol.* 37 (1955): 180–210.

Scott, W. A., and M. Wertheimer. *Introduction to Psychological Research.* New York: Wiley, 1962.

Shaxby, J. H., and F. H. Gage. "The Localization of Sounds in the Median Plane," *Med. Res. Council Spec. Rept.*, Series No. 166. London: 1932.

Shepard, J. F., and F. S. Breed. "Maturation and Use in the Development of an Instinct," *J. Anim. Behav.* 3 (1913): 274–285.

Sherrington, C. S. *The Integrative Action of the Nervous System.* New Haven, Conn.: Yale University Press, 1947.

Shower, E. G., and R. Biddulph. "Differential Pitch Sensitivity of the Ear," *J. Acoust. Soc. Amer.* 3 (1931): 275–287.

Sidowski, J. B. (ed.). *Experimental Methods and Instrumentation in Psychology.* New York: McGraw-Hill, 1966.

Simmons, J. A. "Echolation in Bats: Signal Processing of Echoes for Target Range," *Science* 171 (1971): 925–928.

———, W. A. Lavender, B. A. Lavender, C. A. Doroshow, S. W. Kiefer, R. Livingston, and A. C. Scallet, "Target Structure and Echo Spectral Discrimination by Echolating Bats," *Science* 186 (1974): 1130–1132.

Sivian, L. J., and S. D. White. "On Minimum Audible Sound Fields," *J. Acoust. Soc. Amer.* 4 (1933): 288–321.

Smelser, G. K. (ed.). *The Structure of the Eye.* New York: Academic Press, 1961.

Skowko, D., B. N. Timney, T. A. Gentry, and R. B. Morant. "McCullough Effects: Experimental Findings and Theoretical Accounts," *Psychol. Bull.* 82 (1975): 497–510.

Smith, R. G. "The Role of Alimentary Chemoreceptors in the Development of Taste Averison," *Communications in Behavioral Biology*, part A, 5 (1970): 199–204.

Snyder, S. H. "Opiate Receptors and Internal Opiates," *Scientific American*, March 1977

Sonn, M. *Psychoacoustic Terminology.* Portsmouth, R.I.: Raytheon Co., 1969.

Steinberg, J. C., H. C. Montgomery, and M. B. Gardner. "Results of the World's Fair Hearing Tests," *J. Acoust. Soc. Amer.* 12 (1940): 291–301.

Stevens, S. S. "The Volume and Intensity of Tones," *Amer. J. Psychol.* 46 (1934): 397–408.

———. "The Attributes of Tones," *Proc. Nat. Acad. Sci.* 20 (1934): 457–459.

———. "Tonal Density," *J. Exptl. Psychol.* 17 (1934): 585–92.

———. "A Scale for the Measurement of a Psychological Magnitude: Loudness," *Psychol. Rev.* 43 (1936): 405–416.

——— (ed.). *Handbook of Experimental Psychology.* New York: Wiley, 1951.

———. "Measurement of Loudness," *J. Acoust. Soc. Amer.* 27 (1955): 815–829.

———. "The Direct Estimate of Sensory Magnitudes: Loudness," *Amer. J. Psychol.* 69 (1956): 1–25.

———. "Calculating Loudness," *Noise Control* 3 (1957): 11–22.

———. "On the Psychophysical Laws," *Psychol. Rev.* 64 (1957): 153–181.

———. "Sensory Scales of Taste Intensity," *Perception and Psychophysics* 6 (1959): 302–308.

———. "The Psychophysics of Sensory Function," in W. A. Rosenblith (ed.), *Sensory Communication.* New York: Wiley, 1961.

————. "Neural Events and the Psychophysical Law," *Science* 170 (1970): 1043–1050.

————. "Issues in Psychophysical Measurement," *Psychol. Rev.* 78 (1971): 426–450.

————. "A Neural Quantum in Sensory Discrimination," *Science* 177 (1972): 749–762.

————. "Perceptual Magnitude and Its Measurement," in E. C. Carterette and M. P. Friedman (eds.), *Handbook of Perception*, vol. II. *Psychophysical Judgments and Measurement*. New York: Academic Press, 1974.

————, and H. Davis. *Hearing: Its Psychology and Physiology*. New York: Wiley, 1938.

————, and J. Volkmann. "The Relation of Pitch to Frequency," *Amer. J. Psychol.* 53 (1940): 329–353.

————, J. Volkmann, and E. B. Newman "A Scale for the Measurement of the Psychological Magnitude Pitch," *J. Acoust. Soc. Amer.* 8 (1937): 185–190.

————, F. Warshofsky, and the editors of *Life*. *Sound and Hearing*. New York: Time, Inc., 1965.

Stiles, W. S. "The Directional Sensitivity of the Retina and the Spectral Sensitivity of the Rods and Cones," *Proc. Roy. Soc., Ser. B.* 127 (1939): 64–105.

————, and B. H. Crawford. "The Luminous Efficiency of Rays Entering the Eye Pupil at Different Points," *Proc. Roy. Soc., Ser. B.* 112 (1933): 428–450.

Strasfeld, N. J., and J. A. Campos-Ortega. "Vision in Insects: Pathways Possibly Underlying Neural Adaptation and Lateral Inhibition," *Science* 195 (1977): 894–897.

Stromeyer, C. F., III. "Curvature Detectors in Human Vision?" *Science* 184 (1974): 1199–1201.

Subcommittee on Vision and Its Disorders, National Advisory Neurological Diseases and Blindness Council. *Vision and Its Disorders*. NINDB Monograph No. 4. Bethesda, Md.: U.S. Department of Health, Education and Welfare, 1967.

Swets, J. A. "Indices of Signal Detectability Obtained with Various Psychophysical Procedures," *J. Acoust. Soc. Amer.* 31 (1959): 511–513.

————. "Is There a Sensory Threshold?" *Science* 134 (1961): 168–177.

———— (ed.). *Signal Detection and Recognition by Human Observers*. New York: Wiley, 1964.

————. "The Relative Operating Characteristic in Psychology," *Science* 182 (1973): 990–1000.

————, W. P. Tanner, Jr., and T. G. Birdsall. "Decision Processes in Perception," *Psychol. Rev.* 68 (1961): 301–340.

Tanner, W. P., Jr. "Physiological Implications of Psychophysical Data," *Ann. N.Y. Acad. Sci.* 89 (1961): 752–765.

————, and J. A. Swets. "A Decision-making Theory of Visual Detection," *Psychol. Rev.* 61 (1954): 401–409.

————, J. A. Swets, and D. M. Green. "Some General Properties of the Hearing Mechanisms," Technical Report No. 30, Electronic Defense Group, University of Michigan, Ann Arbor, Mich., 1956.

Tansley, K. *Vision in Vertebrates*. London: Chapman & Hall, Ltd., 1965.

Tavolga, W. N. *Principles of Animal Behavior*. New York: Harper, 1969.

Teevan, R. C., and R. C. Birney (eds.). *Color Vision: Selected Readings.* New York: Van Nostrand Reinhold, 1961.

Teyler, T. J. *A Primer of Psychobiology.* San Francisco: Freeman, 1975.

"The Electric Ear," *Newsweek,* April 1, 1974.

Thorson, J., and M. Biederman-Thorson. "Distributed Relaxation Processes in Sensory Adaptation," *Science* 183 (1974): 161–172.

Thurlow, W. R., and A. M. Small, Jr. "Pitch Perception for Certain Periodic Auditory Stimuli," *J. Acoust. Soc. Amer.* 27 (1955): 132–137.

Thurstone, L. L. "Psychophysical Analysis," *Amer. J. Psychol.* 38 (1927): 368–389.

——. "Phychophysical Methods," in T. G. Andrews (ed.), *Methods of Psychology.* New York: Wiley, 1948.

——. *The Measurement of Values.* Chicago: University of Chicago Press, 1959.

Tobias, J. V. (ed.). *Foundations of Modern Auditory Theory,* vols. I and II. New York: Academic Press, 1970.

Torrey, T. W. *Morphogenesis of the Vertebrates.* New York: Wiley, 1962.

Townsend, J. C. *Introduction to Experimental Methods.* New York: McGraw-Hill, 1953.

Underwood, B. J. *Experimental Psychology,* 2d ed. Englewood Cliffs, N.J.: Prentice-Hall, 1966.

Underwood, H., and M. Menaker. "Photoperiodically Significant Photoreception in Sparrows: Is the Retina Involved?" *Science* 167 (1970): 298–301.

——. "Photoreception in Sparrows," *Science* 172 (1971): 293.

Uttal, W. R. *The Psychology of Sensory Coding.* New York: Harper & Row, 1973.

Van Bergeijk, W. A., J. R. Pierce, and E. E. David, Jr., *Waves and the Ear.* Garden City, N.Y.: Doubleday, 1960.

Waddington, C. H. *Principles of Embryology.* New York: Macmillan, 1960.

Wald, G. "Eye and Camera," *Scientific American,* August 1950.

——. "On the Mechanism of Visual Threshold and Visual Adaptation," *Science* 119 (1954): 887–892.

——. "The Receptors of Human Color Vision," *Science* 145 (1964): 1007–1017.

——, and P. K. Brown. "Human Rhodopsin," *Science* 127 (1958): 222–226.

Wallace, P. "Animal Behavior: The Puzzle of Flavor Aversion," *Science* 193 (1976): 989–991.

Walls, G. L. "Land! Land!" *Psychol. Bull.* 57 (1960): 29–48.

Warren, R. M., and R. P. Warren. *Helmholtz on Perception.* New York: Wiley, 1968.

Wasserman, E. A., and D. D. Jensen. "Olfactory Stimuli and the 'Pseudo-extinction' Effect," *Science* 166 (1969): 1307–1309.

Wasserman, G. S. "Invertebrate Color Vision and the Tuned-Receptor Paradigm," *Science* 180 (1973): 268–275.

Webster, D. B. "Audition," in E. C. Carterette and M. P. Friedman (eds.), *Handbook of Perception,* vol. III. *Biology of Perceptual Systems.* New York: Academic Press, 1973.

Wegel, R. L., and C. E. Lane, "The Auditory Masking of One Pure Tone by Another and Its Probable Relation to the Dynamics of the Inner Ear," *Phys. Rev.* 23 (1924): 266–285.

Wehner, R. "Polarized-Light Navigation by Insects," *Scientific American,* July 1976.

Weinstein, S. "Intensive and Extensive Aspects of Tactile Sensitivity as a Function of Body Part, Sex, and Laterality," in D. R. Kenshalo (ed.). *The Skin Senses.* Springfield, Ill.: Thomas, 1968.

Weintraub, D. J., and E. L. Walker. *Perception.* Belmont, Calif.: Brooks/Cole, 1966.

Weiss, P. *Principles of Development.* New York: Holt, 1939.

Wellington, W. G. "Bumblebee Ocelli and Navigation at Dusk," *Science* 183 (1974): 550–551.

Wendt, G. R. "Vestibular Functions," in S. S. Stevens (ed.), *Handbook of Experimental Psychology.* New York: Wiley, 1951.

Wenger, M. A., F. N. Jones, and M. H. Jones. *Physiological Psychology.* New York: Holt, Rinehart and Winston, 1956.

Werblin, F. S. "The Control of Sensitivity in the Retina," *Scientific American,* January 1973.

Wetterberg, L., E. Geller, and A. Yuwiler. "Harderian Gland: An Extraretinal Photoreceptor Influencing the Pineal Gland in Neonatal Rats?" *Science* 167 (1970): 884–885.

Wever, E. G. *Theory of Hearing.* New York: Wiley, 1949.

———, and C. W. Bray. "Action Currents in the Auditory Nerve in Response to Acoustical Stimulation," *Proc. Nat. Acad. Sci.* 16 (1930): 344–350.

———, and C. W. Bray. "The Perception of Low Tones and the Resonance-Volley Theory," *J. Psychol.* 3 (1937): 101–114.

———, and M. Lawrence. *Physiological Acoustics.* Princeton, N.J.: Princeton University Press, 1954.

White, B. W., F. A. Saunders, L. Scadden, P. Bach-y-Rita, and C. C. Collins. "Seeing with the Skin," *Perception and Psychophysics,* 7 (1970): 23–27.

Whorf, B. L. *Language, Thought and Reality.* Cambridge, Mass.: MIT Press, 1956.

Wilcoxin, H. C., W. B. Dragoin, and P. A. Kral. "Illness Induced Aversions in Rat and Quail. Relative Salience of Visual and Gustatory Cues," *Science* 171 (1971): 826–828.

Wilson, E. O. "Chemical Communications in the Social Insects," *Science* 149 (1965): 1064–1071.

Wilson, M., and the editors of *Life. Energy.* New York: Time, Inc., 1963.

Witschi, E. *Development of Vertebrates.* Philadelphia: Saunders, 1956.

Wolsk, D. "Chemical Sensitivity," in M. Alpern, M. Lawrence, and D. Wolsk. *Sensory Processes.* Belmont, Calif.: Brooks/Cole, 1967.

———. "The Internal Environment," in M. Alpern, M. Lawrence, and D. Wolsk, *Sensory Processes.* Belmont, Calif.: Brooks/Cole, 1967.

Wood, A. B. *A Textbook of Sound.* New York: Macmillan, 1955.

Woodrow, H., and B. Karpman. "A New Olfactometric Technique and Some Results," *J. Exptl. Psychol.* 2 (1917): 431–447.

Woodworth, R. S. *Experimental Psychology.* New York: Holt, 1938.

———. *Psychology,* 4th ed. New York: Holt, 1940.

———, and H. Schlossberg. *Experimental Psychology,* rev. ed. New York: Holt, Rinehart and Winston, 1954.

Woolridge, D. E. *The Machinery of the Brain.* New York: McGraw-Hill, 1963.

Wright, W. D. *Researches on Normal and Defective Colour Vision.* London: Henry Kimpton, 1946.

———. "The Characteristics of Tritanopia," *J. Opt. Soc. Amer.* 42 (1952): 509–521.

Yost, W. A., and D. W. Nielsen. *Fundamentals of Hearing.* New York: Holt, Rinehart and Winston, 1977.

Zawala, A., H. P. Van Cott, D. B. Orr, and V. H. Small. "Human Dermo-optical Perception: Colors of Objects and of Projected Light Differentiated with Fingers," *Percept. Mot. Skills* 25 (1967): 525–542.

Zigler, M. J. "Pressure Adaptation-Time: a Function of Intensity and Extensity," *Amer. J. Psychol.* 44 (1932): 709–720.

———, and A. H. Holway. "Differential Sensitivity as Determined by the Amount of Olfactory Substance," *J. Gen. Psychol.* 12 (1935): 272–282.

Zotterman, Y. (ed.). *Olfaction and Taste.* New York: Macmillan, 1963.

Zwaardemaker, H. *Die Physiologie des Geruchs.* Leipzig: Englemann, 1895.

Zwicker, E., G. Flottrop, and S. S. Stevens. "Critical Bandwidth in Loudness Summation," *J. Acoust. Soc. Amer.* 29 (1957): 548–557.

Zwislocki, J., and R. S. Feldman. "Just Noticeable Differences in Dichotic Phase," *J. Acoust. Soc. Amer.* 28 (1956): 860–864.

author index

430

subject index